Face Masks Hurt Kids

Face Masks Hurt Kids

Allan Stevo

Crafting 52
Chicago • Vienna • Pressburg
New York • San Francisco

ISBN-13: 978-1-953847-15-7

To purchase 10 or more
copies at a time contact
Sales@RadioRemnant.com.

TABLE OF CONTENTS

INTRODUCTION

Face Masks & Courage: Is Family Your Excuse For Cowardice,
Or Is Family Your Motivation For Standing Upright? 1

A Note On So-Called Fact Checkers 5

FACE MASKS DO NOT WORK

Reason 1: The CDC Says Face Masks Do Not Work 11

Reason 2: CDC & WHO Say Face Masks INCREASE Spread Of Disease 17

Reason 3: *New England Journal Of Medicine* Says Masks Do Not Work 19

Reason 4: The FDA Says Face Masks Do Not Work 22

Reason 5: Yes, Data From The Council On Foreign Relations Even Says
Face Masks Do Not Work 23

Reason 6: Many Other Medical Researchers Say Masks Do Not Work 27

Reason 7: Countries With Face Mask Mandates Are Not Better Off
Than Countries Without Them 29

Reason 8: Face Masks Did Not Work In 1918, 1957, 1968, 2002, 2004,
And They Do Not Work Now 31

Reason 9: The SARS Hype Is Severely Blown Out Of Proportion 33

Reason 10: The Flu Is More Dangerous Than Covid & Neither Of Them
Are Stopped By Face Mask Wearing 36

Reason 11: If Face Masks Do Not Work, Then Government And Media
Are Lying To You — A Very Scary Thought For Some 40

Reason 12: You Have Been Lied To This Whole Time, Then Vilified
If You Ask Too Many Revealing Questions About Those Lies 42

Reason 13: If Morality Is Being Argued By Bullies Rather Than Scientific
Debate Being Had By Peers, You Know Something Is Wrong 48

Reason 14: The Rationale "Comply Or Else" Is Such A Monstrously
Bad Rationale, Whenever It Is Used, That It Should Always Trigger
A Lack Of Compliance 54

Reason 15: "The Precautionary Principal" Has Not Been Followed 57

Reason 16: Mandatory Face Masks Harm 1.5 Billion Students 59

Reason 17: Face Masks Are Another Way To Crush Their Spirit 61

Reason 18: Masks Are A Conditioning Tool To Make Children Compliant 64

Reason 19: Compliance To Bad Ideas Is The Last Thing A Free Thinking
Person Wants To Teach A Child 66

Reason 20: You Teach Your Children To Do Things They Do Not Like
And Intuitively Know Are Not Only Uncomfortable, But BAD 68

Reason 21: You Teach A Child That Reason Does Not Matter 70

Reason 22: You Teach A Child Not To Trust You 72

Reason 23: You Raise A Tyrant, A Slave, Or Both, Rather Than
A Healthy And Fully Capable Adult 73

Reason 24: You Sow Seeds Of Harm In The Future 75

Reason 25: You Teach Your Child "Might Makes Right" 77

Reason 26: You Teach Your Child Weakness 77

Reason 27: You Teach Your Child To Lie 80

Reason 28: You Teach Your Child Tacit Approval 81

Reason 29: You Teach A Child To Rat Out Friends, Parents, & Neighbors 82

Reason 30: You Teach Your Child To Be A Person Of Preference
And Not A Person Of Values 84

Reason 31: You Teach Your Child To Misread Romans 13 86

Reason 32: You Are Being Conditioned To View Your Freedom As Selfish 90

Reason 33: You Put Your Child Through A Class On Scientism, Not Science ... 92

Reason 34: Your Child Will Imitate You 93

Reason 35: You Place Your Child In The Hands Of Very Twisted People 94

Reason 36: We Are NOT All In This Together 95

Reason 37: A Tale Of Two Mothers 96

Reason 38: The Boy Who Asks "Why Do I Have To Wear This?" 97

Reason 39: The Mom Who Brought Her Son To The Playground 100

Reason 40: Do Not Look At Masks For Covid Avoidance, Look At Obesity,
Or A Host Of Other Meaningful Comorbidities, But Especially Obesity 103

Reason 41: Obesity Drives Covid 107

Reason 42: Covid-19 Is An IQ Test 108

Reason 43: You Do Not Want To Wear It, They Do Not Want To Wear It 109

Reason 44: Ask These Kids What They Think Of Face Masks 112

Reason 45: Othering Children 116

Reason 46: There Is No Feedback Loop 118

Reason 47: No Informed Consent Is Possible 119

Reason 48: Very Little Data, Very Much Interpretation 120

Reason 49: The Shy Tory Effect 121

Reason 50: The Following List Of Biases 122

Reason 51: If You Want To Make A Sacrifice For Society, Make
A Sacrifice By Being A Member Of The Control Group 127

Reason 52: The Story Of Vioxx 129

FACE MASKS ARE NOT SAFE

Reason 53: This List Of Health Concerns That The Political Establishment, Media Establishment, And Medical Establishment Will Not Talk About 137

PREGNANT MOTHERS, AND DEVELOPING BABIES

Reason 54: Face Masks Hurt Pregnant Women And Their Babies 155

Reason 55: Masks May Cause Mothers To Have Elevated Enough Carbon Dioxide To Prevent Fetuses From Being Able To Clear Carbon Dioxide.......... 157

Reason 56: Face Masks On Pregnant Women During Exertion Should Be Avoided To Protect The Unborn Child 160

Reason 57: Face Mask Material May Cause Birth Defects 162

Reason 58: Face Masks Are Harmful For Babies... 163

Reason 59: Children Are More Vulnerable To Mask Harm Than Adults 164

SOME OF THE HARMFUL COMPONENTS OF FACE MASKS

Reason 60: Graphene In Face Masks May Pose A Particular Risk 169

Reason 61: Inhaled Cotton Fibers Cause Lung Disease 170

Reason 62: Inhaled Synthetic Fibers Cause Lung Disease 172

Reason 63: Inhaled Fibers Cause Pulmonary Fibrosis...................................... 174

Reason 64: Prolonged Textile Face Mask Use May Lead To Respiratory Illnesses Like Those Experienced By Textile Workers In The Third World...... 176

Reason 65: Your Child Inhales Dangerous Chlorine Compounds While Wearing A Face Mask.. 178

Reason 66: Exhaled Air Contains Over 250 Substances Meant To Be Removed From Your Body And Not Breathed Back In 179

BACTERIA, FUNGI, AND VIRUSES
ON THE SURFACE OF FACE MASKS

Reason 67: Eighty-Two Bacterial Colonies And Four Mold Colonies Found On A Child's Face Mask After Eight Hours 183

Reason 68: Face Masks Are Breeding Grounds For Bacteria In A Way Our Unmasked Faces Are Not.. 184

Reason 69: Bacteria On Masks Are Not Benign And Have Been Proven To Be Very Harmful.. 186

Reason 70: Face Mask Wearing Causes Harmful Bacteria To Proliferate Outside The Protection Of The Many Pathogen-Defenses The Body Has 190

Reason 71: The Build Up Of Fungi And Bacteria In Face Masks 194

Reason 72: Face Masks Cause Sore Throats 195

Reason 73: Masked People Get More Fungal Infections Of The Lungs............ 196

Reason 74: Mayo Clinic: Face Mask Wearing Is Leading To An Increase In Staph Infections, As Can Be Expected As They Help Bacteria Access Deeper Quarters Of The Body 198

BONDING, LEARNING, AND THE DEVELOPING MIND

Reason 75: Face Masks Harm A Child's Developing Mind 205

Reason 76: Face Masks Affect A Person's Ability To Think Clearly 207

Reason 77: Face Masks Cause Brain Degeneration 208

Reason 78: Mask Wearing Reduces Attention And Speed In Athletes 210

FACE MASKS DISRUPT COMMUNICATION

Reason 79: Face Masks Are Disruptive To Basic Human Communication 215

Reason 80: We All Read Lips 217

Reason 81: Babies And Children Especially Read Lips 219

Reason 82: Face Masks Act As An Acoustic Filter 220

Reason 83: Face Masks Cause Further Harm To The Mentally Impaired And Hearing Impaired 221

Reason 84: Face Masks Reduce The Ability For A Child To Bond And Reduce The Ability For A Child To Learn 222

Reason 85: Face Masks Harm Relationships 223

Reason 86: Face To Face Contact Is Reduced When Children Wear Masks 224

Reason 87: Face Masks Block Emotional Signaling Between Students And Teachers, Students And Parents, Students And Students, And Between Students And All Other Humans 225

Reason 88: Both Face Masks And Face Shields Cause Fear In Children 227

Reason 89: Masks Are Particularly Harmful On A Person's Wellbeing 229

Reason 90: Face Masks Help You Raise A Sociopath 230

Reason 91: Face Mask Peer Pressure Is So Great That Mask Wearing Is Encouraged Far Beyond The Point Of Harm To The Mask Wearer 231

HARM TO THE HEAD

Reason 92: Face Masks Are Long Known To Cause Headaches 235

Reason 93: Face Masks Trigger Migraines 237

Reason 94: Face Masks Are So Bad For You That The Vast Majority Of Healthy People Get Headaches From Wearing Them 238

Reason 95: Face Mask Wearing Causes Neurological Harm And Cognitive Impairment 240

Reason 96: Face Masks Make Headaches Worse And May Make Other Neurological Pathologies Such As Aneurysms And Tumors Worse 242

Reason 97: What They Are Doing To Your Children Makes Your
Children Stupider And Gives Your Children Learning Disabilities 244

HARM TO THE MIND

Reason 98: The Powerful Impact Of Despair 247

Reason 99: Face Masks Are Psychologically Harmful For You 250

Reason 100: Face Mask Wearing Is Linked To Substantial
Psychological Side Effects 253

Reason 101: Face Mask Wearing Leads To Panic Attacks And
Exacerbates Significant Other Psychiatric Conditions 256

Reason 102: Masks Cause Unstudied Psychological Harm To Children 259

EXERCISE IN FACE MASKS HARMS
BOTH THE HEALTHY AND SICK

Reason 103: CDC And WHO Advise Against Exercising in Masks..................263

Reason 104: Face Masks Are Dangerous When Worn During Exercise 265

Reason 105: Exercising In A Face Mask Will Hurt You...................................266

Reason 106: Exercising With A Mask May *Increase* Infection Rates 267

Reason 107: Even Activity As Simple As Walking Is Made Measurably
Harder By A Face Mask, Even Among Healthy People.....................................268

Reason 108: Exercising In A Face Mask Harms The Sick 270

Reason 109: N95 Wearing Hurts The Sick..271

Reason 110: Simple Activity Is Made Measurably Harder By Mask
Wearing In Unwell People 272

Reason 111: The Overweight, Those With COPD, Lung Disease, Cardiac
Disease, Pregnant Women, And Stroke Patients Must Be Particularly
Cautious Around Face Masks...275

Reason 112: Japanese Government Warns Masks May Cause Heatstroke.........277

Reason 113: Face Mask Fatalities In Kids...279

Reason 114: Exercise With Face Masks Can Be Lethal 281

Reason 115: Mask Wearing Has The Opposite Effect Of The
Health-Promoting Deep Breathing Encouraged In Prayer, Meditation,
And Holistic Healing...282

SURGEONS, HEALTH WORKERS, DRIVERS,
AND CONFLICTED DOCTORS

Reason 116: Surgical Face Masks Were Made For Surgery And Might
Not Even Work For That..285

Reason 117: Face Masks Cause Medical Care To Be Worse For Children 287

Reason 118: Surgeons, Doctors, And Other Medical Staff In
Face Masks May Be More Likely To Harm Patients...288

Reason 119: The Nebulizer Effect 290

Reason 120: Face Masks Impair Cognition Among Healthcare Workers 291

Reason 121: Face Masks On Medical Workers Hurt Kids 292

Reason 122: Face Masks Do Not Bring About Greater "Health"
As Defined By The World Health Organization 294

Reason 123: Reminder: The World Health Organization Even Says
Face Masks May Be Dangerous To Your Child 295

Reason 124: No One Even Uses A Face Mask Correctly 297

Reason 125: Experiments Are Often Done In "Ideal" Settings
And Therefore Carry A Bias 298

Reason 126: Face Masks Are Visibly Misused 299

Reason 127: Mandating Face Mask Wearing Is Unethical 301

Reason 128: Some Doctors Are Conflicted And Unable To Properly
Represent Their Patients' Interests 302

Reason 129: Face Masks While Driving Are A Hazard To Your Children 304

DOUBLE MASKS, CLOTH MASKS, FACE SHIELDS

Reason 130: The Mask Mandate Was Issued Without A Single Scientific
Paper Cited In Support Of Cloth Masks Providing Respiratory Protection 309

Reason 131: Wearing Cloth Face Masks Leads To More Flu-Like Illness
Than Wearing No Face Mask, Causing Exactly The Opposite Outcome
That Mandatory Masking Is Said To Prevent 310

Reason 132: Cloth Face Masks Are Awful 311

Reason 133: Cloth Face Masks Are So Awful That They Should Never
Be Recommended To Prevent The Spread Of A Virus 312

Reason 134: Double Masking May Cause Even Higher Risk Of Infection
To The Wearer 313

MICRO ENVIRONMENTS, DEAD SPACE, OXYGEN,
CARBON DIOXIDE, AND TEMPERATURE STRESS

Reason 135: Years Of Masking Precautions Meant To Benefit
The Wearer Were Thrown Out The Window Suddenly In 2020 317

Reason 136: OSHA Considers The Micro-Environment Of Face Masks
As "Not Safe For Workers" 318

Reason 137: Increased "Dead Space" Can Be Lethal 320

Reason 138: The Many Details Of Breathing Are Not One-Size-Fits-All,
But Highly Individualized, Face Mask Policy Can Therefore Not Be
One-Size-Fits-All 323

Reason 139: Too Much Carbon Dioxide 325

Reason 140: Increases In Exhalation Resistance, Inhalation Resistance,
And Temperature May Be Harmful To One Wearing A Face Mask 330

Reason 141: Masks Induce Thermal Stress & Affect Heartrate, Even Among Healthy Adults, Far More Among Children & The Infirm 332

Reason 142: Hypercapnia 334

Reason 143: Face Masks Increase "Dead Space" 335

Reason 144: Face Masks Increase Carbon Dioxide Dangerously And Decrease Oxygen Dangerously 336

Reason 145: Masks Dangerously Increase Rebreathing Of Carbon Dioxide 338

Reason 146: Increased Dead Space Is Significant, And So Is Increased Breathing Resistance 340

Reason 147: Increased Dead Space Increases Breathing Resistance, Leading To Decreased Gas Exchange Of The Respiratory System — And A Cascade Of Other Physiological Side Effects 342

Reason 148: Suprathreshold Stimuli Can Cause Pathological Consequences, But So Can Subthreshold Stimuli 343

SELF-INDUCED ILLNESS AND EXACERBATION OF ILLNESS

Reason 149: Everyone In A Face Mask Induces A Condition Similar On The Body To Sleep Apnea 349

Reason 150: Exercising In A Mask Induces An Artificial Version Of COPD ... 350

Reason 151: Face Masks Are Definitely Not Suitable For Epileptics 352

Reason 152: Face Mask Wearing Affects The Central Nervous System And May Increase Sleep Apnea 354

Reason 153: Face Masks Harm Cancer Patients 357

THE IMMUNE SYSTEM

Reason 154: Face Masks Weaken Immunity, And Therefore May Make Children *More* Susceptible To Covid-19 361

Reason 155: Masks Reduce Healthy Functioning Of The Immune System 363

Reason 156: Face Mask Wearing Increases Leptin Release 364

Reason 157: Face Mask Wearing May Negatively Influence Metabolism All The Way Down To The Cellular Level 365

Reason 158: Immunity Debt 367

FACE MASK USE HARMS THE MOUTH

Reason 159: Face Masks Harm Teeth And Gums And Cause A Condition Known As "Mask Mouth" 371

Reason 160: Face Mask Wearing Causes "Mask Mouth" And Other Harm 373

Reason 161: Face Mask Wearing Exacerbates Existing Voice Disorders And May Trigger New Voice Disorders 374

Reason 162: Face Mask Wearing Has Caused A New Condition, A Form Of Face Mask-Induced Rhinitis 375

FACE MASK USE HARMS THE EARS AND THE SKIN

Reason 163: Face Masks Deform Children's Ears............................. 379

Reason 164: Face Masks Are Bad For Your Face 381

Reason 165: Face Mask Wearing Harms The Skin............................. 382

FACE MASK USE HARMS THE EYES

Reason 166: Face Mask Use Is Harmful To The Eyes....................... 389

Reason 167: Face Mask Use Impairs Vision 390

FACE MASK USE HARMS THE KIDNEYS

Reason 168: Face Masks Are Hard On The Kidneys.......................... 393

Reason 169: N95 Respirators Are Bad For Your Kidneys As Well.................. 394

FACE MASK USE HARMS THE LUNGS

Reason 170: You Need To Breathe, Everyone Needs To Breathe,
Your Child Even Needs To Breathe 397

FACE MASK USE HARMS THE HEART

Reason 171: Face Masks Affect The Heart.. 403

Reason 172: Face Masks Lead To Exhaustion And Increased Stress
On The Heart 404

ENVIRONMENTAL CONCERNS

Reason 173: Environmental Harm... 407

Reason 174: Face Mask Wearing Comes With Environmental Effects 408

Reason 175: The Great Pacific Face Mask Patch............................... 411

Reason 176: Kids Are Not A Biohazard — Dirty Face Masks On
The Ground Are The True Biohazard 413

FACE MASK USE LEADS TO MASK-INDUCED EXHAUSTION
SYNDROME AND OTHER SYSTEMIC CONDITIONS

Reason 177: Symptoms Of Face Mask Wearing Are Now Being
Blamed On Covid-19 417

Reason 178: The Long-Term Consequences Of Face Mask Wearing
Are Likely Far Worse Than We Can Imagine 419

Reason 179: Face Mask Wearing Creates Symptoms Akin To
"Sick Building Syndrome" 421

Reason 180: Masks Lead To Mask-Induced Exhaustion Syndrome (MIES)..... 423

SUMMARY

Reason 181: Covid Is Hardly More Dangerous Than The Flu, Face Masks
Have No Impact On Respiratory Viruses Anyway, And Masks Are
Measurably Harmful In the Short-Term, Long-Term, And Cumulatively..........427

CONCLUSION

Now What Do I Do?...431

APPENDIX

Acknowledgements 439

Notes 448

Index...492

About The Author 507

Amaryllidi:

May you always
feel my fatherly protection,
my fatherly wisdom, and
my fatherly love,

May you never be
in want of it, and

May you have ample
supply of the fruit of that
to share with
our next generation.

INTRODUCTION

I do not write this to scare anyone. I write this to make it impossible for anyone to say, "Face masks are safe for children and effective at preventing the transmission of a respiratory virus."

Anyone who can say so without reservation is either lying to you or misinformed. Either way, they do not deserve your trust, whether that be family, friend, or doctor.

Use this revealingly difficult time as an opportunity to have a moment of insight into that person's character.

The amount of evidence against the masking of children is enormous and can no longer be ignored. Face masks are not safe for the general population. Face masks are not effective in the prevention of the transmission of a respiratory virus. They are most certainly not safe and effective for our children. Face masks for this purpose are experimental, and the experiment on children, as well as the rest of the population, must stop.

1.) Primarily, 75% of the people who open this book want a list of the harm caused by face masks, so I will give that list to you. Please turn to page 137 to see that list of ways children can be harmed by a face mask.

For more on any of these topics, see the latter two-thirds of the book.

The first one-third of the book is on topics of philosophy around face masking, and the latter two-thirds of the book is on topics of hard science around face masking.

2.) Thump this book on a desk or podium to prove a point.

This book is not a short book. It is made of a size and heft that make it easy and useful to thump on the desk of a bureaucrat to emphasize a point. It is also made for podium thumping. Thumping your Kindle or iPad on the podium just does not carry the same impact.

3.) Skim this book, do not read it beginning to end.

The table of contents is outlined to be clear and to be easily read by you. The index is the same. Each chapter title is written to be clear — no mystery about what is contained therein.

4.) Each chapter can stand on its own.

There is, consequently, some redundancy around the main point of the book: masks are not safe, masks are not effective, masks are not to be worn by the general population, least of all your children.

With that in mind, my suggestion to you: skim the chapter titles and read those chapters that interest you.

5.) Each chapter title tells you what that chapter is about.

Memetics is the study of viral ideas. Quick, clear ideas are the in-demand hallmark of this era in which we live — an era so filled with noise and so little signal, so much data and so little wisdom, so much deceit and so little truth.

Some people get that. Such people are hungry for signal and not noise, wisdom and not data. Each chapter title is meant to be that.

6.) This is an easy, quick read.

It is a long book, with complicated subject matter, laid out for you to read as deeply as you wish. Those who pick it up for two minutes, ten minutes, or ten hours will each get something out of it.

The days since mid-March 2020 have not only brought the most perverse experimentation and neglect to the mainstream of society, it has been done on our most sensitive and precious members of society: our children.

The level of experimentation is sick and rises to what generations, even in the barbaric past, would have deemed child abuse and which I am confident generations of the future will look upon during this twisted age as.

Nothing can be said that justifies this behavior visited upon children.

World War II remains, in memory, as a time of great wrong. Even trusted officials were involved in such wrong — military and civilian alike. Among them were doctors, doctors widely trusted by many. On June 2, 1948, the Doctors Trials at Nuremberg came to a conclusion with the hanging of the doctors found guilty of atrocities perpetrated over years on their fellow man.

The medical experimentation of World War II that led, in part, to the Nuremberg Codes, were a thing many believed had been put behind us.

They had not. Twisted medical experimentation on innocents continues. 2020 is proof of that.

The blame does not stop with officials, however. Public officials are not in charge of our homes. Public officials are not in charge of our families.

Shame on every one of you parents who obeyed and masked your children, and shame on each of you who did not ask the hard questions *before* masking your child.

If you did mask your children in the past, the good news is, you never have to do that again. I am here to help you make sure that barbaric tradition stays in the past, where it belongs.

Thousands have used my work to never wear a face mask again, not for any reason. I have video tutorials that are available free of charge to those who sign up to RealStevo.com, and I have a bestselling book *Face Masks in One Lesson,* which guides you through the process of never wearing a face mask again. It will answer almost any question you can think of on how to stop wearing a face mask. Buy it now and by the time you are five pages into that book, you will want to thank me.

As an additional resource, you can always write me at Allan@ RealStevo.com with any questions you may have.

Really, what it comes down to, though, is resolving to never wear a face mask again and then following through on that.

Again, face masks are a total lie. Anyone, at the time this book went to press, was either mistaken, a liar, or both, if they were claiming that face masks were safe and effective.

Face masks are not safe. Face masks are not effective. Face masks are experimental.

After a quick note about the importance of courage, I will begin addressing how *Face Masks Hurt Kids* with information starting from there: the unsafe, ineffective, experimental face mask debacle of 2020 and 2021.

May a shift in opinion occur so quickly, against mask mandates, that this book becomes unnecessary the moment it hits the printing press.

May that face mask debacle of 2020 and 2021, forever be a part of our past, a shameful moment that we never repeat. May that sentiment be so culturally pervasive that anyone who dares wear a mask, be seen as a dangerous extremist unable to admit how wrong it all was and undeserving of any role of power or influence, least of all in the lives of our children.

I work day and night to bring us to that better place.

Will you join me?

Allan Stevo
August 15, 2021
Rock Snake Lake
Near Swallow Cliff, California

Face Masks & Courage: Is Family Your Excuse For Cowardice, Or Is Family Your Motivation For Standing Upright?

Parents used to stand up in life FOR THE BENEFIT of their kids. They realized that no matter how much money they left their kids, **the inheritance of freedom is worth so much more to a child than the dollars and cents a parent could leave behind.**

Today, so many parents make their child an excuse for why they refuse to stand up in life. They say they are keeping their lips zipped BECAUSE of their child. They are doing it BECAUSE of their child they say.

That is not okay.

There is the story of a Kentucky soccer coach who refused to go masked and refused to enforce the mask. He did not keep quiet because of his daughter. She was on his team. He refused to let her or anyone else wear masks on the field. He stood up because of his daughter. He lost his coveted position as a result.

But because of his courage, he is also the father of the only soccer player in his county who played without a mask through 2020.

There is a father who wrote me from Arizona who did not back down from his values because of his kids. No, he doubled down. When the lockdowns began, this decorated teacher did not put on a mask or mask his two sons. Instead, he quit his job, pulled his two sons out of school and now homeschools them, which is a far more nurturing environment for all three of them. 2020 was a last straw for him, and I bet a blessing in disguise. Who better to rear a child than a parent?

These are heroes of 2020 — not the 16-year-old Trader Joe's bag boy yelling at his 60-year-old elders to mask up, emboldened by the unhealthy public health dictates and the trillion dollar media machine that wants to sell us all manner of bad ideas.

These parents are the leaders of 2020 — not the chattering classes who go on guilt-filled tirades in the media, trying to get regular folks to do the most irregular and unnatural things. That would include placing a ten-cent polypropylene mask from Wuhan on their children's faces and calling that normal. It would include letting a child be put on house arrest and calling that lockdown normal. It would include letting the public health bureaucrats know that every weird experiment on their child, that a bureaucrat could possibly come up with, is an experiment that family will willingly sacrifice their youngest and most precious to.

Those things are not normal.

We are experimenting on our children. We are subjecting our most precious members of society to experimentation that is demonstrably neither safe nor effective.

You tell your child everything that he needs to know about you in a moment like this. Your words mean so little. Your actions say it all.

This is a book chock-full of science, but more importantly it is a book about virtue. If you cannot be courageous in the moments that really matter, then you have no virtue.

All other virtue depends on your ability to walk through life courageously. It is at such moments that your worth to those around you is shown. All your talk of virtue means nothing if your own sense of duty and courage do not undergird that virtue and move you to action.

For this reason, courage has been called the greatest of virtues, for upon courage, all other virtues rest.

I call on you, dear reader, to be as courageous as possible in a moment like this, to err on the side of courage, to err on the side of valor, to err on the side of bravery.

This moment needs that of you. The people around you need that of you.

If you cannot give that, and give that 110%, then you owe those around you the honesty of letting them know that, so that they, at least, can realize that you are not the protector in their lives that they can count on at a moment like this, to be there when all else goes wrong. At least then, they have the clarity to realize that they must step up and protect themselves. At least then, they will not walk alongside you thinking that you have this under control. At least then, they will not be left delusionally thinking that you are watching out for them no matter what.

You can, at least, do them that favor of providing that clarity.

If you choose to walk through this important moment in time as a coward, everyone from the 8-month-olds to the 108-year-olds in your life deserve to know that from you.

The face mask signals exactly that to the world, but your loved ones may not see your cowardice as clearly. As loved ones, they are prone to have more faith in you and may give you the benefit of the doubt. As quickly as possible, you owe them that hard dose of reality that says "I will not be your protector. You are on your own in this fight. My actions may even prove me as a friend to your enemy. I may be someone whose cowardice rubs off on you, undermines your sense of decency, and corrupts your values."

Reality is harsh, and reality is what they need from you now more than ever.

History presents decisive moments. Such decisive moments are looked back on as a moment when everything was able to go so right or in which everything could go so wrong. We are living through a moment like that. The next century of human history may very well be built on the actions taken by individuals in the months ahead.

Act now, for soon that opportunity will have passed.

If you choose to walk through such a decisive moment as a coward, those placed under your stewardship, at least, deserve the honesty of being told that you will not be there for them.

They deserve that much.

It is my hope that you can give them so much more, but perhaps not everyone has that ability at their disposal to look such a moment in the face and stand up tall.

I would not know.

I have many flaws, but cowardice is not one of them.

I refuse to let cowards around me.

I would rather surround myself with those who disagree with me on 75% of issues, but who I know have courage, than to surround myself with those who agree with me 95% and are filled with cowardice.

A coward you can never depend on.

His 95% agreement is in his words alone, but when placed under pressure, you can be certain that he will no longer agree with you 95% of the time. His actions will communicate everything you need to know about him.

The days that have followed since the Ides of March 2020, have told us who the cowards are and who the upright are. Hardly could I have asked for a better gift than the wisdom these days have brought into my life, as the most vocal and outspoken about the topic of virtue cowered.

It quickly became evident who they were. As painful as that realization may have been, that clarity about who was cowardly and who was courageous has truly been a blessing in my life.

"It is just a face mask," is something only a coward or a weasel would say to you. "It is just a face mask," is something that will only be said by someone looking to downplay the role of courage, the role of bravery, the role of valor, the role of wisdom in the world, someone looking to convince you of an agenda that provides you with no benefit.

A face mask says so much. It says nearly everything you need to know about a person. Because if they will cower, their words are worth so little. If all they need is the right reason in order to acquiesce to the unwise, then their wisdom means so little.

I do not care if a man agrees with me, but I care if he is steel-spined enough for his actions to match his words.

Give me a table full of men who agree with me about just a little, but whose actions match their words, and I will trade them for an entire army of the most doctrinaire who lack courage. I will trade them for an entire free state full of the most doctrinaire who lack courage. I will trade them for an entire country full of the most doctrinaire who lack courage.

What will you be?

Will you be a person of faith? A person of values? A person of boundaries? A person of courage?

Or will you be a person of fear? A person of preference? A person obedient and flexible to the world? A person of cowardice?

The choice is yours, but you do not have to say a word. You tell the world everything it needs to know about you when you put a mask on your face.

A Note On So-Called Fact Checkers

Future generations will look upon this book and realize what times we live in today, for a book chapter like this to even have to be written.

Virtually every chapter in this book has material that can be searched for on a search engine and will produce top results that lead directly to so-called fact checking websites. If so-called fact checking websites are the top returns, that is almost a guarantee that the topic is politically controversial and offends some powerful interest.

The major internet search engines likely to produce these inferior results are Bing, Google, Yahoo, Swiss Cows, Qwant, Yippy, Internet Archive, Search Encrypt, Gibiru, Verizon's One Search, Start Page, and Duck Duck Go. Some of these search engines concern themselves with privacy, but produce very bad results, often censored. These results are often not based on the smart and effective algorithm Google was built on, but which produce the results that someone else wants you to see instead. The original Google algorithm was based on the exact opposite concept — showing you the results you want to see. Google has strayed a great distance from its original vision, and even small, scrappy search engines have followed along by providing censored results.

While the so-called fact checkers, likely see themselves as doing sincere and legitimate work, they come from a dishonest starting point — some likely without even realizing it.

Truth-seeking inquiry must begin without a predetermined result in mind other than "seeking the truth." Our society is not built upon that process. Our government and legal system, so dominant in society, are not built upon that process. Our educational system is not built upon that process, and that process is not commonly a part of daily life.

Instead, the very opposite takes place: a search for supporting evidence is pursued under the desire to prove a predetermined point. A search for truth is nowhere involved in such a process. Truth only comes into play as a word applied superficially at the end of the process to help add validity to the claim being made.

This is the equivalent of *Daily Planet* editor, Perry White, telling his reporters, Clark Kent and Lois Lane, "Write an article for me saying that last night's fire did not take place last night," rather than "Go cover the fire that we are getting reports from."

While so-called fact checking websites are far more subtle in their dishonesty, such an egregious example is akin to the process that takes place at so-called fact checking websites.

As such, it can be no surprise that so-called fact checking websites can have articles supporting total falsehoods and often do. Overwhelmingly, that is what exists on so-called fact checking websites. Such websites often have accurate data that is presented, or "spun," in such a way that renders the results inaccurate.

Despite their overwhelming inaccuracy, they also provide a useful purpose, though quite limited in scope. When such articles contain links, oftentimes, one need only click on those links as a researcher to find quality evidence that entirely debunks that so-called fact checker who cites it.

Additionally, so-called fact checking websites can be useful for writers, like myself, seeking to identify, in advance, what narratives will be used to attack the results of truthful inquiry and address those ahead of time.

So-called fact checking websites often come with a headline labelling a specific detail true or untrue, often in salacious and well-marketed ways. While such websites have usefulness, my experience with such headlines — the part of the article most intended to be read and which most people read — is that they are inaccurate 90 to 95% of the time for so-called fact checking articles that I have read.

Given this trend, it is no surprise to me that the topic of virtually every chapter in this book has been "debunked" or will be "debunked" by such websites.

The savvy reader knows this and understands the lack of truthful inquiry that takes place at such websites and throughout the media and society.

Popularity, or lack thereof, does not make truth any more or less accurate. Search engine rank does not make truth any more or less accurate. Appearance as a media talking point does not make truth any more or less accurate. In fact, quite the opposite is more likely to be the case. Truth is unlikely to appear in a media talking point. Half-truth or outright deceit is far more likely to appear there — a condemnable detail of the era in which we live.

As bold truth seekers rise up in greater number and replace those who make a living dispensing lies, such a state of affairs will come to be remedied. That state of affairs may also return one day if truth seekers let down their guard.

Such is the way of the world in this period and in all of history. I ask you, dear reader, to do your part, to be diligent about that, and to as often as possible, seek to identify the truth rather than to identify evidence in support of a point you aim to prove.

That is at the heart of the scientific method. That is at the heart of rational inquiry. Each of us must be comfortable re-examining our own views and holding them up to scrutiny to see if they ring true.

The narrative of the safe and effective face mask does not ring true. Despite that, public health professionals have been slow to address that policy. This indicates a disinterest in the scientific method and a disinterest in rational inquiry. This behavior demonstrates defense of science or the protection of health cannot, at this point, be said to play any role in the mask policies of 2020 and beyond.

FACE MASKS DO NOT WORK

Reason 1: The CDC Says Face Masks Do Not Work

The US Center for Disease Control and Prevention (CDC) has an estimated 15,000 people in its workforce; some 88 of them work on *Emerging Infectious Diseases*,[1] a highly regarded, peer-reviewed journal of epidemiology, published by the CDC.

April 3, 2020 — CDC Face Mask Order

On April 3, 2020, the CDC announced that everyone should wear face masks, wash their hands, and clean surfaces in order to prevent the spread of Covid-19.[2]

CDC 4/3/20: Wear Masks To Fight Covid

On April 3, 2020, the CDC advised, "Everyone should wear a cloth face cover when they have to go out in public, for example to the grocery store or to pick up other necessities."[2] Private and governmental policies across the US and internationally were crafted according to this statement.

CDC 4/3/20: Wash Hands To Fight Covid

On April 3, 2020, the CDC advised, "Wash your hands often with soap and water for at least 20 seconds especially after you have been in a public place, or after blowing your nose, coughing, or sneezing."[2]

CDC 4/3/20: Clean Surfaces To Fight Covid

On April 3, 2020, the CDC advised, "Clean and disinfect frequently touched surfaces daily. This includes tables, doorknobs, light switches, countertops, handles, desks, phones, keyboards, toilets, faucets, and sinks."[2]

May 2020 — Researchers Prove the Opposite

May 2020, Jingyi Xiao, an epidemiologist from the University of Hong Kong, and her colleagues, ran a paper entitled "Nonpharmaceutical Measures for Pandemic Influenza in Nonhealthcare Settings — Personal Protective and Environmental Measures"[3] at the CDC's journal of epidemiology, *Emerging Infectious Diseases*. In this paper they sought to separate myth from reality and to demonstrate what data-driven measures can be helpful in preventing the spread of Covid-19. Xiao's research in the peer-reviewed CDC journal specializing on this topic, showed the opposite of the April 3, 2020, statements from the CDC to be true.

Superior Methodology

Xiao's efforts began with more diligent and rigorous methodology than recent reviewers who came before: "We searched 4 databases[3] (Medline, PubMed, EMBASE, and CENTRAL) for literature in all languages. We aimed to identify randomized controlled trials (RCTs) of each measure for laboratory-confirmed influenza outcomes for each of the measures because RCTs provide the highest quality of evidence."

Throughout 2020, it has been easy for low-quality Covid research to get published and then circulated through the media, entirely out of context. This has been detrimental in a time when high quality and dependable information would be most useful in the protection of life and livelihood in 2020. Consequently, Xiao does not treat every study the same. Randomized controlled trials with laboratory confirmed outcomes were the standard their review of the literature sought. Rather than cherry-picking the studies with fashionable results, they sought truth and quality over political correctness and assessed the gold standard studies. Not surprisingly, in doing so, Xiao produced the exact opposite results of what you would find from Fox News, *The New York Times*, Google, or their many clones.

Xiao, unsurprisingly, reports what researchers of randomized controlled trials with laboratory-confirmed outcomes have long known:

> "Although mechanistic studies support the potential effect of hand hygiene or face masks, evidence from 14 randomized controlled trials of these measures did not support a substantial effect on transmission of laboratory-confirmed influenza. We similarly found limited evidence on the effectiveness of improved hygiene and environmental cleaning. We identified several major knowledge gaps requiring further research, most fundamentally an improved characterization of the modes of person-to-person transmission."[3]

You read that right:
1.) It does not matter if you sanitize surfaces;
2.) It does not matter if you wash your hands;
3.) Masks do not work.

CDC Journal 5/1/20: Sanitizing Surfaces Does Not Protect Against Covid[3]

Sanitizing surfaces is effective for the prevention of gastrointestinal illnesses, but it does not protect from Covid. Xiao writes:[3]

"Although we found no evidence that surface and object cleaning could reduce influenza transmission, this measure does have an established impact on prevention of other infectious diseases."

CDC Journal 5/1/20: Washing Your Hands Does Not Protect Against Covid[3]

Similarly, hand washing is useful for the prevention of gastrointestinal illness, but the laboratory-confirmed, randomized controlled trials show that it is not useful in the prevention of Covid. Xiao writes:[3]

"Hand hygiene is a widely used intervention and has been shown to effectively reduce the transmission of gastrointestinal infections and respiratory infections. However, in our systematic review, updating the findings of Wong et al.[4] we did not find evidence of a major effect of hand hygiene on laboratory-confirmed influenza virus transmission. Nevertheless, hand hygiene might be included in influenza pandemic plans as part of general hygiene and infection prevention."

CDC Journal 5/1/20: Masks Do Not Work[3]

Face masks might help prevent the spread of some infections, but there is no proof that they work with Covid-19 or influenza. Xiao writes:[3]

"We did not find evidence that surgical-type face masks are effective in reducing laboratory-confirmed influenza transmission, either when worn by infected persons (source control) or by persons in the general community to reduce their susceptibility. However, as with hand hygiene, face masks might be able to reduce the transmission of other infections and therefore have value in an influenza pandemic when healthcare resources are stretched."

CDC Journal 5/1/20: Face Masks Do Not Work When Worn By The Sick Either[3]

Some say face masks should be worn by the infected, not the healthy. In doing so, they can prevent infected people from transmitting the virus to the healthy. Xiao found no such evidence of this. Rather than relying on datasets based on questionnaires such as "Did you suffer from the sniffles last week?" Xiao, in examining this issue, only looked at laboratory-confirmed cases and found no proof that people sick with a respiratory virus should wear masks either:

> "There is limited evidence for their effectiveness in preventing influenza virus transmission either when worn by the infected person for source control or when worn by uninfected persons to reduce exposure. Our systematic review found no significant effect of face masks on transmission of laboratory-confirmed influenza."

CDC Journal 5/1/20: Covering Your Mouth Does Not Even Seem To Work[3]

Etiquette in many places says you cover your mouth when you sneeze or cough. Xiao went so far as to investigate this also, finding such respiratory etiquette unhelpful in preventing the transmission of Covid, and encouraging others to take up that area of research:

> "Respiratory etiquette is often listed as a preventive measure for respiratory infections. However, there is a lack of scientific evidence to support this measure. Whether respiratory etiquette is an effective non-pharmaceutical intervention in preventing influenza virus transmission remains questionable, and worthy of further research."

Caveat: Xiao Did Not Look At N95 And P2 Respirators[3]

Focusing on the most pressing matters that relate to the greatest number of people, Xiao looked at face masks and not respirators. Respirators come with their own warning. They, too, require their own hygiene and fit protocol in order or be effective, protocol seldom followed. Xiao writes:[3]

> "We did not consider the use of respirators in the community. Respirators are tight-fitting masks that can protect the wearer from fine particles and should provide better protection against influenza virus exposures when properly worn because of higher filtration efficiency. However, respirators, such as N95 and P2 masks, work best when they are fit-tested, and these masks will be in limited supply during the next pandemic."

Who Is More Credible — Political Hacks or Gold Standard Scientists?

It would look, on the surface, like the CDC is contradicting itself. One organ of the CDC said one thing in April,[2] and another organ said something else in May.[3] This would not be the first confusing message from the CDC. One may feel torn between who to believe. That need not be the case at all.

You have the top brass at the CDC, composed of political hacks saying to wear something, anything, as long as it vaguely resembles a mask. Their statements shift whenever it is expedient to them. Then, in contrast, you have the peer-reviewed scientists pointing to the well-established fact that masks do not work for reducing coronavirus transmission.

I do not know what the political hacks are trying to pull or why, and I do not particularly need to know in order to understand why not to trust political hacks. What I know is that what they are saying is predictably inaccurate. This is the case for much of what political hacks say. Just because it comes from the hacks does not make it wrong, but hacks have a bad track record when it comes to science. They just do not have a primary penchant for truth. If they did, they would not be political hacks.

Face masks do not work in preventing the spread of Covid.[3] The science on that is well-established.

2020 — A Year Of Superstition, Not Science

Many of the weird, OCD, germophobe, anti-social, hypochondriac maneuvers that have become commonplace in 2020 and beyond are rooted in superstition, but not science.[3] While these interventions may be the advice of those reading Fox News marquees or *The New York Times* headlines, they are not data-driven interventions backed by peer-reviewed, laboratory-confirmed, randomized controlled trials. Those trials say something clearly different.[3]

Face mask orders are the territory of the science-denier, the anti-logician, the mob with torches ready to punish Copernicus for applying the scientific method and thinking according to his findings. It is not me saying that. These are the 14 gold standard studies used by Xiao and her research team.[3]

Knowing This, What Will You Do?

Now I have tremendous regard for those who will take this knowledge and evangelize. I also have tremendous praise for those who will take this knowledge and crash the gates. My method has been to encourage people with exemptions to say the words "I am unable to wear a face mask safely."[5] Thousands have successfully used this technique. Millions can successfully use it. One free person at a time, these lockdowns come to an end, not when a blue ribbon committee says they end.[6]

Conclusion: The Experts Know A Lot Less Than They Have Led Us To Believe

Xiao provides a useful slice of humble pie to the people who suddenly became Covid experts[7] and tinpot dictators in the spring of 2020. The aggressive mask-police do not know as much as they think they do. The "experts"[8] that the aggressive mask police are getting their information from do not either.

Unfortunately, this sober appraisal does not sell advertising, fund studies, or make careers, so instead of being the most cited study of 2020, Xiao has practically been ignored.[9]

Perhaps in your own circle of friends, you can change this by sharing her important research.

So many of the bad policies of 2020 and beyond were refuted in the pages of the May 2020 study, yet it was widely ignored. It remains the best paper on the topic of face masks and demands widespread consideration by the medical and public health community.

Reason 2: The CDC And WHO Say Face Masks May INCREASE The Spread Of Disease

Xiao's paper, mentioned in the last chapter, says face masks do not work, but it does not stop there.[1]

CDC Journal 5/1/20: Do Not Wear A Dirty Mask, It Can INCREASE The Risk Of Covid Transmission[1]

Xiao takes it a step further, saying not only may face masks be unhelpful in stopping the spread of Covid-19, but they can actually increase the risk of transmission: "Proper use of face masks is essential because improper use might increase the risk for transmission. Thus, education on the proper use and disposal of used face masks, including hand hygiene, is also needed."[1]

What Is "Proper Use?"

Xiao cites a World Health Organization (WHO) notice from 2009[2] entitled, "Advice on the use of masks in the community setting in Influenza A (H1N1) outbreaks,"[3] which offers some well-established advice for proper mask use. Again, Xiao has demonstrated that proper mask use does not stop Covid-19, but to cite the WHO, the great risk of the mask is that transmission is increased: "Using a mask incorrectly however, may actually increase the risk of transmission, rather than reduce it."

The following from the WHO[4] is listed as behavior that can increase transmission:

- Touching mouth and nose,
- Touching a mask in use,
- Touching a clean mask with unwashed hands,
- Not washing hands every time after touching a dirty mask,
- Wearing a mask that is not new and clean,
- Continuing to wear a mask after it has become damp, instead of immediately replacing it,
- Re-using a single-use mask,
- Not discarding a single-use mask immediately upon removal, as opposed to leaving it in the immediate environment.

Have you seen even one person follow that protocol in 2020? Proper mask protocol does not stop there either. Rather than informing the public that such behaviors may actually help spread Covid, the most vocal, in-

stead, demand that everyone be masked, regardless of the potential negative impact it may have in increasing the transmission of Covid-19.

Reason 3: *The New England Journal Of Medicine* Says Face Masks Do Not Work

On May 21, 2020, seven weeks after the CDC's April 3, 2020 face mask recommendations were released, *The New England Journal of Medicine* addressed the foolishness of mandatory masking of the general population:[1]

> **"We know that wearing a mask outside healthcare facilities offers little, if any, protection from infection.** Public health authorities define a significant exposure to Covid-19 as face to face contact within six feet with a patient with symptomatic Covid-19 that is sustained for at least a few minutes (and some say more than 10 minutes or even 20 minutes). The chance of catching Covid-19 from a passing interaction in a public space is therefore minimal. **In many cases the desire for widespread masking is a reflexive reaction to anxiety over the pandemic."**

Emphasis has been added in this quote and the following quotes. The same article goes on to theorize when masking may be helpful in hospital environments before going on to warn of the necessity to recognize limitations associated with possible benefits in that environment as well.

> "What is clear, however, is **that universal masking alone is not a panacea.** A mask will not protect providers caring for a patient with active Covid-19 if it is not accompanied by meticulous hand hygiene, eye protection, gloves, and a gown. A mask alone will not prevent healthcare workers with early Covid-19 from contaminating their hands and spreading the virus to patients and colleagues. **Focusing on universal masking alone may, paradoxically, lead to more transmission of Covid-19 if it diverts attention from implementing more fundamental infection-control measures."**

In couched language, the same authors go on to say, that while a mask may have no "technical" benefit on the spread of disease, the mask may have a psychological benefit, by being a visible reminder to others that people must fearfully avoid each other.

> "There may be additional benefits to broad masking policies that extend beyond their technical contribution to re-

ducing pathogen transmission. Masks are visible reminders of an otherwise invisible yet widely prevalent pathogen and may remind people of the importance of social distancing and other infection-control measures."

The same piece, almost shockingly honest for *The New England Journal of Medicine,* goes so far as to call the mask being pushed upon billions harmfully and ineffectively "a talisman."

> "It is also clear that **masks serve symbolic roles.** Masks are not only tools, they are also talismans that may help increase healthcare workers' perceived sense of safety, well-being, and trust in their hospitals. **Although such reactions may not be strictly logical, we are all subject to fear and anxiety, especially during times of crisis.** One might argue that fear and anxiety are better countered with data and education than with a marginally beneficial mask, particularly in light of the worldwide mask shortage, but **it is difficult to get clinicians to hear this message in the heat of the current crisis.** Expanded masking protocols' greatest contribution may be to reduce the transmission of anxiety, over and above whatever role they may play in reducing transmission of Covid-19. The potential value of universal masking in giving healthcare workers the confidence to absorb and implement the more foundational infection-prevention practices described above may be its greatest contribution."

The idea of scientific consensus on the topic of masking has been heavily pushed in politics, media, and society. There is no consensus. Dissent has poked through repeatedly despite the very heavy handed censorship by government and corporations alike.

Just as Jingyi Xiao indicates, in the CDC's peer-reviewed journal of epidemiology, *Emerging Infection Diseases*, masks offer "little if any protection."[2]

Quite logically, seeing such rampant nonsense as the mandatory masking of society, these sober commentators in the same *The New England Journal of Medicine* article, took it further and offered cautionary words: **"Widespread masking is a reflexive reaction to anxiety over the pandemic."** It is not wise. It is not sound. It is not well thought out. It is reflexive, like a blink or a flinch or a shiver.

These are quite critical words and from a well-respected source. Like Xiao, these sober words, too, fell on deaf ears and were largely censored.

Sober researchers were writing about how ineffective masks were to anyone who would listen. Were you listening?

Reason 4: The US Food And Drug Administration Says Face Masks Do Not Work

A brilliantly written California lawsuit of 2021, *Jennifer Guilfoyle v. Austin Beutner* [1] points out how even the FDA is clear that masks are not for "infection prevention or reduction."[2]

Face masks are not FDA approved, which would require a far more stringent process. Face masks are merely authorized under an "Emergency Use Authorization."

In the Emergency Use Authorization, which authorizes general emergency use of face masks, the FDA stated that it "would misrepresent the product's intended use" to state that it "is for use such as infection prevention or reduction."[3]

The FDA, furthermore, in a document entitled "Enforcement Policy for Face Masks and Respirators During the Coronavirus Disease (Covid-19) Public Health Emergency (Revised)" clearly states that face masks are not intended to reduce or prevent infection.[4]

Reason 5: Yes, Data From The Council On Foreign Relations Even Says Face Masks Do Not Work

The Council on Foreign Relations, an organization dedicated to making others live less free lives, even found it important to conduct a study on face mask effectiveness and compliance.

It is an organization imbued through and through with a spirit of control and most certainly not a spirit of charity. When the CFR is studying masks, one can almost be certain that the study is not about a charitable interpretation of helping others live more helpful and prosperous lives.

In a September 2020 paper entitled: "Microbial challenges from masks," Boris Borovoy et al. uses the CFR study alongside readily available public data to demonstrate the ineffectiveness of face masks:"[1]

"In July 2020, the Council of Foreign Relations conducted a survey of 25 countries, with the following question to their citizens:

"'Have you always worn a face mask outside the home in the last seven days?' The 'Yes' responses ranged from 1% in Finland and Denmark, to 93% in Singapore.[2]

"We then examined each of the same 25 countries for prevalence of mask use versus Covid-19 deaths per 1 million population. This data was gathered from Worldometers statistics.[3] That data is shown in Table 1, also represented in Graph 1."

Table 1

* % mask use over Jul 6-12, 2020 from CFR survey
** Covid deaths per 1M pop, at 10/7/2020 from Worldometers

	*	**
Singapore	93	5
Philippines	92	54
Brazil	90	694
UAE	89	44
India	88	76
Spain	87	696
Mexico	86	637

Hong Kong	85	14
Thailand	82	0.8
Indonesia	80	42
Italy	79	597
Saudi Arabia	79	142
Malaysia	76	4
Vietnam	68	0.4
China	67	3
United States	65	653
Germany	63	115
Taiwan	59	0.3
France	52	497
United Kingdom	22	625
Australia	12	35
Norway	3	51
Sweden	3	582
Denmark	1	114
Finland	1	62

Graph 1

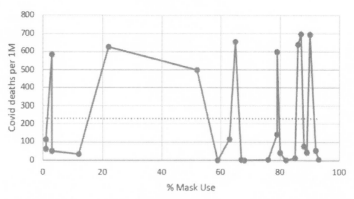

Covid deaths per 1M pop, at 10/7/2020 from Worldometers

Borovoy identifies in this data no correlation between Covid death rates and face mask use (Emphasis added):

> "**As we see from the above data, there was no significant correlation with mask use and either increase or reduction of deaths from Covid-19; thus masking could not have caused a significant reduction in deaths.** In fact,

two of the countries with the highest Covid-19 deaths also had high rates of mask use: Spain at 87% mask use and Brazil at 90% mask use. Again, masking could not have caused a significant reduction in deaths."

While there is no correlation between mask use and deaths, Borovoy identifies a correlation between mask use and PCR test rates that is counter to the main stream narrative:

"Another table presented from Worldometers data also demonstrates the rate of positive Covid-19 PCR tests per one million population in the same 25 countries surveyed. This data is reported in Table 2 and Graph 2."

Table 2

* % mask use over Jul 6-12, 2020 from CFR survey
** Total + PCR tests per 1M pop, at 10/7/2020 from Worldometers

	*	**
Singapore	93	9866
Philippines	92	2998
Brazil	90	23378
UAE	89	10264
India	88	4938
Spain	87	18654
Mexico	86	6146
Hong Kong	85	385
Thailand	82	52
Indonesia	80	1151
Italy	79	5525
Saudi Arabia	79	9661
Malaysia	76	431
Vietnam	68	11
China	67	59
United States	65	23385
Germany	63	3708
Taiwan	59	22
France	52	10006
United Kingdom	22	8006
Australia	12	1063
Norway	3	2742
Sweden	3	9557

| Denmark | 1 | 5297 |
| Finland | 1 | 1993 |

Graph 2

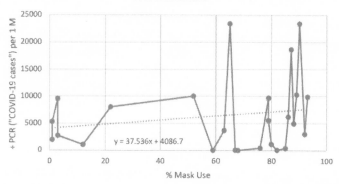

Total + PCR tests per 1M pop, at 10/7/2020 from Worldometers

Borovoy identifies a trend in this second set of data (Emphasis added):

> "Contrary to data in table 1, we do see a significant trend in table 2. Curve-fitting a trend line, we see a positive slope for this line of 37.536. That is, **for every increased percentage point of mask use in a country, there were an average of 37.536 additional positive PCR tests per one million population.** This shows that masking has not accomplished the advertised function of reducing the number of positive PCR tests, but rather seems to be correlated with an increased number of positive PCR tests for Covid-19."

To allow Borovoy to state this even more clearly:

> "Mask use does not decrease the number of positive PCR tests, mask use actually <u>INCREASES</u> the number of positive PCR tests."

Are you starting to see a trend here?

If you scratch the surface a little, it becomes evident that face masks have been known to not work against the transmission of a respiratory virus. All anyone needed to do to figure that out was to turn off the media, stop listening to politicians, and to find some quality research. That research has been readily available.

Reason 6: Many Other Medical Researchers Say Face Masks Do Not Work

The last few chapters demonstrate that face masks do not work. This information is not new information.

The face mask is an enduring example of that. It has been observed that the politics of science is so ingrained in the field that "Science only changes one dead scientist at a time." Hopefully, the face mask debacle of 2020 and 2021 is the last hurrah for the superstitious practice of masking. Below are further examples of other medical researchers saying face masks do not work. Emphasis has been added below.

Tom Jefferson in the April 7, 2020 article "Physical interventions to interrupt or reduce the spread of respiratory viruses. Part 1 — Face masks, eye protection and person distancing: systematic review and meta-analysis,"[1] writes:

> "There was **no reduction of influenza-like illnesses** when healthcare workers or the general population wore masks."[2]

Jeffrey D. Smith, in the article "Effectiveness of N95 respirators versus surgical masks in protecting healthcare workers from acute respiratory infection: a systematic review and meta-analysis," published on March 7, 2016, writes that face masks:

> **"Did not show any benefit against the transmission of acute respiratory infections**."[3]

Faisal bin-Reza, in the December 21, 2011 article "The use of masks and respirators to prevent transmission of influenza: a systematic review of the scientific evidence," writes the wearing of face masks:

> "Resulted in **no significant difference** in the incidence of laboratory confirmed influenza."[4]

N.J. Mitchell and S. Hunt, in the July 18, 1991 article "Surgical face masks in modern operating rooms — a costly and unnecessary ritual?" writes:

> "This study found **no difference in wound infection rates** with and without surgical masks."[5]

Seongman Bae et al. in the April 6, 2020 article "Effectiveness of Surgical and Cotton Masks in Blocking SARS–CoV-2: A Controlled Comparison in 4 Patients," writes:

"Neither surgical nor cotton masks effectively filtered Sars-Cov-2 during coughs by infected patients.[6]

Neil W. M. Orr, in the November 1981 article "Is a mask necessary in the operating theater," published in *Annals of the Royal College of Surgeons of England*,[7] writes that they:

"Found no difference in wound infection rates whether or not surgeons wore surgical masks."

Göran Tunevall wrote a paper called, "Postoperative wound infections and surgical face masks: a controlled study," which was published in *World Journal Surgery* in 1991. The author noted **the use of masks in surgery were found to slightly increase incidence of infection over not masking** in a study of 3,088 surgeries. The surgeons' masks were found to give no protective effect to the patients.[8]

Let me repeat the finding of that last one: Masks are so counterproductive that if you are having a surgery and your surgeon wears a mask, you are *more likely* to get an infection than if he does not wear a mask.

The idea of face masks as a mere talisman and ineffective against disease transmission has been demonstrated repeatedly.

Old habits die hard though.

Reason 7: Countries With Face Mask Mandates Are Not Better Off Than Countries Without Them

Across American states, and in countries around the globe, there were variables worth studying regarding why some states were hit harder in 2020 and 2021 with reported cases of Covid-19. Face masks, however, were not one of the variables.

Topics of study that have shown some early promise and may be worth further consideration by researchers include: season, latitude, sunlight exposure, skin melanin levels, EMF waves, obesity, comorbidities, sugar consumption, diet and nutrition, faith, mood, personality, outlook, fitness level, age, blood serum vitamin D levels, available treatment options, presence of a patient advocate, heart disease, and willingness to take authority over ones health and wellbeing.

There is no consistency that proves the efficacy of face masks in 2020 and 2021 against the spread of a respiratory virus, which is exactly what the best research of the past 40 years on the topic would predict.

As the Association of American Physicians and Surgeons points out:[1]

> "Holland's Medical Care Minister Tamara van Ark says 'Despite a global stampede of mask-wearing, data show that 80-90 percent of people in Finland and Holland say they 'never' wear masks when they go out, a sharp contrast to the 80-90 percent of people in Spain and Italy who say they 'always' wear masks when they go out. 'From a medical point of view, there is no evidence of a medical effect of wearing face masks, so we decided not to impose a national obligation.'"[2]

Comparisons of countries and states have repeatedly shown that face masks are not what separates places with high Covid-19 impacts from places with low Covid-19 impacts.

With these real world results repeatedly showing that face masks are not the variable, we are left with many meaningful data sets that show that face masks do not prevent the spread of a respiratory virus. Anyone suggesting otherwise is doing so contrary to the available evidence. Face masks do not work to prevent the spread of a respiratory virus. If face masks do not work, then there is no reason to wear them to stop the spread of a respiratory virus.

Given the fact that face mask wearing is so harmful on the wearer, they must not be worn at all, least of all out of obligation to the debunked theory that they are effective at stopping the spread of a respiratory virus.

Reason 8: Face Masks Did Not Work In 1918, 1957, 1968, 2002, 2004, And They Do Not Work Now

There were influenza pandemics in the years 1918, 1957, 1968, 2002, 2004. Face mask use did not work during any previous pandemic to stop the spread of respiratory viruses because face masks do not stop the spread of a respiratory virus.

This is true no matter who wore them. It is true no matter what powers are inaccurately ascribed to face masks.

The same is true today.

Kai Kisielinski, in an April 20, 2021 article, in *International Journal of Environmental Research and Public Health*, entitled "Is a Mask That Covers the Mouth and Nose Free from Undesirable Side Effects in Everyday Use and Free of Potential Hazards?"1 writes:

> "The history of modern times shows that already in the influenza pandemics of 1918–1919, 1957–58, 1968, 2002, in SARS 2004–2005 as well as with the influenza in 2009, masks in everyday use could not achieve the hoped-for success in the fight against viral infection scenarios.[2,5] The experiences led to scientific studies describing as early as 2009 that masks do not show any significant effect with regard to viruses in an everyday scenario.[3,6] Even later, scientists and institutions rated the masks as unsuitable to protect the user safely from viral respiratory infections.[4,7,8] Even in hospital use, surgical masks lack strong evidence of protection against viruses."[2]

What we have here is a preference for tradition over science, a preference for superstition over wisdom, a preference for the status quo over genuine evidence based inquiry and practice. Face masks do not work to prevent the spread of a respiratory virus. Rhetoric does not change that fact. Marketing does not change that fact. Talking heads cannot change that fact. That fact does not change no matter how many times the anti-science crowd claims to be following the science.

We now have data more than a century old that show that face masks do not work to prevent the spread of a respiratory virus during pandemics. We have data that say they are not effective against Sars-Cov-2. We have data that says they do not work to prevent the spread of a respiratory virus in non-pandemic settings either. There is a phrase that has been a useful talking point from the anti-science crowd during 2020 and beyond: "Your mask protects me and my mask protects you." While that sounds catchy, the years of data and research show that your mask does not help me and my mask does not help you.

In fact, there is overwhelming evidence that your mask is harmful to you and my mask, if I ever wore a mask, would be harmful to me. Furthermore, your mask may be harmful to me and my mask may be harmful to you.

Not only that, as Kisielinski points out, we have an absence of data for the usefulness of face masks in hospital settings. As the latter pages of this book show, there is even a strong argument to be made for masks to be removed from hospital settings, since masks are both harmful for the wearer AND for those around the wearer. This is especially true when the wearer is operating heavy machinery or engaging in complex tasks such as those required to treat a patient safely and effectively. Hospital care teams that were once unmasked have suddenly all been masked. This has been done despite the fact that there is a lack of evidence to support this behavior and substantial evidence against this behavior. Despite the constant insistence on "evidence based medicine," so few talking heads are interested in this data. Consequently, a very dangerous situation has occurred as untrustworthy people in positions of authority make foolhardy proclamations over the population entirely contrary to available evidence.

The impact a face mask has on the cognition of the wearer and the impact that creates on the patient in a hospital setting is a major unaddressed public health concern that has emerged since the Ides of March 2020.

A century of sporadic data and two years of very precise, carefully collected, readily available data now shows this to be the case: face masks are not safe, face masks are not effective.

Reason 9: The SARS Hype Is Severely Blown Out Of Proportion

Not only do face masks not work, but Sars-Cov-2 did not turn into the virus it was promised to be.

Baruch Vainshelboim writes in "Face masks in the Covid-19 era: A health hypothesis:"[1]

> "On January 30, 2020, the World Health Organization (WHO) announced a global public health emergency of severe acute respiratory syndrome-coronavirus-2 (Sars-Cov-2) causing illness of coronavirus disease-2019 (Covid-19).[2] As of October 1, 2020, worldwide 34,166,633 cases were reported and 1,018,876 have died with virus diagnosis. **Interestingly, 99% of the detected cases with Sars-Cov-2 are asymptomatic or have mild condition, which contradicts with the virus name (severe acute respiratory syndrome-coronavirus-2).**"[3] (Emphasis added)

Vainshelboim's point is important.

How "severe" can an illness be, if better than 99% of people recover fully, with most never even realizing they are sick?

Given Vainshelboim's observations, would not a more truthful name for this be "very mild and relatively harmless respiratory condition?"

That would not sell the public on a host of things that a scarier sounding name helps to sell, such as media advertising, pharmaceutical interventions, and big government projects.

So a deceitful name, effective at tricking people and altering behavior to the benefit of special interest groups is preferred over a truthful name? Do I pretend to know the motivation of the people involved? Certainly not. Vainshelboim clearly points out, however, that a deceitful name has been preferred over a truthful name. That alone is a cause for alarm.

Not only is Vainshelboim pointing out the lack of severity of this illness for better than 99% of people, if you set aside the narrative and look at published scientific data, the head of the US National Institute of Allergy and Infectious Diseases (NIAID) Anthony Fauci is saying the same. Vainshelboim prefaces this and quotes Fauci as he compares Covid-19 to a seasonal flu:

> "Although infection fatality rate (number of death cases divided by number of reported cases) initially seems quite high 0.029 (2.9%),[3] this overestimation related to limited

number of Covid-19 tests performed which biases towards higher rates. Given the fact that asymptomatic or minimally symptomatic cases is several times higher than the number of reported cases, the case fatality rate is considerably less than 1%.[4] This was confirmed by the head of National Institute of Allergy and Infectious Diseases from US stating, 'the overall clinical consequences of Covid-19 are similar to those of severe seasonal influenza,' [4] having a case fatality rate of approximately 0.1%."[4-7]

The United States recorded cases of people who died *with* Sars-Cov-2 rather than dying *of* Sars-Cov-2 in 2020 breaking with past practice.

Rather than being a great killer of people, Sars-Cov-2 was predictably present in sick people and not the cause of death for sick people or healthy people. Prior lifestyle decisions and pre-existing conditions were the killers. The fraudulent US death numbers from 2020 and beyond have included reports of death *with* Sars-Cov-2 not *from* Sars-Cov-2. This is a crucial distinction that cannot be overstated.

As a result, a total fraud has been perpetrated on trusting people by the public health institutions. Vainshelboim continues:

"In addition, data from hospitalized patients with Covid-19 and general public indicate that the majority of deaths were among older and chronically ill individuals, supporting the possibility that the virus may exacerbate existing conditions but rarely causes death by itself.[8,9] Sars-Cov-2 primarily affects respiratory system and can cause complications such as acute respiratory distress syndrome (ARDS), respiratory failure and death."[2,8]

In the midst of this, Vainshelboim points to the ineffectiveness and harm in using face masks, which is the exact opposite approach one would take if one wanted to keep a population healthy:

"It is not clear however, what the scientific and clinical basis for wearing face masks as protective strategy, given the fact that face masks restrict breathing, causing hypoxemia and hypercapnia and increase the risk for respiratory complications, self-contamination and exacerbation of existing chronic conditions."[10-14]

Vainshelboim takes a special look at sufficient oxygen supply, needed by all of us, denied to those in masks.

"Of note, hyperoxia or oxygen supplementation (breathing air with high partial O2 pressures that above the sea levels) has been well established as therapeutic and curative practice for variety acute and chronic conditions including respiratory complications.[11,15] It fact, the current standard of care practice for treating hospitalized patients with Covid-19 is breathing 100% oxygen.[16-18] Although several countries mandated wearing face mask in healthcare settings and public areas, scientific evidences are lacking supporting their efficacy for reducing morbidity or mortality associated with infectious or viral diseases.[10,14,19] Therefore, it has been hypothesized: 1) the practice of wearing face masks has compromised safety and efficacy profile, 2) Both medical and non-medical face masks are ineffective to reduce human-to-human transmission and infectivity of Sars-Cov-2 and Covid-19, 3) Wearing face masks has adverse physiological and psychological effects, 4) Long-term consequences of wearing face masks on health are detrimental."

Instead of acknowledging how minor of an illness Covid-19 has been, the narrative keeps shifting as if the goal is not to recover, but as if the goal of it is something else.

We flattened the curve. We stopped the spread. We reduced cases. We got the test numbers up. We got the case numbers down. We got into the right color zone.

The goal posts are constantly shifting. When the goal posts are constantly shifting, there is no way you ever reach them. The only way to end this, is for each of us, to put an end to it in our own lives: not an end to Covid-19, an end to this foolish pursuit of constantly moving goalposts.

That is how every lockdown has always ended, that is how every bad, oppressive imposition upon a free people has always ended: with individuals determining individually to no longer comply, one person at a time. That is how this will end as well.

The Vainshelboims of the world are playing their part in ending it.

But they cannot bring it to an end in your life. That is up to you as an individual.

What are you waiting for?

Reason 10: The Flu Is More Dangerous Than Covid & Neither Of Them Are Stopped By Face Mask Wearing

Making sense of basic Covid statistics is not so complex. Much of the data is widely available and only requires the user to be willing to challenge the talking heads in the media and to insist on seeing the data. For whatever reason, politicians and media figures are so eager and willing to contradict what available data is saying. One example is in the case of the risk of Covid-19 to a child or anyone a child comes in contact with.

As a caveat, merely because data is posted on a government website does not make that data accurate. A great deal of effort is put into making some of the data appear accurate, though it is inaccurate. Even inaccurate data, skewed to look much worse than it is, can be read with a critical eye to arrive at a more truthful interpretation.

It is said that "A man with experience is never at the mercy of a man with a theory."[1] Chris Wark, who notably beat stage 3 colon cancer in 2004 without chemotherapy, is a researcher and blogger on the topic of health, nutrition, and natural therapies. His experience with the medical industry as a patient with a death sentence gives him a special passion for getting to the truth that many physicians and researchers, unfortunately, do not have. Wark writes:

"Children have a 99.997% Covid-19 survival rate.

They have a higher risk of death from the flu.

Let us review the data from the CDC:

In the 2017/2018 flu season (Nov-March), 643 children (under 18) died.[2]

In the 2018/2019 flu season, 477 children died.[3]

In the 2019/2020 flu season, 434 children died.[4]

Comparatively, 423 children have reportedly died of Covid-19 as of 8/11/21.[5]

That is less child deaths from Covid-19 than from each of the last three flu seasons.

But wait...

The 423 reported deaths in children from Covid-19 is over a period of 20 months (since January 2020), not over a 4-month winter flu season.

This means the risk of death for children from Covid-19 per season is even lower than the flu, perhaps half as low.

And the CDC's Covid-19 death count includes 18 year-olds, whereas the CDC's seasonal flu death count does not. It's ages 0-17.

This suspicious CDC reporting inconsistency skews the Covid-19 'childhood death' numbers higher to those who are not paying attention (everyone).

After some digging, I found *Statista* reporting 349 Covid-19 deaths in children ages 0-17 through August 4th.[6]

This more accurate number reduces children's actual risk of death compared to previous flu seasons EVEN FURTHER.[7]

It is important to keep in mind that children who die from the flu or Covid-19 often have serious pre-existing conditions.

Children with co-morbidities have nearly double the risk of severe Covid-19 than healthy children. And children with underlying conditions including obesity were found to have nearly triple the risk of Covid-19-associated death.[8]

Dr. Marty Makary's team at Johns Hopkins found a mortality rate of ZERO among children with no pre-existing medical conditions[.9]

Based on this data, the logical, rational conclusion is:

Children have a higher risk of dying from the flu than from Covid-19.

And thankfully, both risks are extremely low.

If you are not concerned about children dying from the flu, you should not be concerned of children dying from Covid-19.

Children have proven to have strong innate immunity. They are safe, resilient and not at a risk of dying worthy of any potentially harmful intervention.

Furthermore, if a child passes Covid-19 to an adult under 70, that adult's survival rate is 99.85%.

Children should not be afraid of Covid-19, or each other, and we should not either.

— Chris Wark

#FactsOverFear"[10]

Covid is not the great danger it is said to be in the media, by public health officials, and by politicians.

Nationally syndicated radio host Kate Dalley goes on to tell a story of her own experience, which points to treatment, as a problem, rather than a virus as the problem. In an August 6, 2021, broadcast entitled, "Our First Hand ICU Story — What is ACTUALLY Killing People In The Hospital," Dalley tells her experience with her own husband in the hospital with a case of pneumonia that was diagnosed as "Covid pneumonia."[11]

Dalley theorizes this was likely what was described as pneumonia in the past, and that because of the high rate of false positive Covid tests, this has come to be an acceptable diagnosis that places a patient on a high intervention tract and ultimately leads to death by over-treatment.

Dalley's horror story anecdotally identifies a major cause of "Covid" death as over-treatment. It is iatrogenic death, or death caused by the process of medical examination and treatment. Iatrogenic death is death by doctor.

Dalley's claim rings true in my own life. In November 2020, two friends entered the hospital. The one with less severe symptoms put himself at the mercy of the medical system and obediently followed the instructions of the doctor. Kenneth lasted less than two weeks before they pulled the plug on him. The one with more severe symptoms, left the hospital when they suggested ventilation as an option, insisting instead upon alternative treatments and lots of rest. Nick is alive and is today healthier than he has been in a long time.

Dalley describes a story repeated thousands of times over 2020 and 2021, except for many patients, they did not have a well-informed and assertive advocate at their bedside the way Kate Dalley's husband did. In fact, during the early days of Covid, no one was allowed at a patient's bedside, which meant that treatment was often pushed upon patients with little recourse. Dalley's case is echoed in the experience of many. Though her husband, by her estimate, did not need to be admitted to the ICU, that was exactly where they were pushed into. Intubation and mechanical ventilation was also repeatedly pushed upon them. They successfully prevented mechanical ventilation from taking place. All treatment protocol not recommended by the CDC was discouraged by doctors. What sounded like it could become a true tragedy ended up as a success, with Dalley telling the story by which they dictated her husband's treatment through a protocol of oxygen, high dose intravenous vitamins, and rest. Within three days, her husband was well enough to walk out of the ICU.

Perhaps it is not Covid-19, a variation on the common cold, that is leaving so many dead. Perhaps the treatment protocol is off target. Perhaps the lockdowns enfeebled the elderly who lived active lives, enfeebled the elderly far more than any cold virus could have. Perhaps the inaccurate testing led to a crisis that would not have existed if there had not been any test — yes, maybe no Covid test would have been better than the testing protocol we had in 2020 and 2021. Perhaps the early 2020 vital records reporting change of definition from dying "from Covid" to dying "with Covid," made our statistics on Covid deaths so wildly unreliable by artificially increasing Covid deaths, to the point that even George Floyd was a "Covid" death. Perhaps the altered ICU policies have led to full ICUs. Perhaps hospital restrictions have caused harm to millions of others depending on routine care. Perhaps the face masks do no good and actually harm the wearer.

I have not dug into the research on most of these topics above, but I know the research on face masks very well. They do not work to stop the spread of a respiratory virus. Face masks harm the wearer and those around the wearer.

If you were not wearing a mask before April 3, 2020, when the CDC told you to put a face mask on, there is no scientific reason to have been wearing a mask since April 3, 2020. In fact, with more information at our disposal, we can now clearly see that there is less reason than ever to wear a mask. They simply do not work. This book goes further to elaborate how very harmful they are for you and for your children.

Reason 11: If Face Masks Do Not Work, Then Government And Media Are Lying To You — A Very Scary Thought For Some

If we are being told to wear masks, and masks do not work, then we are being lied to. We are being lied to by doctors, dentists, family, pastors, friends, media, government, schools, employers, employees, businesses, and did I mention media, and government too.

That is a discomforting thought.

I can see why it is easier for some to just lie to themselves and to say they are not possibly being lied to by these institutions.

As Denis Rancourt points out in his February 22, 2021, "Review of scientific reports of harms caused by face masks:"[1]

> "There have been no less than 15 policy-grade Randomized Controlled Trials (RCTs) with verified outcome, in healthcare, community, and general-population settings. All but the most recent one have been analyzed in published formal systematic reviews. All 15 studies find that no reduction in risk of being infected can be detected with statistical significance. This means that any benefit is too small to be detected by science.

> "The government claims that masks work are in effect disingenuous propaganda, improperly relying on substandard and irrelevant studies.

> "Therefore, the presumption that masks work is incorrect. It is disproved by science: Any risk reduction is too small to be detected using usual and established statistical criteria."

This is very strong language from a relatively sober researcher. Other scientists are so flummoxed by the decision to mask the population that they call for "urgent research."[2] Rancourt continues:

> "A total of 343 healthcare professionals on the Covid-19 front lines participated in this study [New York City]. 314 respondents reported adverse effects from prolonged mask use with headaches being the most common complaint (n = 245). Skin breakdown was experienced by 175 respondents, and acne was reported in 182 respondents. Impaired cognition was reported in 81 respondents. ... Some respondents experienced resolved side effects once

masks were removed, while others required physical or medical intervention."

Study authors further conclude:

"Prolonged use of N95 and surgical masks by healthcare professionals during Covid-19 has caused adverse effects such as headaches, rash, acne, skin breakdown, and impaired cognition in the majority of those surveyed. ..."[3]

They are not saying "mask more people." They are not saying "make sure you mask the children to protect them." They are not saying "we need stiffer fines for non-compliance." They are screaming "WHAT ARE YOU DOING?!?" as loudly as a researcher who does not want to be fired tomorrow can scream it.

What are YOU doing?

These courageous scientists are trying their best, but they cannot stop this without you. It stops one person at a time, one family at a time.

You must lead your own life.

You must commit to never wearing a mask again, and you must prevent your child from ever being forced into one.

If you lead, the politicians, the media talking heads, and the heads of institutions will all eventually follow, or they will all eventually be replaced.

No other option is possible, but that process will likely take a very long time. Change happens one person at a time and starts with you leading in your own life by making change happen in your own life. You do not have to wait for anyone. It starts as soon as you say it starts.

Why not let that be this very moment?

Reason 12: You Have Been Lied To This Whole Time, Then Vilified If You Ask Too Many Revealing Questions About Those Lies

It goes further. Not only do masks not work, not only are you being lied to about it, you are being vilified, cancelled, gaslit, made to seem like a crazy person if you are one of the people who refuse to lie to themselves and instead, ask pointed, revealing questions. Asking pointed, revealing questions is exactly what people tend to do once they are tired of being lied to.

If the lies about face masks were isolated to simply face masks, an argument could be made for there being a small misunderstanding of the science on this one topic that got misconstrued during the fear and concern following the Ides of March 2020.

Only by taking the topic out of context could such a statement be made.

To contextualize this a little, it is evident that at every turn, people portrayed as trusted experts were duplicitous in their switching of science for politics. They operated not out of a focus on wisdom or data, but out of a spirit of control and the provocation of fear.

San Francisco was the epicenter of the March 17, 2020 lockdown and is the home of a globally recognized public health department known for its comfort and eagerness to experiment on its obedient populace. In a truly amazing summary of the Covid lies of 2020 and 2021, in a piece entitled "The War on Reality," Alex Gutentag, a public school teacher, writes from San Francisco, California:

> "Experts have consistently taken an imprecise approach to statistics, changed their minds, and withheld information while claiming the mantle of 'scientific consensus.' Over the summer of 2020, the WHO quietly changed its definition of herd immunity from protection acquired through both natural immunity and vaccination to one acquired only through vaccination. Similarly, in December 2020, Fauci declared that he was changing his estimate for vaccination rates needed to achieve herd immunity from 60% to 90%."[1]

There was no science behind the WHO decision. In fact, all signs indicate that naturally acquired immunity is superior to vaccine acquired immunity, in terms of length of immunity and quality of immunity. Additionally, there was no science in Fauci's December 2020 determination.

There is no science that says 90% of a population should be vaccinated to achieve herd immunity. In fact, 0% can be vaccinated and herd immunity can be achieved naturally as humans have always done with all diseases until recently and continue to do so with all but a tiny fraction of diseases. Gutentag illustrates Fauci's lack of reliance on science:

"When asked for a scientific rationale, Fauci said he changed the percentage based purely on polling that indicated more Americans were willing to take the Covid-19 vaccine.

"When lockdowns failed to yield meaningful mitigation results, public health agencies that had previously recommended against masking changed their position."

Gutentag goes on to expand on further inconsistencies in "the science" cited by public health officials. This is "science" which is not very scientific in its approach.

"Although simulations[2] suggested that 80% mask compliance would do more to stop the spread of Covid-19 than lockdowns, regional analysis in the United States does not show[3] that mandates had any effect on case rates, despite 93%[4] compliance. Moreover, according to CDC data, 85%[5] of people who contracted Covid-19 reported wearing a mask.

"Research has shown that once unquestioned rules like 6 feet[6] for social distancing are arbitrary and not actually associated with lower transmission. Reporting of death and hospitalization rates was also inexact, and mass asymptomatic testing distorted public understanding of the virus. Ninety-five percent[7] of Covid-19 deaths had an average of four related underlying conditions and the CDC's death count includes 'deaths involving unintentional and intentional injury.' As a result of testing children hospitalized for unrelated conditions, the number of pediatric Covid-19 hospitalizations was exaggerated by at least 40%."

Not only were the intrusive solutions proposed based on cherry picked bad science, but they did not at all work and led to further distortion of the Covid-19 scare. Gutentag turns her attention to the awful use of the PCR tests for Covid-19 diagnosis.

Without this fraudulent use of a PCR test as a diagnostic tool, the public health crisis of Covid-19 would not have existed because the numbers overstated by the test used to diagnose healthy people would never have been considered Covid cases. Nor would it have been used to highlight Covid as the key concern for sick people with other more pressing medical concerns.

To cite an example that is hard to state too frequently, under the definition of Covid-19 adopted in the US, George Floyd, a man who died on the streets of Minneapolis on May 25, 2020, in a death widely viewed by the world, is a Covid-19 death, having tested positive weeks earlier on April 3, 2020.[8] Gutentag continues about the fraudulent PCR test:

> "The PCR testing protocol for Covid-19 was based on a paper by Christian Drosten, which was peer-reviewed and published within just two days in a journal on whose editorial board Drosten sits. The method was created 'without having virus material available,' using instead a genetic sequence published online. The PCR test amplifies genetic material of the virus in cycles but does not determine whether a case is infectious. A higher number of cycles indicates a lower viral load. The cycle threshold for PCR tests used in the US was usually limited at 37 or 40, highly sensitive levels. In July 2020, Fauci remarked that at these levels, a positive result is 'just dead nucleotides, period.'"[9]

As if this were not already bad enough, the CDC stepped into create an apples and oranges scenario so that data from 2020 and 2021 of unvaccinated individuals could never be compared to vaccinated individuals to prove effectiveness or ineffectiveness of a Covid shot.

If honesty were the goal, why would the CDC deny public health researchers that basic tool for determining the effectiveness or ineffectiveness of a vaccine? Gutentag continues:

> "For vaccinated Americans, the CDC has lowered the cycle threshold for 'breakthrough infections' to only 28 cycles[10] and announced that post-vaccine cases will only be counted if they result in hospitalization or death.[11] CDC Director Rochelle Walensky stated that vaccinated Americans who died and tested positive for Covid-19 merely died 'with' Covid-19, not 'from' Covid-19. This method of tallying would eliminate many pre-vaccine cases. It is also likely

that 85%-90%[12] of tests that are positive at a cycle threshold of 40 would be negative at a cycle threshold of 30.

"Despite this lack of accurate data, authorities have consistently scapegoated members of the public as 'anti-maskers' or 'anti-vaxxers' responsible for prolonging the pandemic. They have used divisive messaging and disorienting scare tactics in order to justify months of Covid-19 restrictions that were based on dogma, not on science."

Gutentag describes the approach as "saving lives by killing people," and perhaps a little too generously describes this utter deceit and murder as "scientific inversion," though she elaborates in a way that minces no words:

"Our current state of scientific inversion has sown intense division in the US and threatens to rip apart the social fabric. For the past 16 months, the public has been told that it is our duty to serve the needs of medical institutions and personnel, not the other way around. Effective low-cost therapeutics like ivermectin were dismissed in favor of a vaccine program that transferred billions of dollars from taxpayers to pharmaceutical executives and shareholders. Critics of measures like school closures were accused of far-right white supremacy, even though these measures were most damaging to working-class people and minorities. Deadly policies were portrayed as lifesaving, and public health protocols caused immense clinical damage."

Some benefited by using the medical industrial complex to make a pretty penny in 2020, while others lost out. Gutentag touches on just a tiny fraction of the severe harm caused by allowing government to be hijacked for use in this scheme:

"A few people have benefited from this war on reality while many have paid a heavy price. In 2020, workers lost $3.7 trillion,[13] while billionaires gained $3.9 trillion[14] and 493[15] new individuals became billionaires. During this same period, decades of progress against diseases[16] like malaria and tuberculosis were reversed. Disruptions to health and nutrition services killed 228,000 children[17] in South Asia. Globally, the impact of lockdowns on health programs, food production, and supply chains plunged millions[18] of people into severe hunger and malnutrition.

"In the US, we are facing a crisis of cardiovascular[19] disease and undiagnosed cancer.[20] Unemployment shock will cause 890,000 additional deaths[21] over the next 15 years. Overdoses from synthetic opioids increased by 38.4%,[22] and 11% of US adults[23] considered suicide last June. Three million[24] children disappeared from public school systems, and ERs saw a 31%[25] increase in adolescent mental health visits."

Are these mistakes? Or are these crimes? Was there malice? Was it intentional? How could it have been anything else and continued for so long and in so many ways. At the time of this book's printing there is still a war being diligently fought against any parent, researcher, politician, teacher, or doctor who would dare speak up and demand the scientific method be followed and the risks and rewards thought through. For doing so, for merely speaking such words, lives are being ruined. Gutentag continues:

"Now, the stories that were used to justify these hardships are continuing to unravel. Many of the people responsible will insist that the second-order consequences are the horrible symptoms of a magic virus and that the mistakes made in handling such a crisis were inevitable. But preventing young children from reaching crucial developmental milestones in the face of mounting evidence is not just a 'mistake.' Forcing hospital patients to die alone without saying goodbye to their families is not just a 'mistake.' Pushing millions of people into poverty and starvation is not just a 'mistake.' These are crimes.

"Basic civil, human, and economic rights were violated under demonstrably fraudulent pretenses. The sacrifices we thought we were making for the common good were sacrifices made in vain. Unlawful lockdowns demoralized the population and ruined lives. The tragic reality is that this was all for nothing. The only way to prevent these events from recurring is to exhaustively investigate not just the origin of the virus, but every corrupt and misguided decision made by politicians, NGOs, public health organizations, and scientific institutions made since its fateful emergence."

Gutenberg stops with a call for investigations. Every person who implemented these policies, no matter how great the cost to society, must be removed from any position of public trust and never again granted funding, let alone ever allowed to hold any role of trust. The lies of 2020 and 2021 are so grand and so egregious. The harm committed must be recompensed.

We must not ever let this go until justice has been done and a full accounting of the ills of 2020 and 2021 has taken place.

The perpetrators realize the harm that will come to them if they lose after so egregiously betraying trust by bringing mass death and harm to the United States and this world, in a never before seen global operation of unprecedented scale.

Thank you to Gutentag for speaking up. This San Francisco school teacher is an unsung American leader and hero who demands praise for the role she has played in 2020 and beyond.

Reason 13: If Morality Is Being Argued By Bullies Rather Than Scientific Debate Being Had By Peers, You Know Something Is Wrong

No two people find agreement on all topics. Consequently, a back and forth conversation between two people with different views is a normal part of life in civil society.

"What should we have for dinner?"

"Who shot, J.R. Ewing?"

"What happened to the nose of the sphinx?"

These are just a few of the many questions that will forever get people with strongly held beliefs ready for a debate.

While debating such topics may provide some entertainment, it is important to keep in mind how important some topics are for determining the quality of life for large swaths of the population.

Debates in the field of medicine have very real consequences.

Because such topics have consequences, we are told it is acceptable to censor debate that one finds disagreeable. It is considered noble, moral in fact, to silence an opinion deemed "dangerous," "misinformed," or "wrong."

In a free society, there is an easy way to destroy ideas that are dangerous, misinformed, or wrong — do the hard work of proving them wrong.

That is what this book is.

That is what many books throughout history have been.

Only those who are unable, or unwilling, to prove their ideas right are eager to censor. Never will a truth teller who believes in a free society be found engaging in censorship.

No matter the excuse given for censorship, it is harmful to a society. It curtails freedom.

Certain behaviors — among them theft, murder, slavery, rape, censorship — are not acceptable, regardless of the explanation.

Free and open debate must be had in every field and unceasingly. Seldom is anything actually "settled," seldom is there actually "consensus." Such terms are inherently deceitful. To make such claims, one would need to obtain a list of all scientists (no such list could ever possibly exist) and to poll them all on a topic (a poll that would not possibly be answered).

To be unwilling to have a debate is the height of arrogance. In academic settings, seldom is anyone able to win a debate, but unwilling to have a debate. Unwillingness to debate almost always stems from an inability to prove a point.

Therefore, the months since the Ides of March 2020 have been filled with censorship. People unable to win a debate did their best to silence all debate and labelled their opponents "dangerous," "misinformed," or "wrong."

Such behavior effectively proves how wrong the views they possess are. It is bullying behavior. Bullies do not bully because it is just. Bullies bully because they are too insecure to win at a fair match.

American society was bullied for a time. Free people were silenced. That period is rapidly coming to end and it is looking increasingly likely, as this book goes to press, that there are bullies from 2020 and 2021 who will be relieved from duty and will see the inside of a jail cell.

No less would be demanded by the tree of liberty.

Every single time someone avoids debate, you should ask yourself "What are they so insecure about?"

Every single time someone seeks to censor another, you should ask yourself, no matter what excuse they give "What are they so insecure about?"

The answer is almost always: YOU.

They do not want to silence the speaker as much as they want to cover YOUR ears.

They do not want to end conversation as much as they want to stop you from hearing the conversation.

Because once you hear the "wrong" conversation, once you get the "wrong" ideas in your head, they know they will not be able to get them out of your head.

The more you hear the conversations, the more likely it is that their hold over you, their false authority over you, disintergrates.

The only way that they can control you is by keeping you ignorant.

Censorship has nothing to do with Julian Assange, Donald Trump, or Robert Kennedy. Censorship has everything to do with you.

They need you to never read the things you are reading in this book. They need you never to share these ideas with others. They need you to never act on them.

Because if you do, their days are numbered.

I turn on the television and I hear the most ridiculous ideas, as if I live in clown world. I speak to normal people who refuse to wear a mask and not a one believes the ideas on the television. I even talk to abnormal, obediently masked people and if they will let their guard down for a bit, it becomes clear that they do not believe it either.

But they are scared. Terrified. So full of fear about what it means for the narrative to be wrong.

So they hold firm, certain that one day it all crumbles, doubling down, tripling down, hoping today is not the day. Praying to their dark lord to give them one more day.

The day of reckoning is coming.

You are mighty. There are too many cracks. The truth is flooding out every which way. The narrative cannot be maintained.

It is coming.

Every day it becomes more and more clear.

Every day since very early 2020, it has become more and more clear.

This was their last stand and they are getting so much mileage out of it. But, do not think that it is done.

There is so much fight ahead, and they know if they give up it may not be so pretty for them this time around.

Every time I see someone try to censor another person, all of this goes through my head in the moment between me seeing the weak attempt and me laughing a laugh of victory over such a fear filled, miserable person seeking to silence a free man in a free land.

How good that laugh feels.

Jenin Younes recounts for the *American Institute for Economic Research* a most exciting tale of censorship and deceit watched by many over the course of 2020:

> "The speed with which mask-wearing among the general public transitioned from unheard of to a moral necessity struck me as suspicious. After all, if the science was as airtight as those around me claimed, surely masks would have been recommended by January or February, not to mention during prior infectious disease outbreaks such as the 2009 swine flu. It seemed unlikely that the scientific proof became incontrovertible sometime between late February and late March, particularly in the absence of any new evidence surfacing during that time period.[1]

> "Perhaps none of this is particularly surprising in this hyper-political era. What is shocking is the scientific community's participation in subverting evidence that does not comport with the consensus. A prime example is the Institute of Health Metrics Evaluation's ("IHME") rather

astounding claim,[2] published in the journal *Nature-Medicine* and echoed[3] in countless articles[4] afterward, that the lives of 130,000 people could be saved with a nationwide mask mandate."

When that "science" was demonstrably debunked, no retraction occurred, instead the lie was allowed to be repeated over and again with little protest from its original editors. Younes continues with a story of outlandish and public intellectual dishonesty from figures who present themselves as upright scholars.

"As my colleague Phil Magness pointed out[5] in an op-ed in *The Wall Street Journal*, the IHME model was predicated upon faulty data: it assumed that 49% of Americans were wearing masks based on a survey conducted between April and June, while claiming that statistic represented the number of Americans wearing masks as of September 21. In fact, by the summer, around 80% of Americans were regularly wearing them. (Ironically, had Dr. Fauci and the Surgeon General not bungled the message in March, mask use probably would have reached much higher rates much earlier on).

"This called into question the accuracy of the 130,000 figure, since many more people habitually used masks than the study presumed.

"Although Magness contacted *Nature-Medicine* to point out the problem, after stalling for nearly two weeks, the journal declined to address it. Needless to say, the damage had been done: newspapers such as *The New York Times* undoubtedly would fail to correct the error and any retractions certainly would be placed far from the front page, where the initial article touting the IHME figure appeared. Thus, as expected, the unfounded claim that 130,000 lives could be saved with a nationwide mask-mandate continues to be repeated, including by president-elect[6] Joe Biden[7] and National Institutes of Health Director Francis Collins.

"That the science behind mask-wearing is questionable at best is further exemplified by a letter[8] to the editor written in response to Magness's article. Dr. Christopher Murray acknowledged that rates of mask-wearing have steadily increased, but then concluded that masks should be used because they are 'our first line of defense against the pandemic' and current IHME modeling indicates that 'if 95% of US residents were to wear masks when leaving home, we could prevent the deaths of tens of thousands of Americans' because 'masks work,' and 'much deeper pain is ahead if we refuse to wear them.'

"None of this accounts for the failure of either *Nature-Medicine* or the IHME modelers to recognize and correct the error. Moreover, neither the IHME modelers nor Dr. Murray provide any evidence that masks work. They assume masks are extremely effective at preventing spread of the coronavirus, and then claim that the model is correct for that reason. This sort of circular reasoning is all-too typical of those who so vociferously insist that masks are effective without going to the trouble of substantiating that contention — or differentiating what is likely a modest benefit from mask-wearing in specific indoor locations and around high-risk individuals from the media-driven tendency to depict masks as a silver bullet for stopping the virus in all circumstances."

Younes aptly sums up this demonstration of scientism as the opposite of science. Younes concludes:

"This is not science: it is politics, and those within the profession who have refused to examine their confirmation biases, or manipulated the evidence to score political points, are utterly unqualified for the job."

This insightful commentary from Younes quite appropriately begs the question "If they are unqualified for their jobs, then why do they have those jobs?" Many must be removed from positions of trust and punished for their behavior since the Ides of March 2020. I would like to encourage you, dear reader, to take it a step beyond that, however.

These are not jobs in the traditional sense. These are not people hired to perform a task. It goes beyond that. They are hired to manipulate public opinion from their roles in positions of public trust. They are marketers disguised as scientists, salesmen disguised as doctors, politicians disguised as researchers. They are acting outside of the bounds of ethical behavior and are tasked with lying to the public, perpetrating a great fraud with every sentence that come from their mouths. Yes, some people should lose their jobs.

This points to a larger problem, however. A massive managerial class presides over society. It is so large as to be stultifying. Everywhere one turns, there is that managerial class making life more difficult. It goes beyond party lines. Within the United States, the American uniparty favors the expansion of the managerial class. Internationally, the party of Davos favors the expansion of the managerial class.

The managerial class has lost its sense of duty to the people that class once claimed to serve. They are not able to be called public servants any longer, except in the most deceitful applications of that term. It is not a few hundred or a few thousand deceitful people in positions of trust who must be removed, it is an entire way of viewing society that must be done away with.

A very top heavy managerial class exists to make work for themselves, create purpose for themselves, and to expand authority for themselves all the while doing so with no overarching moral or ethical guidance and at great cost to all other people walking the earth. They even make life more miserable for themselves as individuals, with the exception of a very small few within the managerial class who are well insulated from the inconveniences of life.

We have finally reached the height of bureaucracy long warned of by modern thinkers, a system in which no one is accountable and in which no one is empowered to stop missteps of the system. It merely perpetuates itself unchecked. Younes is right. Such people are unqualified for their jobs. More importantly, the system of bureaucratic rule by a managerial class is unfit for the tasks we have assigned it. "Firing" means to keep the job, but to switch the person in the job. A more precise term developed by members of the managerial class is more befitting in this scenario — "lay off" — because it refers to getting rid of both the person *and* the job.

Evidenced by the atrocities from the Ides of March 2020 to the present, it is not so much that individual people need to be fired, but that a whole industry needs to be laid off. Our managerial class, our technocratic class, our bureaucratic class have to go. They were once a minor annoyance but have now become a hazard to life and liberty, perhaps a hazard to life and liberty worse than any that humanity has ever known.

Reason 14: The Rationale "Comply Or Else" Is Such A Monstrously Bad Rationale, Whenever It Is Used, That It Should Always Trigger A Lack Of Compliance

When it comes to face masks, virtually any consideration of the risk to your child versus the reward is entirely discouraged. Any parent being discouraged from asking this question is being consequently reminded how important that question is and how untrustworthy anyone who can give such orders should be considered.

As Boris Borovoy et al. write, in the October 2020 paper "Microbial challenges from masks,"[1] the harm of masks had been very lightly researched. This lack of research prior to mandating masking is significant, especially given the known harm that was already understood to be possible. Borovoy writes:

> "In this paper, the second in our series, we continue our examination of the potential hazards of masks, in which we now turn attention to microbial contamination from masks and mask use, changes in oral and nasal microbiota, and potential risks to the lungs and other organ systems from microbial factors. Because widespread masking is a very new societywide experiment, the impact of this experiment, the obstruction of airways from free breathing and a typical air exchange interplay with oral microbiota is not yet known. Furthermore, the effects of such changes in the lungs and beyond are not yet known. This paper will explore some considerations of these changes, by examining mask effectiveness against transmission, historical evidence of epidemiology from the 1918-1919 pandemic, microbial contamination, respiratory disease and the role of oral bacteria in systemic disease; and infections involving fungi, yeast, and molds. Compiling statistical and scientific evidence from these subjects alone should help equip any individual with adequate information on risks and benefits when choosing whether to wear a mask."

Masks do not work and are harmful to yourself and others when you wear them. The evidence for that is so apparent. For anyone to attempt to silence the transmission of that evidence, let alone silence the asking of basic questions on the topic is such a red flag that should, on its face, trigger a disinterest in complying. Borovoy writes:

"Masks have been shown through overwhelming clinical evidence to have no effect against transmission of viral pathogens.[2] Penetration of cloth masks by viral particles was almost 97% and of surgical masks was 44%.[3] Even bacteria, approximately ten times the volume of coronaviruses, have been poorly impeded by both cloth masks and disposable surgical masks. Face masks became almost ineffective after two hours of use, and after 150 minutes of use, more bacteria was emitted through the disposable mask than from the same subject unmasked.[4] One must wonder, if new masks worn by healthcare workers, that are soiled by wear during a work shift, transmit more bacteria to patients than from an unmasked healthcare worker, then what is happening to the lungs of the mask-wearer?"

How could such data not be headline news? How could such data instead be enough to cause the bearer of such information to be banned, seen as a social, political, and professional pariah? Borovoy continues with such inconvenient truths, pointing to the fact that even among healthcare workers masks hardly make sense:

"Use of personal protective equipment (PPE) has long been debated for healthcare workers regarding their interactions with patients who are carrying highly pathogenic organisms, and this study found about half of even trained healthcare workers in clinical settings make at least one protocol deviation in donning and doffing PPE.[5] Certainly the general public without such training is likely to have a higher rate of similar or more egregious errors in PPE protocol. Masks have been determined to be unnecessary even in surgical settings, and of no benefit in preventing infections.[6] In fact, 'The rate of wound infections [while unmasked] was less than half what it was when everyone wore masks.' Oral microbial flora dispersed by unmasked healthcare workers standing one meter from the workspace failed to contaminate exposed plates on that surface.[7]

"Let us also examine the entire surface area of the masked person when considering that person's potential for transmitting pathogens. Face masks generally only cover the lower half of the face, which we know from studying burn victims is less than 2% of the entire body surface area.[8] We know that numbers of airborne bacteria expelled from the upper airway are insignificantly small compared with the volume of bacteria shed from the skin.[9] The shed from the skin of mask wearers was found to create more contamination than from non-mask wearers, presumably due to shifting, wiggling and increased rubbing and exfoliation."[10, 11]

Why was "comply or else" so frequently the mandate of 2020 and 2021? Because if anyone gave a person like Boris Borovoy ten minutes in the mainstream each night, the fear-fueled pandemic would be over more quickly than it began, the harmful lockdowns that cost more blood and treasure than any virus would promptly end, and the nonsense around masks, Covid injections, or any other one-size-fits-all approach would quickly come to an end.

Reason 15: "The Precautionary Principal" Has Not Been Followed

The precautionary principal states that officials should err on the side of caution when mandating a health approach to one patient, or to a whole population.

It is rooted in the concept of medical ethics that a doctor is to do no harm. This goes back at least 2,500 years.[1]

That was done away with around the time of the Ides of March 2020. To this very moment, it has not been revived, though it is now abundantly apparent that Covid was not the great harm we were told it was going to be in March 2020.

Only with certainty that the cure will not be worse than the disease, does the precautionary principle let an ethical physician proceed.

We learned in 2020 how few ethical physicians there were. They feigned expertise on things they knew nothing about. They do not today repent, and let us get past the harm of their lies, instead doubling down. They claim consensus of scientific opinion when the exact opposite is true, and they today censor those truth tellers who call them on their lies.

They lied outright about the science, as well, and called upon their stenographers in the media to do the same, to this day not seeing to it that the record is corrected, instead leaving the greatest amount of rubbish and detritus out there to confuse any person with a diligent interest in determining the truth.

The time for calling this all a mistake has passed.

Nothing but the greatest malice is now behind the most pivotal events of our day, as unsafe and ineffective masks are pushed upon children alongside far worse unsafe and ineffective one-size-fits-all approaches.

Scientific knowledge was said to be lacking when this all began.

That is a lie, and it is even more of a lie today.

There was dissent about the lockdown, the face masks, the mRNA shot from the first moment they were discussed.

Scientific knowledge was abundantly available, and those with the knowledge were promptly silenced.

Was the precautionary principle at least turned to? No. It was thrown out the window.

Bioethics writer Anne Zimmerman illustrates an argument that was used to entirely invert long standing medical ethics by claiming that the non-interventionist "do no harm," now means all intervention can and must be taken by physicians, public health, and society as long as it is done in the name of preventing harm. Zimmerman argues:

> "The precautionary principle in mask-wearing when waiting for explicit scientific evidence is unwise."[2]

Medical ethics be damned. Why not just throw principle to the wind and do whatever we feel to a naive and trusting people.

A good reason not to do that is because when people figure out they have been had, they will want retribution.

The medical community thinks Americans do not have that in them.

In February 2020, Denis Rancourt of the Ontario Civil Liberties Association wrote in "Review of scientific reports of harms caused by face masks,"[3]

> "Following the precautionary principle, government has the onus to demonstrate absence of significant anticipated harm, prior to imposing a measure, especially with a personal medical measure applied to the general healthy population.
>
> "The precautionary principle was not followed for masks in the Covid-19 pandemic."

That can still be said today. Except, as the days go on, the evidence mounts that face masks are not safe and are not effective, yet policy makers double down stubbornly, showing they will be unwilling to back down until made to back down.

The time will soon come when they have no choice but to back down.

Reason 16: Mandatory Face Masks Harm 1.5 Billion Students

Mandatory masking hurts children around the world. You can have a marked impact in changing that in the world around you. Denis Rancourt of the Ontario Civil Liberties Association writes in "Review of scientific reports of harms caused by face masks:"[1]

> "Along with other measures of physical distancing and economic lockdowns, school closures were implemented during March 2020 affecting more than 1.5 billion students (children and adolescents) around the globe.[2] These closures of schools lasted for a few weeks only (as in Denmark) up to several months (in Italy and many other countries;[3]) and led to marked decreases in educational gains,[4] hunger (because school meals were no longer served), increases in child abuse (because children were no longer observed by school staff), and, in general, the risk of 'scarring the life chances of a generation of young people'[5] (because of the long-term psychological, physiological, educational and even economic burden,[6] that societies put on their most vulnerable members[7])

> - Wearing masks may have physical side effects.
> - Face masks impair face recognition and face identification.
> - Face masks impair verbal and non-verbal communication.
> - Face masks block emotional signaling between teacher and learner.

> "Given these pros and cons, it is not clear whether face masks should play a major role in educational settings in times of the current viral pandemic. ... This matter should be discussed urgently, since it globally affects more than 1.5 billion students, teachers, and school staff directly, and, in addition, their families indirectly."[8]

Many children are harmed by mandatory masking. It is time to make that number one less. You may not be able to singlehandedly impact 1.5 billion children, but you have the power to impact the children in your life who are in your care. Those are the children that you are responsible for the wellbeing of, not the other 1.5 billion. All that is required of you is resolve and bravery. If you are determined to never let yourself or your child be masked again, neither you nor your child will ever be masked again.

Reason 17: Face Masks Are Another Way To Crush Their Spirit

I taught for several years after college. Sometimes, after long days of teaching, I would watch the film *Dead Poet's Society* and gather inspiration.

> *"You must strive to find your own voice because the longer you wait to begin, the less likely you are going to find it at all."*
>
> — *Dead Poet's Society*

I was, by many measures, an unorthodox teacher and I was good at getting the message through.

> *"No matter what anybody tells you, words and ideas can change the world."*
>
> – *Dead Poet's Society*

I assigned five essays a week many weeks, sometimes six — to fluent 13-year-olds learning their second, third, or even fourth language in my classroom.

> *"When you read, do not just consider what the author thinks, consider what you think."*
>
> — *Dead Poet's Society*

Parents would tell me things like "You do not just teach our children, you teach our children to think."

> *"I brought them up here to illustrate the point of conformity: the difficulty in maintaining your own beliefs in the face of others."*
>
> – *Dead Poet's Society*

Students left my tutelage able to think and able to write. Few teachers can say that.

> *"We do not read and write poetry because it is cute. We read and write poetry because we are members of the human race. And the human race is filled with passion. And medicine, law, business, engineering, these are noble pursuits and necessary to sustain life.*

*But poetry, beauty, romance, love, these are what we
stay alive for."*

– Dead Poet's Society

Let us face it, by and large, teachers are not inspiring.

I know the teachers' union propagandists would like you to believe
otherwise, but ask a high caliber teacher how most teachers stack up. A lot
of them are duds, and the teachers I worked with were even of a higher
caliber than most, but still many of them ended up being duds. For whatever reason, that is who gets attracted to teaching — lots of duds.

The Episcopal school children near my house eat lunch in the local
park. The lunchtime rule is "No talking when your face mask is off." The
teacher is forever scolding the boys on either shutting their mouths or getting their face masks back on. Can you picture that? Some washed up
middle aged video gamer spending half an hour of his day feeling big in
life by scolding a bunch of ten-year-old boys not to speak as they enjoy a
sandwich outside on a park bench next to their best chum.

The French bilingual school in town puts kids in face masks AND face
shields. They need to wear both at the same time. Though the children are
hardly obedient to their parents (internal/familial authority), they are infi-
nitely obedient to their teachers (external authority). That is exactly the
wrong obedience to have. Teenage years are tumultuous without that parental bond. Modernity teaches it is best to put a child in day care and get
the parents back to work as soon as possible after a child is born. Put two
parents in fifty hour a week jobs for the next twelve years and even if their
marriage survives — a source of the child's sense of security — the children are unlikely to have much of a bond with either parent.

With little or no meaningful bond between parent and child — only
authority — the parent's job in the teenage years is not to walk alongside
a child as a trusted advisor. How could it be? There is no bond, so there is
no trust. Instead, the parent has to figure out methods of control, methods
of exerting authority. A lot of that looks like spirit-crushing torment. If the
infant child could predict the future, he would beg his parents to stay
home more: which he did, every time they left for work for some period
of time and left the kid with strangers, usually itinerant strangers, who
moved on so quickly that no bonds could form with any adult in the
child's life.

Kids are happy at 2-years-old, 5-years-old, and 7-years-old. By 18-
years-old they are not. Someone — often the parents — messed them up,

but the extension of parental authority — the school — is what does it worst of all.

Misbehavior and disobedience in school practically has to be encouraged unless you want your children messed up.

But again, we have the conflict between authority and bondedness. Control and trust. Force and love. Manipulation and conversation. A stranger is almost always going to give a kid the former, a parent can build a relationship in which the latter is the norm, but so many parents are too busy for that to happen. The trendy notion of "quality time" replaces the real variable: quantity time. Kids end up with strangers at school bossing them around and practical strangers at home doing the same.

Can it be any surprise that children get run down by modern life?

By 18-years-old, so much of their energy has been sucked from them. And why? Because no one cared enough to stay home instead of playing big shot in the boardroom.

The face mask becomes another lever of compliance, in a world full of people who do not want to build a bond and just want something from that kid. Often they want to exert authority and little else.

Reason 18: Face Masks Are A Conditioning Tool To Make Your Child More Compliant

Masks help teach a child to pervert the thought process: scientism replaces the scientific method.

Authority replaces thought.

Falsehoods replace reality.

But they do not just make a child stupid and dishonest, they also make a child more obedient.

There is an ugly trend in American life, which can generally be called "behaviorialism." It can be generally grouped as treatment that researchers like B.F. Skinner paid to his lab rats, that he brilliantly "trained" to run a maze in order to get a piece of cheese. This field did not start with him, nor does it perfectly grow out of his work, but he is an excellent example.

Some people say this an awful lot: "I do X to get Y" or "I do X to avoid Z."

This is pursuit of pleasure and avoidance of pain.

People train themselves in all kinds of way. Training is for animals. Training is not for man. The rationale behind any attempts at "training" man should be carefully examined and not easily acquiesced with, let alone automatically acquiesced with.

Compare the above rationale of avoiding pain and pursuing pleasure to this: "I do X, because I know it to be good," "I do X, because it is in line with my values," or "I do X, because I want to."

There are far better reasons than the pursuit of pleasure and the avoidance of pain to engage in an activity.

To use risk and reward as the only basis for an activity is a method of conditioning. Skinner had rats, Ivan Pavlov had dogs.

The animals were "conditioned" or trained to have a certain output in response to a certain stimulus.

It feels an awful lot like intelligence, or sentience, or even eerily human. It is not.

A human has free will. A human has a moment to pause and reflect between input and output. A human is not a robot, nor is a human an animal. A human is quantifiably different.

Robots and animals may be able to do things humans cannot. That is okay. That does not make them human.

That moment of decision between input and output, the moment of thought, judgement, the moment that theologians call "free will," is such an important part of what makes us human.

So much of our humanity resides in that moment and the ability to build upon it.

Any external "training" or "conditioning" that seeks to automate that moment should be greeted with great suspicion.

Any opportunity that seeks to grow that moment should be seen as an opportunity to edify the person.

Wonderful things are built upon the foundation of that moment.

School bells, unsolicited alerts from electronic devices, and traffic tickets, are examples of conditioning in the world around us. They are unavoidable when interacting with a world that adores behavioralism, which is to say a world that sees you as a programmable robot or a trainable animal and not as a human with free will.

Face masks are another conditioning tool imposed by the outside world. They are a conditioning tool that you can choose to place on your child, or not. I strongly discourage conditioning tools around children. From the moment life begins, I encourage the full recognition of them as humans and no less.

That is what a child is and no conditioning tool is to be appended to a child's face or the face of any other human.

You broadcast so many negative messages about yourself to the world when you put on a face mask. You broadcast those messages tenfold — about yourself, your family, and your children — when you put that face mask on a child.

Reason 19: Compliance To Bad Ideas Is The Last Thing A Free Thinking Person Wants To Teach A Child

Your child needs to be incredibly obedient to father and mother — no asking three times.

To the rest of the world, your child must not be obedient. It is a rough world out there. Obedience is not the way to excel in it. Obedience is the path to mediocrity.

Are you attempting to raise a mediocre child?

Unless that is your aim, it is vital for you to both teach your child how to be disobedient to bad orders and to model this for your child.

Compliance to bad policy corrupts those who follow that policy.

"We are just following orders," is not a legitimate explanation. It is neither moral nor ethical. "I am on a need to know basis," is not a tolerable response.

Only in the military, during time of war, in very specific circumstances, is "need to know" acceptable. Instead of keeping those firm limits on a policy like that, we have allowed the idea of "need to know" or "just following orders" or "stay in your lane" to creep into all areas of life.

That is not acceptable.

You must always know the consequences of your actions. You must always understand what it is you are working toward, even if you only play a small role.

It is unacceptable to do otherwise.

Feigned ignorance is no excuse for bad behavior. It is a lie.

Participating in bad, corrupts he who participates. From birth onwards is the time to teach and model this for your child, by not participating in bad.

Never comply. Willingly cooperate. Withdraw your support as soon as the mission goes astray — even if it is only your tacit approval you are withdrawing. Yes, even your tacit approval in the face of evil, your silence in the face of evil, even that speaks volumes.

"Well, I was just a clerk," or "I was just following orders," does not cut it, nor does "I was just a shareholder with limited liability."

All around us are tricks people use to avoid responsibility for the things they do. Take no part in those. Take full responsibility. Model that for your child.

Let your child grow up with a very clear understanding of that concept, so clear that he can see and avoid those without that same understanding, can see them from a mile away. Help your child have an allergy to compliance with bad. Help your child know a love to cooperate with good.

The face mask is a tool of compliance that no child should have anything to do with. Furthermore, no child should ever see a parent having anything to do with that tool of compliance, lest that child be irreparably harmed by that demonstration of cowardice.

Reason 20: You Teach Your Kids To Do Things They Do Not Like And Intuitively Know Are Not Only Uncomfortable, But BAD

I want to raise children who are independent thinkers and who can process their feelings with relative ease.

I want to raise children who develop their natural passions, excel from a young age, and learn to take on responsibility early. By 18-months-old, a night and day difference already exists with some children raised this way.

For reasons like this, I turn to thinkers like:

Maria Montessori,
Magda Gerber,
Emmi Pikler,
Roslyn Ross,
Stephan Molyneux,
John Holt,
Norman Vincent Peale,
John Taylor Gatto,
Marshall Rosenberg,
Laura Markham,
Aletha Solter,
Pam Leo,
George Clason,
Robert Kiyosaki,
Sally Fallon Morell,
Thomas Cowan,
Suzanne Venker,
Thomas Szasz, and
Robert Mendelsohn.

Free, successful, happy, healthy adults do lots of what they want and very little of what they do not want. Anyone doing otherwise is doing it wrong. Childhood is not just preparation for adulthood, it is also its own stage of life.

There is no reason to create a lifestyle in which your child is doing what he does not want. Children are very intuitive, far more intuitive than most adults, especially if you help them develop that rather than learning to disregard that side of themselves. Also they are able to be supremely rational, especially if you help them to develop that side of themselves.

Parents who have no idea what I am talking about are missing out on an important part of their child, by not nurturing the rational in him and expecting more.

The face mask is more of that low standard way of looking at a child and treating a child, when the opposite is needed — high standards. Teach your child to do what is right from birth, and expect the best from him. Giving him inferior and excusing your own poor decisions by saying "He is just a child," is wrong.

Your child deserves the best. That does not mean he deserves what is lavish. It means he deserves the best behavior around him, and he deserves the best behavior expected from him.

That is what giving a child your best means.

Reason 21: You Teach A Child That Reason Does Not Matter

"Why do I have to wear it?" is an inevitable question from a child about a face mask.

A parent can lie and say "Because, it is good for you," "Because I love you," or "Because it is safer."

The first and last are total lies. The second option is pure manipulation. A child will eventually see through all three. Just because an adult is so comfortable lying to oneself does not mean that adult's child will be.

Lie: Because It Is Good For You

A face mask is not good for a child. A face mask does not prevent the spread of a respiratory virus even when used in ideal conditions by trained professionals. A face mask does even less when worn by average people in the ways common in 2020 and beyond. A face mask may even help to *spread* disease, per the World Health Organization's 2009 guidance on that topic.[1-3] This only takes into consideration the idea of spreading a respiratory virus to others or protecting themselves from respiratory virus. It says nothing of the other hundreds of things that could go wrong in a child's body as a result of wearing a face mask and make him unwell.

Lie: Because It Is Safer

No one is safer from respiratory viruses in a face mask. Anyone who says this to a child is lying.

Lie: Because I Love You

I feel bad for the child who asks for reasonable evidence and gets maternal or paternal manipulation in response. Please never respond to any question with this answer.

If you want to express love, do it after answering the question. Do not silence a budding brain, a budding conscience with such nonsense. If you can avoid doing that, you will spend a lot less time alone in your golden years.

If you cannot, well, that is a bed you make and will almost certainly lie in, as a result of your manipulation.

The real answer to the child's question is "Because I am a coward," "Because I will not stand up to evil, even if it means you may be injuried by that evil," or "Because we are told to."

These answers are at least honest.

Honesty gives a child the chance to understand rather than live longer in darkness.

To have a cowardly parent and one who lies about his cowardliness are two giant strikes against a child that will almost assure him that he starts life behind his peers.

Lies from a parent can be very hard for a child to get past. The child will spend time behind the dark veil of dishonesty and will have the additional burden of the parent-child bond devalued by the dishonesty.

If you are going to be a coward, at least do your child a favor and be an honest coward.

Reason 22: You Teach A Child Not To Trust You

As an adult, you have skills to handle emotions. You can take a deep breath and box them up for later or chose to let them all out now. You have a lot more ability to manage those emotions.

Children do not.

Children feel emotion 100%. Sad is felt 100%. Mad is felt 100%. Frustration is felt 100%. Betrayal is felt 100%.

Children do not know who to trust and intuitively know they need safety: not just physical safety, but also emotional safety. They are very intuitive on how to find that. It is a protective sixth sense of theirs.

Adults, after decades of learning to push down their natural and protective feelings tend to miss this about kids.

Whether or not you are empathetic enough to recognize this does not change this fact about your child.

Each time you put a child in a face mask, you wear away at their certainty that they are safe with you.

At least this is true, unless you can really do a number on them and brainwash them into believing one of the many lies around face masks.

That is unlikely. Eventually, they will catch on and it will come to harm the relationship. Everyone is entitled to mistakes, but you cannot let mistakes continue endlessly and still pretend they are mistakes. That too is a lie and one rooted in malice.

The quicker realized truth can be brought in, the better it is for the parent-child bond, and the better it is for the child's wellbeing.

Reason 23: You Raise A Tyrant, A Slave, Or Both, Rather Than A Healthy And Fully Capable Adult

By putting a child in a face mask against his will, you teach a child that individual wants do not matter.

You teach a child specifically that *his* individual wants do not matter, and you teach a child by extrapolation that the individual wants of others do not matter as well.

Some parents have never forced a child into a car seat. A parent can be a pushover in such a scenario, or a parent can do the hard work of learning to communicate with a child at a young age, work that bears fruit quickly.

This becomes evident when an 18-month-old is able to do better with conversation and negotiation, though largely pre-verbal, than the far-more-developed, though in some ways less emotionally mature, 18-year-old, whose parents have put little effort into this topic.

It shows when a parent has wasted eighteen years with a child, and it also shows when a parent has made the most of eighteen months.

Children raised to communicate rather than to rely on force, learn communication and trust from a very young age.

How do children learn to rely on force? By watching their role models, who are often their parents.

Other children spend an entire childhood being forced into car seats, literal and proverbial. And their adulthoods look a lot like that too: either they spend a lot of time forcing others into car seats or they spend a lot of time being forced into car seats. Maybe both.

While you may offer many words that teach morality opposite to this and a higher morality than this, it is with your actions that you truly communicate your morality to your child. Actions outweigh all words.

The bullying begets bullying. You teach a child who you refuse to communicate with how to obey, but you deny that child the opportunity to learn the peaceful interaction of grown adults.

You teach a child that might makes right.

If that is the basic moral system you instill in a child, you teach him to be a controlling tyrant, you teach him to be an obedient slave, and you likely teach him to alternate between the two based on environment, but you do not teach him how to be a thinking, unique, mature individual.

You let him out into the world without that skill set, a skill set the world has little incentive to teach your then grown child.

Such evil you do to a child when you force a mask upon him against his will, but that is hardly the greatest problem in your relationship.

If you will force a mask on your child against his will, you have much bigger problems, both as a parent and as a person.

May all that you have sown into the fertile ground of your child come back to you many times over. I pray that you have sown blessings and not curses into that fertile ground.

Reason 24: You Sow Seeds
Of Harm In The Future

You undermine the sense of trust your child has for you, you devalue your own parental authority, and connection to the child. This may not seem like much when the child is 5 or 7 or 9-years-old, but when that child is 15 and does not have a solid parental bond to cling to when life is hardest, he will have many other influences to turn to: teachers, pastors, coaches, counselors, or the most common and worst place teens turn — peers.

The peers with the most certainty in their voice are often the least trustworthy, yet the peers with the most certainty in their voice is exactly the peers a teen tends to turn to.

You set the stage of their teenage years during their childhood. Is the relationship going to be solid when they are a teen or challenged? The foundation for that is laid long before they are a teen.

And this is not for you, quite honestly. The teenage years may be troublesome for you, no matter what. This is for them. They can make some really awful mistakes when they do not have a parent to turn to. If the relationship is not in place to overcome all the strife that the teenage years bring, the bond will not be enough to bring them home for advice.

Seldom do parents realize how their childhood neglect of their children — as they let strangers raise their kids — leads to teenage distance from a parent.

The face mask is another way society drives a wedge between parent and child.

Until April 3, 2020, almost no one wore a mask. After April 3, 2020, almost everyone wore a mask. There will be a day of reckoning. Society will come to its senses. The mask will likely come to be seen as a massive over-reaction brought about by a trendy culture with endemic low self-esteem.

I do not know when that will happen. If it happens when your child is a teen, your child may see you as a total cretin and power freak who manipulated him for pointless reasons. That would be deserved, and it might be a good defensive mechanism that your child stops trusting you, making it hard for you to do that level of harm to him again.

However, if that does not describe you, this is a good time to make that clear. For your child's benefit, he cannot go into his teenage years with such concrete justification of what a fraud you are if you are not actually a fraud.

Wait too long, and no amount of words will be able to reverse that trust in you that the imposing of the face mask denied him.

Reason 25: You Teach Your Child "Might Makes Right"

"Why do I have to wear a face mask?" your child may ask.

If your answer is "Because those are the rules," you will have merely taught your child that might makes right. That is the morality you bow down to.

One day he will be bigger than you, more independent than you, and more gutsy than you. If that is the morality you taught him as a child, do you expect him to suddenly bring a different morality to the relationship once you are the weaker party?

Best wishes with that.

On the other hand, if you truly believe that the best morality is might makes right, then the face mask is perfect for you. You could hardly choose a better tool for teaching that to your child.

Reason 26: You Teach Your Child Weakness

Are you going to be flexible or strong?

The goal is not "to break" a child, like one breaks a horse. The goal is not to train a child, the way one trains a dog. The goal is not to "harness" a child, the way one does to a wild falcon.

These methods — in which the person with the right commands and a handful of food are able to step in and be the nearly interchangeable master to that animal — may be fitting for an animal, but they are not fitting for a human.

The goal is to teach a child to be obedient to, or cooperative with, the right people — to parents and others who exhibit virtue — and to be supremely uncooperative with all others.

Children, as early as possible in life, need to know to be supremely uncooperative with even those trusted few, even their parents, when they go outside of the bounds of virtue.

This is an important crux. This is an important distinction between raising someone obedient to all authority, or raising someone obedient to his examined values.

I do not, for a moment, pretend this is easy. Nor do I pretend it is the way of the world, but training an adult to be an obedient sheep begins at birth, just like allowing a child to grow into a courageous lion of virtue begins at birth.

I very intentionally use the word "allow."

At an early age, preverbal, a child knows how to identify virtue and challenge its inconsistent application. I have no question when allowed to grow into a lion of virtue, many children will do exactly that. On the other hand, to grow into an obedient sheep takes training.

It is worth noting that some people in your child's life do not want your child to be a lion. It makes that person's life harder. That person does not want it for your child now, and that person does not want it for your child later. One of the most fundamental measures of how well a person honors freedom is if he can lead free people. Few school teachers can. They seek to break your child as they break a horse. Few bosses can. Few political leaders can. So many want to lead the obedient and compliant. To lead a free man they say is like "herding cats."

In reality, it is like herding lions. Lions do not *need* to be herded by you, they do not *want* to be herded by you, and may react quite ferociously if they sense you trying to herd them.

Those weak souls used to herding sheep should NEVER be left alone with a child. The inevitable outcome is that they will seek to "break" the child.

If the child ever recovers, many unhappy years will be spent trying to find the lion cub that once grew in him.

Yes, I truly mean "allowing a child to grow into a courageous lion of virtue begins at birth."

So much of modernity seeks to disallow this.

The intent is not to let a child run wild. That is a great evil committed against that child. The intent is not to submit a child to obedience. That, too, is a great evil committed against that child. The intent is to teach a child to know and love virtue and to voraciously and fearlessly oppose its opposite. That is the heart of wisdom. That is the kernel of adulthood.

Age does not qualify one as a man. Youth does not disqualify one from being a man. To be a man, more is needed than mere age or biology.

No obedient sheep is a man.

Yet, some thirteen-year-old lions are men.

Reason 27: You Teach Your Child To Lie

As is a theme of this book — actions speak louder than words.

We know conclusively that the masks do not work to prevent the spread of respiratory viruses such as Sars-Cov-2.

We know masks work for all kinds of other things, such as causing children to be sick, spreading disease, spreading cowardice, and letting your child know you will not be there to protect him from bad in the world.

Masks are great for all of that.

If you know masks do not work to prevent the spread of respiratory viruses, and you say that you and your child must wear a mask to protect against the spread of respiratory viruses, then you are lying. You are acting out a lie. When your children see that, no matter how many times you tell them "Do as I say, not as I do," they will see you lie and are very likely to internalize that morality. Best case scenario, they will not grow up broken and demoralized, but will instead struggle with the disquiet and reject you as an immoral liar.

That is the best case outcome of you so brazenly and unapologetically lying to a child over and again. The far-more-likely outcome is that he will grow demoralized by your behavior and have long lasting consequences because of it.

In all likelihood, if you are strapping a mask on a child's face, having the child messed up probably does not bother you too much. You have other priorities that do not involve putting the best interest of your child first and do not involve doing the hard work to uncover the truth.

Reason 28: You Teach Your Child Tacit Approval

Though not often called "a lie," tacit approval is one type of lie.

Tacit approval is the act of remaining silent as a lie is told in front of you, or even nodding your head. It is silence, or nodding, in response to immoral behavior in your presence that violates your own values. It is the act of telling yourself and others that everything happening around you is okay.

The world needs brave men of valor and wise women of virtue who will stand up to lies told in their presence, to the breaking of values in their presence, to unethical and immoral behavior in their presence.

Childhood is the training ground for adulthood. As early in life as possible, a child must be introduced to virtue and valor, from birth ideally.

Not only by words, but in deed, as well. Never should a parent ever demonstrate tacit approval for evil in the presence of a child, no matter the age of the child.

Putting a mask on a child, and wearing a mask in front of a child is exactly that: the tacit approval of a lie.

Reason 29: You Teach A Child To Rat Out Friends, Parents, Neighbors, And Strangers

In some places, you get a real whooping if you rat anyone out to authority for any reason.

It takes a special kind of person to rat his brother out to his parents instead of dealing with it between themselves.

It takes a special kind of person to rat the bully out to the teacher instead of dealing with it.

With words, with fists, with wiles, whatever it may be, not turning to authority teaches you to figure out problems better and to communicate better.

The mask is a way to break that down and to teach a child to rat people out.

There is a new type of accusing look that some children give to the unmasked. It was not an accusing look that existed prior to 2020. The look demonstrates a mighty corruption of the child.

The term "tattle-tale" refers to someone who takes an age appropriate challenge and refuses to embrace it, choosing instead to bring the matter to an authority figure.

At the heart of this term is a hesitation to be courageous, a hesitation to say "I have got this, and come what may, everything will be alright."

As children are increasingly "raised" by mothers they never see, in homes populated by distant male role models, if a stable man is even present at all, who can possibly fault a child for being unable to say "I have got this, and come what may, everything will be alright."

That may be the case for an 18-month-old, an 18-year-old or even an 80-year-old. A basic sense of security is developed at a young age and in the familial bond, though it can, of course, be developed later in life and in other ways, or degraded. He who can interfere with that sense of security has done all he needs to in order to turn a person to authority when placed under pressure, rather than having the confidence and wherewithal to handle a matter on his own.

A tattle-tale is not merely one who goes to an authority figure, it is one who goes prematurely, refusing to handle a matter well within his level of ability.

One does not always know what one's abilities are, of course. An adventurous spirit, undergirded, by self-confidence, helps a person grow more quickly. A spirit lacking in that, will grow more slowly in his individual capacity, perhaps not growing at all in some areas, always needing to turn to authority in those areas, when he is, in fact, perfectly capable of handling the matter.

A tattle-tale is not only ugly because he cannot be trusted and gets people in trouble — sometimes people deserve to get in trouble. A tattle-tale is ugly because he simply cannot be trusted. He lacks the self-confidence that undergirds all virtuous behavior. He shows that by so regularly turning to authority to handle what he could handle perfectly fine on his own.

Authority figures who want to see that person grow, abhor this behavior and want the individual to take on as much responsibility as he can and to grow accordingly. This is the case at every stage of human development.

Authority figures who crave power and do not desire the growth of that individual, appreciate this behavior and will encourage it.

That is where we now find ourselves. A growing list of behaviors that fit in a category of "If you see something, say something," are foisted upon our children as normal. It is not normal. It is sick.

Normal is for a healthy child to want to take on as much responsibility and challenge as possible and to report back about his failings and accomplishments later that day at the dinner table.

Abnormal is to go through the day, looking for reasons to report others to an authority figure.

Sure, there are all kinds of people who use the word tattle-tale, rat, stool pigeon, because they do not want to get into trouble for the bad that they have done, but it is about far more than that.

Being a tattle-tale is bad for the tattle-tale. There are times to judiciously turn to authority. We are far beyond that point. The trend in society is to constantly turn to authority rather than to take ownership over a situation.

There are many ways by which that sense of personal responsibility and sense of ownership are chipped away at. They must all be avoided: among adults and children alike.

Reporting non-compliance with one-size-fits-all health mandates is a recent and powerful trend in a long line of trends that have the long-term impact of further enfeebling children on the road to adulthood.

Reason 30: You Teach Your Child To Be
A Person Of Preference And Not
A Person Of Values

Would you steal a candy bar?

Would you steal a candy bar if you knew no one would catch you?

Would you steal a candy bar in San Francisco, where everyone is doing it, no one is allowed to catch you, and the police are told to stand down?

Would you steal a candy bar in San Francisco if I gave you a million dollars to do so?

Here we have the answer to whether you are a person of preference or a person of values, and if not stealing is one of your values.

A person of preference prefers to behave in a certain way and not behave other ways. A person of values does not transgress his values under any circumstances.

A person of preference is flexible about his ethics and morality depending on the circumstances. He is just waiting for the right reason to be flexible about the stances he takes.

A person of values is solid in his values. His values exist independent of circumstances. The right reason cannot be invented to turn him away from them.

Some may call a person of preference "pragmatic." They erroneously define pragmatism as dealing in reality rather than ideals. Pragmatism instead means dealing in that which is sensible and realistic rather than that which is theoretical. The truth is, that there is hardly anything more realistic and sensible than following one's well-grounded values.

The face mask indicates a great deal about your values and even if you have any values at all.

A person who never wears a face mask for any reason is a person who will be able to say "No!" to all one-size-fits-all public health mandates. No reason will be good enough for him to flex on his values. A person who wears a face mask, even for "just a minute," even "just to get through the door," is a person who will do far worse — it only takes the right rationale.

He who will wear a mask will also take a Covid shot. The mechanism of compliance is the same, and really, it is far easier to get a Covid shot — it only takes ten seconds of weakness. Yes, he who will wear a mask will also take a Covid shot; he just has not heard the right rationale yet.

A great deal of effort has been spent since the Ides of March 2020 to "break" people of values and to prove to them, and to society, that they are morally relativistic creatures, that they are people of preference only and not people of values.

Before I take this too far and perhaps overly glamorize this topic, let it be known that the world has no use for a person of values. They only need a person of preference. A person of values can be a very prickly and unpleasant predictable person for the world to deal with. The world has no need for a person of values, until a true crisis exists, at least. At a moment like that — perhaps this very moment we live in being an example — a person of values is the only one with solid footing to weather the storm.

He was made for a time such as this, whereas, everybody else is left utterly clueless.

Determine to be a person of values and not a person of preference. That test is before you every time you are told to mask up.

Reason 31: You Teach Your Child To Misread Romans 13

You speak loudly with your actions. No matter what your words are, you actions speak so much more loudly.

Romans 13 is often presented as a guide for the cowardly Christian. Only out of context can it be read so. In context, the text so clearly says to do what is moral at all times. No child should be taught the bootlicker, out-of-context, reading of Romans 13.

Romans 13 Does Not Apply To Covid-19

In the United States, we do not have one government. We quite specifically have checks and balances between branches (examples include the checks and balances laid out in the US Constitution, or through the seizure of judicial power that took place with *Marbury v. Madison* in 1803), checks and balances between state and federal (as stipulated in the Tenth Amendment), checks and balances between local and federal (through the existence of sheriffs, or with the existence of home rule communities), checks and balances between individuals and federal (as indicated by concepts such as jury unanimity or jury nullification, voting, civic participation, lobbying, civil disobedience, the right to redress grievances contained in the First Amendment, the Second Amendment's implicit threat from an armed citizenry, or even Thomas Jefferson's November 13, 1787 letter to William Stephens Smith[1] in which he praises the tax protest commonly known as Shay's Rebellion), and numerous other checks and balances.

For all of its messiness, that befuddling bureaucracy of conflict appears to be part of how our government was intended to operate.

A president would like you to believe that he is in charge, a congressman would like you to believe that his body is in charge, the courts the same, the governor the same, and yet others may say a cabal, a special interest group, or the deep state runs the whole operation. In reality, no one is in charge.

Governmental factions were intentionally established by the founding fathers to constantly battle against each other in a separation of powers. This is defense of freedoms by self-entangling bureaucracy. It is a reason that the utilitarian libertarian shibboleth of "efficiency" may reduce freedom. Unfortunately, that bureaucracy spends a lot of time cooperating across its various parts, which is to the detriment of the free man, rather than fighting each other, which would be in the interest of greater liberty.

This proves 234 years of critics accurate that the US Constitution has been used as an instrument of tyranny.

Elusive Authority Renders Romans 13 Irrelevant

The amorphous "authority," in the United States, includes the above factions, established as various checks and balances.

There is no single government in the United States and there is no single voice for the country. There are 1.) settled matters of consensus, 2.) contested matters of consensus, and 3.) matters on which no consensus exists.

This system of elusive authority renders Romans 13 irrelevant, until a settled consensus can be nailed down on a particular topic.

For all its flaws, the US Constitution, by design, makes that consensus hard to nail down. It makes the defining of authority nearly impossible.

Some commentators address this by asking what constitutes moral authority, and defining it as "That which is in line with the US Constitution," but that does not go far enough. To be in line with the Constitution is so amorphous a concept, even from a strict reading. Some place that alongside two other amorphous concepts — individual conscience and natural law — both useful despite their amorphous nature. There is no need to even push this issue, though, until a determination has been made about what "Caesar" is really saying.

Romans 13 Is A Text On Moral Obligations,
Not A Guide To Civic Participation

Romans 13 says nothing about whether you may ask for an audience with Caesar to discuss an edict and to inform him of his edict's unintended consequences. It says nothing about what to do if the courts do not agree with the executive. It says nothing about what to do if the legislature does not agree with the governor. It says nothing about what to do if the public health technocrat does not agree with a member of the judiciary.

We do not have a Caesar in the year 2020 or any other clear unitary figure. We have a political class, many competing layers of government, and a population that has cooperative streaks and uncooperative streaks, with varying claims to authority. Before compliantly shuttering their churches beginning on the Ides of March 2020, the pastors did not even do the most basic work to make sure that the right hand of Caesar agreed with the left hand of Caesar. Nearly two years later, as this book goes to print, there are churches that remain closed.

I am not suggesting rebellion. This is a far cry from that. To even think that some cowardly church leaders would do anything of the sort is preposterous — they did not even bother to bow to their almighty Caesar and ask for permission to make sure that all the parts of great Caesar's government, source of temporal truth and authority, were in agreement. They did not seek meetings with the Governor. They did not seek meetings with the President. They did not seek meetings with judges — also known as lawsuits. They did not seek for all of these parties to get on the same page with each other. The duty of a responsible citizen in the United States is to exert some pressure on the system in order to bring about communication across these parts. The many parts of our adversarial system will barely communicate without some provoking.

A bold, anti-bootlicker reading of Romans 13 is suitable for an edict from a unitary king or a statement rooted in governmental consensus, but we have neither in the case of Covid-19.

Churches Did Not Behave Pro-Actively Enough To Trigger Romans 13, They Merely Treated Press Releases As Gospel

From the Ides of March 2020 onward, many churches refused to provide the very minor level of resistance to figure out what the government was even officially saying. Many churches simply accepted the press release of some relatively minor pettifogger with a government sinecure and elevated that to the official word of the United States of America or the official word of their state or their county, and then using the lens of Romans 13 effectively elevated that press release to the official word of God. Louis XIV, who saw himself as a God-like figure, said "I am the state." Many local pastors said "The unsigned county press release is the state." To some extent, they even said "The unsigned county press release is *superior* to the Word of God."

When their country needed them to aid the government by applying some minor pressure, American clergy largely refused. They pretended that abrogating their civic duty, was the same as performing their civic duty. Even a bootlicking reading of Romans 13 calls on them to fulfill this civic duty, for without it, there is often no way to even know what government authority is instructing you to do. Unfortunately, for those who seek to be both a good citizen and a compliant human, the American system does not provide well for this. It requires pressure, often from the actions of individual citizens, to achieve consensus among the disparate branches. To be a compliant human is to fail as a good citizen.

Romans 13 is not instruction to sit on the sidelines. Romans 13 does not instruct a pastor to blindly follow the unsigned press release. A pastor, a church council, and the elders of a faith community are entrusted with protecting the church for their short time on this earth and passing on its teaching to the succeeding generations.

After they have performed their civic duty of getting agreement from government, then they may do what many brave-spirited commentators suggest and evaluate the morality of the request, because until then, there is no official government edict to follow. Taking a press release from a minor pettifogger with a government sinecure, made into a false idol, and given far more loyalty than such a document could possibly deserve, is an error of many who so easily fall into the trap of seeing democracy as a god, to reference the insightful Hans Herman Hoppe,[2] a god which predictably fails.

The Romans 13 Test Was Not Triggered By The Covid Response

To use the judicial parlance of our day, the "test" of Romans 13 is not even triggered until an authoritative government edict is determined. That determination takes some resistance to arrive at.

The pastor seeking to be obedient to the governmental authority of our day, must do the basic work of bringing the authorities in line with one another. The lazy compliance we have seen from some ecclesiastical bodies does not fulfill even their own reading of Romans 13, for it ignores the nature of American government.

I am grateful to all who provide anti-bootlicker readings of Romans 13, but until the disparate parts of government are brought in line, on a specific topic, no application of such a reading is possible.

Reason 32: You Are Being Conditioned To View Your Freedom As Selfishness

There is no us. There is you and the people you choose to associate with. There is me and the people I choose to associate with. Those people and I arguably have an "us." The guy on the TV and I do not have an "us."

If you can be confused about that detail, all manner of ill can befall you. If you can stay firm about that detail, such ill cannot befall you. Reject all claims strangers have that you are part of their "us." You simply are not.

Around the Ides of March 2020, a new era of harm was ushered in, harm that was able to occur because people were willing to believe that some public health bureaucrat, who they had never even heard of, was now more a part of their "us," than their neighbor, friend, or child. In fact, the stranger even got to command the "us."

You are an individual. You get to make choices for yourself. That is how life works. That is the natural state of man. Nothing selfish or unselfish about that. It is reality. That is how freedom works. That is how society works. That is even how God works. Upon that concept of free will and individual autonomy are greater things built.

An anti-social element in society seeks to tear that all down.

They seek to tear down the foundations of society by saying if you make your own decisions, and your neighbor makes his own decisions, then that is "bad." Instead, a third person, or group of people, needs to be given all the control to make all the decisions, they claim. That is not how our culture works, that is not a good idea, and it is frankly sociopathic. I have yet to find even a single example of a government doing that on a wide scale without creating the most awful human misery.

Are you selfish for wanting to make your own decisions? Is your neighbor selfish for wanting to make his own decisions?

No, in fact, I would like to commend you for protecting society from the most awful centralized, totalitarian control by simply saying "No, thank you. I will be making decisions for myself. Have a nice day."

So much good in the world is protected by people doing exactly that. Doing so creates a healthy boundary around your mind, your life, your home, and your family. It protects that which is valuable from the control of those who cannot possibly value it.

Are you the selfish one? No. You are the freedom fighter, protecting the good of society in this psychological war being waged.

You are a hero for defending your boundaries. Thank you.

Reason 33: You Put Your Child Through A Class On Scientism And Not Science

Science is the practice of the scientific method. The scientific method is the process of following these steps or steps like these:

Observe.
Hypothesize.
Test the hypothesis.
Theorize.
Share results.
Invite others to duplicate results.
Share feedback.
Repeat the process unceasingly.

Anytime anyone says the phrase "settled science," they are not speaking about science, but about a narrative. Science is a process. There is no end to that process. There is no destination, no terminus, no laurel on which to rest, no ability for a matter to be settled.

A ten-year-old may come along and upend five hundred years of so-called "settled science" by simply asking questions and disproving a hypothesis.

Scientism is an obedience to authority so austere in its devotion that it causes its adherents to repeat a narrative, opinion, or perspective and to mislabel it as science.

Science, again, is a process.

The questioning of an idea is a fundamental concept to science and the scientific method.

The fanaticism of scientism is so extreme in its almost religious devotion, that the questioning of sacred ideas is firmly prevented.

Reason 34: Your Child Will Imitate You

Poet Milan Rufus writes:

Mind your kids,
you adults.
They are gathering your pollen,
those little bees from God.
They will seal it into their little bodies.
They imitate you.
They are the most exact living
little mirrors of you.

Their shape is from your anvils.
They live from your bread.
One day they will be exactly like you.
So be humane to each other.[1]

Children should not be masked by you. Neither should they see you in a mask.

To do so is to teach them to do wrong.

Everyday be doing two things:

As an adult, be moving toward the person you want to become. Never stagnate. Always be moving toward that person you want to become — that even better version of yourself. This is not to say you should be unhappy with who you are and what you have, but to always be striving for greater excellence.

As a parent, be the person you want your child to model: using the language patterns, using the thought patterns, making the decisions judicious, wise, appropriate, upright, acting as if your child were witnessing every moment, which they so often are, whether you realize it or not.

In that context, is not the refusal of a face mask a no-brainer? Are not there so many other no-brainers? Where you have the dogged will to do right, courage, resources, and know-how will follow.

Reason 35: You Place Your Child In The Hands Of Some Very Twisted People

There are people in the world who do not wish well for your child. They do not wish well for you either. You are harder for them to manipulate. Your child is not. They may not necessarily want *harm* for anyone, but the best interest of your child is not a primary concern to them.

This inevitably leads to reduced benefit to your child, if allowed to be influenced by people like this.

Parents are the decision maker for a child. No one else. Honor that policy in your family, and it will help protect your child.

Draw the firmest of boundaries around that, and do not let anyone cross that without feeling the greatest wrath from you.

That means until he is eighteen-years-old, **NO ONE** talks medicine with him unless you are in the room.

No one. No exceptions. And your child is not the decision maker. You are. No exceptions.

Once a third party places this wedge between you and your child, greater wedges can easily be formed, and your child may wind up dependent on some bad people for his medical decisions. This much will certainly be true: they will not put your child's interests first the way you, as a parent, will.

Take any incursions on your parental authority very seriously. This matters now even more dearly than it has ever mattered. Please take the gravity of this situation and the severity of these times seriously. Much worse is being planned for you and your family. To refuse to draw an impenetrable boundary here and now is foolhardy.

Reason 36: We Are NOT All In This Together

"We are all in this together," is a phrase developed by public health researchers to tug at your heart strings. Millions of dollars were spent training the people who developed that phrase.

That is the case with many public health messages that are intended to appear organic. Implausibly, they are adopted by many mouthpieces all at once.

Far from being organic, it was developed with the intent of it having maximum impact.

Coca-Cola or Pfizer spends a great deal of money on messaging meant to convince you to pump their high fructose corn syrup or their pharmaceuticals into your child's body. Public health researchers do exactly the same. They do it with a similarly high level of sophistication. The only difference is that they pretend to have your child's best interest at heart. That is not at all the case. When you read an advertisement from Coca-Cola or Pfizer, you know exactly that neither Coca-Cola nor Pfizer put the best interest of your child first. The same should be presumed of public health researchers. They have an agenda. Their agenda, in fact, tends to be far more pernicious than any agenda from Coca-Cola or Pfizer, companies that simply want to make a few dollars. Public health researchers are motivated by much more than money.

We are not all in this together. Life has never worked that way. You are in it with the people you choose to be in it with. That is it.

No one can force you into being his teammate. You get to choose your teammates, and they get to choose you. That is it.

When a vaccine, a lockdown, a face mask order goes wrong and you end up with an injured child, you will see how not in it together we all are. Try to get a penny from them, try to get an ounce of sympathy, try to even be believed by them that your child has been injured by their insane policies — these people who claim to be in it together with you. It will not happen.

Make decisions for you and your family as if you and your family are all alone, as if only your family's interests matter, and as if all liability falls on you, because that is the reality of the situation.

Reason 37: A Tale Of Two Mothers

In early 2020, I encountered two mothers, and I quickly realized I was encountering these personality types of mothers over and again.

One, generally speaking, had an approach of filling her child up with fear of the world and fear of all that was not like her. Such a child may end up with generational wounds, wounds likely generational prior to the mother's own neuroticism and passed along through the family. She was miserable. Her son was miserable. And the father, tellingly, did not go to the park with them.

Another mother, generally speaking, was a most wonderful woman with a happy child, a happy husband, a happy dog, happy friends, and happy family who liked to be at the park all together being happy. She made it look effortless. As the weight of 2020 came down on her and her family, she flourished all the more emotionally and the family prospered.

I spent a lot of time in the park during lockdown, often spending hours a day of family time there. I like to observe my surroundings. I watched a lot of families. The dynamics were hard to miss.

These two mothers represent extremes, but every parent tends towards one of these extremes: teaching a child that the world is a place to be feared, or teaching a child that life is a blessing to glory in.

The two are exclusive. Some parents would like to pretend otherwise, but that is simply not the case. Such confidence and faith cannot co-exist alongside such a state of terror about the world.

Welcome the one, and you get rid of the other. Get rid of the other, and you welcome the one.

I do not know why it works that way, but it does.

You get to decide what kind of parent to be. You get to decide what kind of experience of the world you want to give your child. You get to decide if your curses will be generational.

The decision rests on you every morning, in fact every moment, you get to decide to continue on the same path or to do it differently.

The tales of these two mothers show that face masks on your child are about so much more than just face masks, even if just for a minute, even if just to get through the door.

A face mask on your child broadcasts volumes about you.

Reason 38: The Story Of The Boy Who Says "Why Do I Have To Wear This?" To His Mother

This is for the kid who yelled at his mom over the leaf blower, "But if no one else is wearing a face mask, *why do I have to*?!"

My phone said it was a sunny 61 degrees out. Most of the people in that park that morning were in short sleeves and shorts.

Some had jump ropes, some had weights, some were walking their dogs, others were talking on the phone. It being lockdown, some of these activities had moved outside to the park.

From your gait, you looked like a healthy kid who loves both sun and fresh air. Some kids these days can barely walk, they get so little exercise.

You were maybe as young as ten-years-old and having started your growth spurt, or perhaps as old as thirteen, but not having started a spurt yet, starting to get independent in your thoughts.

But not that independent yet, for your mother had wrapped you head-to-toe in a track suit that matched her own. She had you in full sunglasses that matched her own. Your full, oversized cloth face mask matched her own as well. You wore similar baseball style caps. Even your hair, on the longer side, and of similar color, would have matched hers, had hers not been up in a ponytail.

It was your internal terrain, though, that did not match hers. I heard you say as you walked into the park, "But if no one else is wearing a face mask, *why do I have to*?!"

I called out to you "Great questions. Great question. You need to protect the mind that asked that question."

You flipped around and faced me. Your mother's tightening physiology was unmistakable through her tracksuit.

I blurted it right out. I am sorry to have interfered in your mother's parenting, but I remain happy that my first instinct was to blurt out truth where there is so little and to praise the youngin' who refuses to be conned.

I kept walking toward my task in the park. You kept walking toward yours.

Fifty others must have been in that park that morning when you walked in. There were many corners of the park in which to avoid a person. Not a single person, other than the two of you, was wearing a mask. The news, of course, claimed our city was 95% masked. Not true. About thirty minutes later, another man came into the park and was wearing a mask. Later, another man would come in wearing a mask around his neck.

Though this city remains on full lockdown and the politicians and media tout the high level of compliance, there is clearly so little compliance.

Your mother instructed you to avoid me if you wanted to stay in the park. You wisely avoided me. I would not have spoken to you again.

Out of an abundance of caution, your mother soon, perhaps within two minutes of your entry, got you out of the park of unmasked people.

She will have a hard time keeping you in that track suit for much longer. She will have a hard time keeping you in that face mask for much longer. But she will have her ways. If she is a good mom, she will start to make way for you to develop your own ways, and will answer your questions with the best amount of reason and evidence she can muster. It is hard. Kids ask some pretty devastating questions. We cannot always be perfect parents.

If she is a bad mom, she will give you answers like "Because I say so," and will enforce it with the amount of power she has over your food, water, housing, and general happiness. She may even be physical in her approach toward your questions. Though you are already about 3/4 her size, a hand slap from a parent you love can surely still send you reeling: emotionally and physically. That will not always be the case. And I doubt she hits you for such questions based on your comfort questioning her as glibly as you did. She, at least, does not hit you in public.

Parents are never perfect. Perfection is not needed from a parent or anyone else.

Ahead of you is a magnificent life, if you let it be. Ahead of you is a magnificent period of intrigue and growth, if you let it be. We have a few assets in life that mean much to us in the grand scheme of things. One of them is the space between our two ears.

You have reached an advanced age without that asset being molded into subservience — either to your parents or your peers. Congratulations. Now, is when the world starts to move into overdrive. The next ten years they will do all that they can to acculturate you.

Wind up on the other side of that crucible with a mind disobedient, and you will be richly rewarded for being one of the few who was able to accomplish that.

It will come at you in different ways in the succeeding decade. Bullies of all sorts will want to bend your will to theirs. Do not stand for it, and you will be one of the few who succeed through that crucible. The good news is that this segment of life will be nothing like the first two decades.

And another reprieve will come to you in the next decade. By this time, most militaries and government agencies will stop seeing you as so desirable. You will have largely lost the ability to be shaped by them.

If you can make it to your forties, society really backs off. The cake is baked. You are who you are. The fight to submit your mind to the will of another never comes to an end, but a little reprieve comes and rewards start to stack up.

Among those rewards are that your acquaintances start self-selecting, if you have not already chased off the facile-minded.

There is a lot of good news. You have made it through the worst. Many tyrants through the ages wanted you early in life. Some said they could shape you by five-years-old, others said they could shape you by seven-years-old. The foundations in life are set during this time. New foundations can always be built, but for many, these early years are so informative about how the rest of this time goes.

And you, dear masked young man, are maturing beyond the period of the first crucible. You have failed the test of acculturation. You have become your own person, able to blurt out his own thoughts to a figure of authority.

It was not the most original thought "If they do not have to do it then why do I?" but it was a good start. From a starting place like that, you could turn into one of the snitching Karens of the world or a disobedient Henry David Thoreau.

That choice is your own.

If it is to be a Thoreau, you have come to the right place.

Reason 39: Thank You To The Mother Who Brought Her Son To The Playground

In West Coast lockdown land, where everyone is said to be compliant, I saw a miserable looking old man taking photos of children and parents who were having an amazing time together at an officially closed playground.

Locked in for more than a week, in March 2020, the parents had enough and took the children out to play.

It was a joy to behold, watching grandmother doing her laps, dad chasing the sons around, leaping over slides and other obstacles as they played tag with the hulking man, boys laughing hysterically, mother looking on from the park bench. A small sign had been posted at the park. It labeled the playground officially closed because of Covid-19. The next day barricades were put into place, intending to more seriously keep people off the playground.

For a moment, I thought about confronting the miserable old man, with a power play that is perhaps the only remaining thing worse than a corona lockdown violation: he was photographing children.

You could see the old man raging on his face at the idea that a child would be playing in a closed playground during the corona hoax, as he snapped photos, his musculature growing more tense with each movement.

Perhaps this rat-faced man reads his corona fear porn each morning at *The New York Times*, *Slate*, *Wired*, or some other publication that can do no better than party line for even 1-in-1000 articles. Sometimes thought slips through.

Perhaps he was the one who complained so mightily to officials that the barricades went up around a children's playground the next morning.

As fun as he might be to dislike, that miserable man is not the great enemy. That miserable editor at *The Times* or *MIT Tech Review* or every other bootlicking establishment rag is not the great enemy.

Author Alan Moore wrote in the early 1980s:[1]

> *"Because while the truncheon may be used in lieu of conversation, words will always retain their power.*
>
> *Words offer the means to meaning, and for those who will listen, the enunciation of truth. And the truth is, there is something terribly wrong with this country, is not there?*
>
> *Cruelty and injustice, intolerance and oppression.*

And where once you had the freedom to object, to think and speak as you saw fit, you now have censors and systems of surveillance coercing your conformity and soliciting your submission.

How did this happen?

Who's to blame?

Well certainly there are those more responsible than others, and they will be held accountable, but again truth be told, if you're looking for the guilty, you need only look into a mirror.

I know why you did it.

I know you were afraid.

Who would not be?

War, terror, disease. There were a myriad of problems which conspired to corrupt your reason and rob you of your common sense."

The enemy is inside. The enemy is he who does not defend his own boundaries. He is an enemy to himself.

At the park one morning, long after the corona barricades went up, long after the social distancing placards became the norm everywhere you turned, after the frightening national face mask advisory went into effect, I saw a simple act of courage.

It was 8 a.m., an hour before the newly installed corona park rangers got out of bed to begin their rounds of the playgrounds, when I saw a mother doing what was once the most natural thing possible: taking her son to the playground.

It was natural before it was deemed both illegal and immoral.

A young family, in an urban area, with a small apartment. What else are you supposed to do on day 20 of the 2-week lockdown? You could cower at home. You could let the kids run on the narrow, hypodermic needle-filled, excrement-filled, and broken bottle-filled left coast sidewalks. You could also just go to the park.

In our era, the cautious feminine reigns supreme. Prevention of chance, socializing of risk, elimination of hazard, "responsible regulation," and loss mitigation are all the rage. To advocate otherwise in life, and especially as a parent, is to risk being labeled negligent. The once strangely antiseptic, tabloid-worthy notion of "the boy in the bubble" has become the American ideal for how childhood should look. Occasionally, a careless oaf of a father[2] is allowed to roughhouse. But not the mother. And certainly not outside during corona madness in West Coast lockdown land.

But there she was.

Here was a mother bucking that, taking her son to the playground. A profile in courage, in the midst of corona.

And before long, the father followed with their dog, who was also happy to get out.

They ran about the morning park, availing themselves of the beautiful playground that everyone else was too gullible and cowardly to visit. Dozens of parents an hour would pass through that park just a few weeks earlier.

This was courage in a city of cowering people, going through every which means of contortion in order to comply: the face masks that do not work, the social distancing that does not work, the quarantines which do not work, the shameful "essential workers only" mandate which evokes brownshirts asking for papers justifying your very existence.

Even the USSR had no massive peacetime lockdown of hundreds of millions like this. The atheist communists could not manage to close churches like America has done. Not even the most ardent Marxist-Leninists seemed able to bring an economy to a halt like what has happened in America: destroying lives and livelihoods along the way. And to help us feel not utter derision, but to instead feel thankful for it all, billions of dollars[3] have been spent these several months on corona fear propaganda, engineered by the masterful psychologists that we call the free press.

In the midst of that, a mother and a father courageously determined they would reject that distraction and instead live their lives.

Courageously, they stepped out to go to the park. Courageously, they stepped out of the house to live their lives.

And I want to thank them.

Because courage is contagious.

Reason 40: Do Not Look At Face Masks For Covid Avoidance, Look At Obesity, Or A Host Of Other Meaningful Comorbidities, But Especially Obesity

J.B. Pritzker has been the Governor of Illinois through Covid. He has the highest body mass index of any US governor, empirically making him the most obese US governor[1] during Covid.

Governor Pritzker spends a considerable amount of time talking about his desire to protect the people of Illinois from Covid.

Covid would be a perfect time for Governor Pritzker to focus on approaches to public health that save lives during Covid, instead he has focused on face masks and lockdowns, neither of which work.

A far more meaningful factor to draw his attention to would be diet, exercise, and obesity.

For whatever reason, the most obese governor in America did not want to talk about that.

I lost some weight during Covid-19. I have made it a point to keep myself and those around me healthy. There are things you can do to take control of your life and protect you from Covid-19 and other problems during this time. Face masks are not one of them.

In the article "Why Covid-19 is more deadly in people with obesity – even if they are young,"[2] dated September 8, 2020, Meredith Wadman writing for *Science* points out that obesity plays a huge role in Covid-19 outcomes:

> "in the first meta-analysis of its kind, published on 26 August in *Obesity Reviews*, an international team of researchers pooled data from scores of peer-reviewed papers capturing 399,000 patients. They found that people[3] with obesity who contracted Sars-Cov-2 were 113% more likely than people of healthy weight to land in the hospital, 74% more likely to be admitted to an ICU, and 48% more likely to die."

Wadman states that obesity plays a role in hospitalization as well:

> "The largest descriptive study yet of hospitalized US Covid-19 patients, posted as a preprint last month by Genentech researchers, found that 77%[4] of nearly 17,000

patients hospitalized with Covid-19 were overweight (29%) or obese (48%)."

Wadman delves into some of the reasons why obesity plays such a role:

"The biology of obesity includes impaired immunity, chronic inflammation, and blood that is prone to clot, all of which can worsen Covid-19."

About the physical pathologies related to people with obesity, Wadman goes on to explain:

"The physical pathologies that render people with obesity vulnerable to severe Covid-19 begin with mechanics: Fat in the abdomen pushes up on the diaphragm, causing that large muscle, which lies below the chest cavity, to impinge on the lungs and restrict airflow. This reduced lung volume leads to collapse of airways in the lower lobes of the lungs, where more blood arrives for oxygenation than in the upper lobes. 'If you are already starting [with] this mismatch, you are going to get worse faster' from Covid-19."

Obesity creates mechanical problems with the lungs and as Wadman points out, also causes problems with the blood, making Covid more lethal for the obese:

"Other issues compound these mechanical problems. For starters, the blood of people with obesity has an increased tendency to clot – an especially grave risk during an infection that, when severe, independently peppers the small vessels of the lungs with clots.[5] In healthy people, 'the endothelial cells' that line the blood vessels are normally saying to the surrounding blood: 'Do not clot,' says Beverley Hunt, a physician-scientist who's an expert in blood clotting at Guy's and St. Thomas' hospitals in London. But 'we think that signaling is being changed by Covid,' Hunt says, because the virus injures endothelial cells, which respond to the insult by activating the coagulation system.

"Add obesity to the mix, and the clotting risk shoots up. In Covid-19 patients with obesity, Hunt says, 'You have got such sticky blood, oh my — the stickiest blood I have ever seen in all my years of practice.'"

Wadman describes how in the obese, important immune system tissue is replaced by fat cells, thereby weakening the immune system:

> "'Immunity also weakens in people with obesity, in part because fat cells infiltrate the organs where immune cells are produced and stored, such as the spleen, bone marrow, and thymus,' says Catherine Andersen, a nutritional scientist at Fairfield University. 'We are losing immune tissue in exchange for adipose tissue, making the immune system less effective in either protecting the body from pathogens or responding to a vaccine,' she says.

> "The problem is not only fewer immune cells, but less effective ones,' adds Melinda Beck, a co-author of the Obesity Reviews meta-analysis who studies obesity and immunity at the University of North Carolina, Chapel Hill. Beck's studies of how obese mice respond to the influenza virus demonstrated that key immune cells called T cells 'do not function as well in the obese state,' she says. 'They make fewer molecules that help destroy virus-infected cells, and the corps of 'memory' T-cells left behind after an infection, which is key to neutralizing future attacks by the same virus, is smaller[6] than in healthy weight mice.'

> "Beck's work suggests the same thing happens in people: She found that people with obesity vaccinated against flu had twice the risk[7] of catching it as vaccinated, healthy weight people. That means trials of vaccines for Sars-Cov-2 need to include people with obesity, she says, because 'coronavirus vaccines may be less effective in those people.'"

Wadman points out, how obesity leads to further inflammation, an issue for Covid patients:

> "Beyond an impaired response to infections, people with obesity also suffer from chronic, low-grade inflammation. Fat cells secrete several inflammation-triggering chemical messengers called cytokines, and more come from immune cells called macrophages that sweep in to clean up dead and dying fat cells. Those effects may compound the runaway cytokine activity that characterizes severe Covid-19. 'You end up causing a lot of tissue damage, recruiting too many immune cells, destroying healthy bystander cells,' says Il-

hem Messaoudi, an immunologist who studies host responses to viral infection at the University of California, Irvine. Of the added risk from obesity, she adds: 'I would say a lot of it is immune-mediated.'"

Covid is not lethal because it is from a lab, Covid is so lethal because Americans are so willing to lie to themselves. Being fat is really unhealthy for you. Really. Masks do not change that. Lockdowns do not change that. House arrest does not change that. Church closure, school closure, and declaring people non-essential does not change that.

Nope. Being fat is really unhealthy for you, and if you cannot be honest about that, you have got a large, unhealthy population bringing about its own demise, all the while telling lies about how masks and experimental shots are the real solution.

Masks and experimental shot are both unsafe and ineffective. That has been what so much research over the past year has unquestionably proven. We should not be experimenting in this way upon ourselves. However, what we know for certain works against Covid and against many other diseases to keep people healthy and to prolong life is to live life more healthfully.

Losing some weight seems to be one of the most meaningful solutions to Covid. Healthy people get sick less. Healthy people get less sick. Healthy people die less.

77% of Americans are overweight or obese. Obesity is a big deal when it comes to Covid.

So why would you let anyone lie to you about a mask rather than talking about the real issues at play: poor health, bad diet and nutrition, lack of exercise, comorbidities, and age drive virtually all illness, Covid-19 being among them.

Masking merely starves a person of oxygen and does much further harm. Lockdowns starve society of freedom and prosperity, alongside further harm. Obesity is a serious topic to talk about. Masks do almost nothing positive and make an illness-prone obese person at greater risk of sickness, isolation, and harm. Lockdowns deny the obese freedom and prosperity.

Obesity is a real problem, causing greater death. No one is dying from a lack of a face mask or a lack of a lockdown.

Reason 41: Obesity Drives Covid

Looking at Covid deaths in the US versus Asia, Simon Denyer and Joel Achenbach writing for the *Washington Post* point to obesity as a possible driver:[1]

> "There is something else that many Asian countries have in common — much lower rates of obesity than in the West. Obesity is a leading risk factor for serious Covid-19 illness. Just over 4 percent of Japanese people are classified as obese, and less than 5 percent of South Koreans. That compares with 20 percent or more in Western Europe, and 36 percent of people in the United States, according to the World Health Organization."

At risk of being called fat shamers, even the *Washington Post* will point out the obvious — unhealthy people — the obese among them, are the cause of illness in themselves, not a lack of face masks.

Reason 42: Covid-19 Is An IQ Test

Having made it this far into a list of problems associated with mask wearing, one can credibly point to Covid-19 as an IQ test.

The prolific Dr. Vernon Coleman points this out in the article, "Proof That Face Masks Do More Harm Than Good:"[1]

> "There is absolutely no scientific reason for mask wearing under any circumstances. The Covid-19 hoax is an IQ test. Anyone who wears a mask after studying the evidence has clearly failed the test."

This is a valid piece of criticism to keep in mind. If you are buying into the face mask hype, you are failing the IQ test. Demand better of yourself.

If those around you are buying into the face mask hype, they are failing the IQ test. Surround yourself with better. As painful as it may be, now is a period in time that is so powerfully throwing in our faces what the people around us are made of.

Those are the people we have chosen to surround ourselves with or who we have tacitly allowed ourselves to be surrounded by. We can take this moment as the gift that it is, or we can ignore that gift and pretend that there is no consequence to being surrounded by such challenged people.

Demand better of yourself. While it is never painless to demand the best for yourself and all you surround yourself with, in living memory it has never been more obvious. Consequently, it has never been easier to do than it is now.

Reason 43: You Do Not Want To Wear It, They Do Not Want To Wear It

You may not want to wear a face mask. That is, for some reason, not a permissible answer in the present milieu. It is the answer that should be most acceptable though, both from a rights perspective and from a medical perspective. In the United States, you are not to be forced to do that which you cannot do safely, unless you are harming someone else.

Therefore, the public health profession has created the lie that by you not listening to them, you cause harm to someone else. It is a foundational, anti-social canard from the public health field. They are always on the lookout for ways that you harm others, because that allows them to seize additional control. Seizing control has always been the prime agenda of the public health profession.

If you have an intestinal bug and shake the hand of another, he may get that bug. Yes, he may, if he does not wash his hands before eating. The public health industrial complex is forever finding excuses to build multi-million dollar and billion dollar government programs when the real answer is that those who do not want an intestinal condition need to wash their hands.

There is nothing collective about that. But, the public health profession, a fundamentally collectivist and very political profession — seeks these opportunities to chip away at individual freedom.

Public health is the very opposite of medicine.

Not wanting to do something is your right. Your medical concerns are your business. The medical concerns of another are that person's business. The two do not have anything to do with the other.

If you do not want to wear a face mask, you do not have to wear a face mask. That is how Western society works. That is how life in a free country works. Those seeking to make any land less of a free country are welcome to utilize their passport and go elsewhere less free and convince people there to live under tyranny and the poverty that tyranny inevitably brings — an approach the public health community is internationally famous for.

This country, however, is quite satisfied with its very expansive concept of individual freedom based on the individual man, woman, and child being made in the likeness of God.

That takes hard work to secure and can make collectivists uncomfortable, but it is nonetheless work we free people do each and every day by living our free lives. Among these methods, are the constant refusal to wear the face mask under any circumstances.

There is a very powerful and important case to be made based on individual liberty for why no one should ever be forced to wear a face mask, and there is also a strong medical case to be made.

A medical approach you do not believe in, is an approach that will fail you. Some part of you must trust in the approach. Some part of you must believe in the possibility. There is medical utility in a patient's approval of the approach. Belief in an approach is meaningful, trust in a doctor is meaningful, emotional investment in the appropriateness of the path forward is meaningful.

Placebos do work.

There is more than biology, chemistry, and pharmacology behind the effectiveness of a treatment. Room must be left for matters of psychology as well, and room must be left for matters of faith in the outcome.

Microscopic focus on his own self-interest, myopic focus on his own beliefs in what is right, can leave a doctor unable to recognize this and unable to effectively treat a patient who refuses to be a passive observer in his care, but instead seeking to be the most active participant.

Such a patient will not stand for answers like "You will take this approach because I say," or "This is good for you, because I have a white coat."

Some doctors do not possess the proper psychology to treat a thinking and insightful patient. They lack the basic philosophical ground to recognize the sanctity of the individual patient. They, likely, even lack the humbleness required of good bedside manner with a patient who is active in his own care.

As medicine increasingly moves away from one doctor and one patient, toward 20 or 30 person rotating care teams, the importance of the patient being active grows and the disinterest of a doctor in dealing with an active patient grows as well.

This approach to medicine encourages one-size-fits-all approaches, while it discourages individual treatment.

Yes, many doctors do not like the idea of you saying that a valid medical argument is "I do not want to wear a face mask, because I know it does not work," but that is one of the most legitimate reasons you can possibly give.

Poorly trained in understanding a patient as a human, discouraged by training from doing so, disincentivized from doing so, it can be no surprise that doctors do not like your insistence of being treated as an individual human made in the likeness of God.[1]

The moment you realize you are dealing with such a doctor, is a great time to find a new doctor, a new hospital, a new way of looking at medical care.

You deserve no less, you wonderful being made in the likeness of God.

Reason 44: Ask These Kids What They Think Of Face Masks

A surprising realization occurs to any parent who makes a shift and says "I am not going to bend my children to the will of the world. If anyone will bend, it will be the outside world who will bend to the will of my family."

Suddenly, once that shift is made, a child's opinion needs to be sincerely sought. You do not need to read piles of medical literature to understand that face masks are awful for children. You can just ask them, and anyone who is willing to listen will quickly realize that children are saying loudly and clearly that they cannot wear a face mask safely. Even children who seem totally fine, may have stories like this, though, as the existence of sub-threshold stimuli demonstrates, feeling fine does not prove the absence of harm. Quite the contrary is, at times, true, in fact.

On Tuesday, August 3, 2021, a few children addressed their school board in Arroyo Grande, California. I will let them speak for themselves. Here is what 10-year-old Riley Stark said that night:

> "Hi, my name is Riley Stark. I am 10-years-old. I will be going into 5th grade at Dorthea Lange this year. Last year I lived out of state and I was able to play sports and attend school full time, in person the entire year. Where I lived, kids under 10 did not have to wear a mask, but I was forced to at school because I went to a school that was only grades 3rd through 5th and they did not want it to be confusing when some kids wore them and some kids did not. This was the only place I was forced to wear a mask. My brother, who was in 1st grade, did not have to wear a mask at his school. Pretty much no one did.

> "Being forced to wear a mask to be able to go back to school was stressful. Teachers were constantly yelling at us to pull up our masks. They did not want us to touch each other or be within 6 feet of each other at first. We had plastic dividers between us a lunch. I felt like I was in prison. I was always on edge. I was also confused. They would yell at us, but then they would touch us or hug us or have their masks down. I would see them outside of school and they did not wear masks, not even to school sporting events. Once, my principal even gave me a hug and said, 'Oh just

go sanitize your hands.' I may be a child, but I am not dumb. It was easy to see through the 'do as I say not as I do' talk.

"The first month of school, I was so stressed out and had so much anxiety, I had to sleep in my parent's room. My mom had to give me melatonin and lay with me, because I felt like I was being choked by a mask. I felt like it was still on even when it was not. I had to take constant mask breaks every day, because they made my migraines so much worse.

"Masks were, and are still, a constant stress for me. They are for so many kids, but so many will not speak up. When in class, we were asked to write an essay about what was the one rule we wish we could change. My friend in my class said she wished we did not have to wear masks because people were so sad because of them. There have been so many times I would pull up my mask and cry behind it, and no one would know.

"I feel that masks should be a choice, we should not be forced. We also should not be called names or made to feel bad about it either. Myself, my brother, and my sister all went to school last year full time, played all the sports we normally do and none of us got Covid. No one I know did. There was very few in our entire district that did. My class was never even quarantined, and this was before teachers and adults started getting vaccines. Now teachers and adults have vaccines.

"If there is one thing I have learned this last year, it is that adults and teachers have not done such a great job at leading by example. We have always been taught in school not to give in to peer pressure. We were taught that we are in charge of our own bodies, we need to do what is right for us, and it is ok to think different than others. But now they are being hypocrites. You should not say one thing and do the exact opposite. Thank you."

This was a heartfelt piece of writing from a little girl that surprised many who listened, because of how adeptly she was able to communicate the harm in her own life being caused by masking.

Here is what her sister, 13-year-old Mahdyson Stark said that same night:

> "Hi, my name is Mahdyson Stark. I am 13-years-old and I will be attending Mesa this year as an 8th grader. Last year I lived out of state and I went to school full time. I was also able to attend sports.
>
> "We always had to wear masks and social distance, which made me feel like I was contagious or something, like no one wanted to be around me. But that was not all, after running we would have to put on our masks which was a struggle in itself. Just wearing a mask makes me feel like trapped and even when I am not wearing a mask it still feels like I am wearing one.
>
> "Last year after school, I would come home very sad and angry. Just the little things make me lash out at someone. I should not have to be home in order to learn mask free. I have a 504 plan[1] and online learning was very challenging for me the couple months I had to do it. I did not have the help I needed. I was very angry and frustrated most of the time and I fell even further behind. It left me in tears, not to mention you cannot hear what people are saying when they wear a mask you cannot see their face. Some of my teachers did not even recognize me when they saw me with a mask, how are they going to know if I am having a hard time or if I am sad.
>
> "Wearing a mask also got me hurt. I fell down the stairs multiple times at my old school. I could not see when looking down most of the time. I would like you to consider making masks optional. We know when we are sick, we can be responsible. Junior high is stressful enough without masks, you do not need to add to it. Thank you."

The past month since the Ides of March 2020 have been another exercise in teaching a child to ignore his wants and needs. This is one of many ways modernity encourages a child to grow into an adult willing to ignore his own wants and needs and to live life forever obedient to some illegitimate authority figure.

Ask your kids to sit down and write about their experience with a mask. If you have an open and honest relationship, if the cognitive decline caused by mandatory masking has not already gotten to them, and if the brainwashing of 2020 and 2021 has not already gotten to them, you might be surprised at how similar your own child's experience is to the experience of these two girls who cared enough about the topic to address their school board on the matter

Reason 45: Othering Children

Does a child need any more reason to have to concern himself with fitting in or not fitting in?

Does anyone in modernity, especially a child, need any further excuse to be less authentic, less himself?

I would say no. I would say modernity saps so much individual power from people that only those who strive for the highest level of authenticity are able to reach such a state.

A face mask on a child is yet another way that modern life "others" children, makes a child into the outsider, tells a child that they do not belong, and that conformity is the only hope of feeling like one belongs. To "other" someone is to make a person into an outsider.

Conformity to what? In traditional cultures, which nearly all humans lived in up until a century or two ago, conformity was the path to wisdom and survival.

Many thousands of cultures and subcultures have existed on this planet. Overwhelmingly, they are gone. They did not survive the process of adapting, whether that be 100 years ago, 1000 years ago, or far longer than that.

The cultures that survived are the cultures that, by definition, where able to pass life wisdom and survival skills to the members of their society.

Until very recently, culture changed very slowly. Conforming to a culture helped one survive, since culture that was passed on was successful. Culture and tradition that was not successful died away.

In contrast, we have a continued encouragement to conform to others in society, but we have constantly shifting social morays. Consequently, so much that people are expected to conform with is new, trendy, and most certainly not tested over time as a means for survival.

There was a time in which conformity helped guarantee survival, but today an empty shell of conformity remains. Since there is no wisdom behind it, it is conformity for the sake of conformity and not conformity for the sake of survival. The habit remains, but the purpose is gone. The façade remains with no structure, no foundation, no purpose beneath — an empty show of virtue with a rotten core.

Notably, throughout all human history, that which is new, almost exclusively, is not helpful to survival. That which is new is quite notably harmful to human survival.

This push for conformity, this comfort with othering children that mandatory masking brings is not encouraging of survival, but discouraging of it.

Masking is exactly the kind of trendy, untested, harmful behavior that has caused thousands of other cultures to disappear and is the opposite of the behavior that has allowed the few hundred present-day cultures to remain.

Nothing about human history suggests masking to be a wise survival strategy.

Nothing about human history suggests trendiness to be a wise survival strategy. Everything about human history indicates wisdom, time tested, of the ages to be the wisest of survival strategies.

Are you following the wisdom of the ages as much as you can during these tenuous times? Or are you following what is trendy, easy to follow, and that which is done in the interest of conformity?

The more you can do the former, the greater the chance of survival you can offer yourself, your family, and those around you.

Some families do not stop there — they are not satisfied with mere survival. They rely on the wisdom of the ages to ensure prosperity — conformity to trends has little to offer on either of these topics — survival and prosperity.

Be wise in your life and courageous in your representation of the righteous, and you will live a good and honorable life, a life that the worldly trends of this era are useless in edifying.

Reason 46: There Is No Feedback Loop

Mandatory masking of the population is a population-wide experiment. When running an experiment you want to make sure you have a way to record results: you want a feedback loop for receiving feedback and logging the data so you can eventually interpret the data.

An experiment is being run on society right now, but there is no feedback loop.

Literally no one in a position of authority is listening to the feedback loop, and if you insist they listen, you are punished for it.

Feedback is the only honest reason for an experiment: you are testing for a result and eager to find the result, whatever the result may be.

As parent-after-parent is suddenly learning this year: no one in authority wants to hear your experience with face masks unless they are positive.

Artificially biased feedback is not honest feedback.

On its face, you should never take part in an experiment with no feedback loop. Such an "experiment" is not an experiment at all, but a method of control. No one can control you who you do not permit to control you. Do not allow yourself to be controlled by such manipulation.

Reason 47: No Informed Consent Is Possible

You can not have informed consent without being informed. You cannot be informed without information. Critical information about mask mandates is prevented from being disseminated and discussed.

We are not able to have a fully informed conversation on this topic. We are not even able to determine how many of the reasons listed in this book are able to hold up under testing. The best we can hope for is loose conjecture to determine if a society-wide experiment on masking is killing and maiming people.

Do we not deserve better?

We have the resources to have better. We simply do not seem to have the will to demand better.

Informed consent is not some pointless theory. Informed consent is a process for protecting humans from those who would carelessly experiment on them. Informed consent is a process of defending human happiness, life, and liberty.

Informed consent is required of all medical interventions — face masks being one example. All of the one-size-fits-all public health mandates of 2020 and beyond are other examples. No informed consent has been allowed to take place

Reason 48: Very Little Data, Very Much Interpretation

The very basics of science are being ignored with masking. Data is being supplanted by interpretation.

Examples of data may include:

The sky is illuminated.

The air is 73°F.

My tongue has taste buds.

Interpretation may start the same way as the above examples, but contain a term like these after that phrase:

Because ...

Therefore ...

That is why ...

Which means ...

Terms like these indicate the insertion of an interpretation or opinion and are separate from pure data.

The face mask debate is full of interpretation by officials and is very, very light on the necessary predecessor to interpretation: study, feedback, data collection, and further study. The scientific method is built upon this. Unwarranted interpretation, politicization, politically or financially motivated interpretation, as well as manipulation and threats towards those who disagree, are not part of the scientific method.

Lots of empty talk, very few useful numbers are at the heart of face masks policies.

This, on its face, presents an objection to all who attempts to interpret data to you, especially those who interpret it with an intent to convince you to behave a certain way. Such behavior is outside of the bonds of science and should be flatly rejected as incredible and dishonest.

Reason 49: The Shy Tory Effect

Science magazine pointed to a flaw in the social sciences: results tend to under-represent so-called conservative views.[1] "Traditional," "conservative," or "status quo" views exist in every field.

In 1805, pirates from the Barbary Coast were seen as antagonistic enemies by some in the United States. It would be hard for anyone living in 1805 to make sense of why that was not the case in 1905 when Spaniards were seen by some as enemies or 2005 when Afghanis were.

At any given time there is a status quo view. The Shy Tory Effect exists in the social sciences: a bias toward change. It is described in political polling. Pollsters are more likely to under-represent conservative or "Tory" views politically, to use British vernacular, and to over-represent non-conservative views.

In masking, or in any aspect of health or nutrition, this can be understood to represent a bias toward the trendy: those who seek to rely on what has worked in the past and is therefore well tested are more likely to be under-represented.

Those who push for untested ideas are more likely to be over-represented.

Research in the social sciences has a bias towards change rather than a "bias" toward divulging the truth.

This is a hard point to take into account too often.

There is a bias toward trendiness, even in studies. On its face, this provides a challenge to all behavioral psychology, social science, and public health policy — public health mandates included.

Since they have a bias toward the trendy, they have this additional obstacle in identifying truth and wisdom through their research. Outsiders look at these fields and see that quite clearly. Insiders have a hard time and tend to believe a great deal of their own nonsense. This brings considerable conflict. Reckless societal distruction and human misery, then, has resulted in the Ides of March 2020 — face mask policies being but one example.

Reason 50: The Following List Of Biases

All research must foremost be logically sound and philosophically sound in its design or else its outcome will be needlessly biased and perhaps even inaccurate. Below are a list of biases that have run amok over the last year of claims made about Covid-19 and the allegedly necessary public health interventions. Even one of these may traditionally, if severe enough, be enough to discredit the work of a researcher and send them back to the drawing board, though identifying these biases honestly and accounting for them goes a long way.

Contrary to that intellectually honest behave, since the Ides of March 2020, public health officials have practically had a contest to see how many of these biases and fallacies they can cram into a body of research and into each policy recommendation white paper.

Confirmation Bias — Focusing on outcomes that align with expectations. Data may therefore be interpreted to support a hypothesis or dismissed if it opposes a hypothesis.

Conformity Bias — This is pressure to be like those around you. It can often be described as peer pressure.

Halo Effect — Encountering positive information about a person makes you value their opinion more.

Horns Effect — The opposite of Halo Effect, hearing something bad about a person causes you to value their opinion less.

Both of these — Halo Effect and Horns Effect — are examples of **Reactive Devaluation** — We judge an idea based on how we feel about a person with the idea.

Ad Hominem Fallacies arise from this — the tendency to attack the person with the idea and not the idea itself.

Anchor Bias — Being unable to let go of a specific piece of information and thereby building an understanding around that not necessarily relevant piece of information. This is particularly harmful with overspecialization and lack of research outside of one's field.

Authority Bias — A piece of information is more cared about because it comes from an authority figure.

Overconfidence Bias — Being too confident in ones own ability. This often leads to being wrong.

Bandwagon Effect — One tends to believe in something because others believe it.

Groupthink — The goal is to avoid conflict, and pursue harmony, so a working group ultimately ends up with weird and disparate outcomes or results, far different from anything a single member of the group would individually consider to be good work. Some would call this compromise, a more correct description of it is awful output.

Ambiguity Effect — If the benefit is clear one is more likely to want that outcome and will take risk accordingly, however if the benefit is unclear one will be less likely to pursue that outcome and less like to take a risk at achieving it.

Curse of Knowledge — The better informed will not listen to the less informed. This is an inability to put oneself into the shoes of another. The more educated one is, the harder it becomes to empathize. This is a common outcome of knowledge accumulation and education. It is a problem with placing decision-making into the hands of the most knowledgeable — they tend to lack empathy. Almost all political debate since 2015 has fallen into these two camps. 1.) I know more than you; you must listen to me. 2.) You do not understand me, and your solution does not work for me.

Observer-Expectancy Effect — A researcher believes X will happen, thereby influencing research towards X outcome. This may be overt or subconscious.

Compassion Fade — A preference for easily identifiable, easily recognizable sources rather than less personal data sets, despite the fact that the less personal data sets may be even more effective at getting to underlying truth.

Law of the Instrument — To he who has a hammer, everything looks like a nail.

Ostrich Effect — Burying one's head in the sand in response to criticism, rather than embracing criticism as an opportunity to more ardently pursue truth.

Stereotyping — Taking a set of characteristics and using them to create an artificial problem that does not exist. Applicable example: If Sars-Cov-2 causes Covid-19 and breathing is one way that a virus is transmitted, then restricting breathing will lead to less virus transmission.

Illusory Correlation — Just because a solution looks like a solution, does not mean it actually is a solution.

Framing Effect — The answer is based on how research is framed rather than what truth is.

Sponsor Bias — Did a participant know who was funding the study? Did they research it? What impact may that have had? Was a participant motivated by strong feelings about a research sponsor.

Habituation Bias — Asking a series of questions similarly, may lead to similar answers.

Many aspects of bias related to the asking of questions exist, which is why headlines of a study should be dismissed until methodology is looked at. Reading the fine print of a study is vital.

Habituation Bias is a variation of the more broad **question-order bias**, by which answer to a question may change based on how the question is asked.

This is related to **wording bias**, such as those used intentionally by push pollsters to see to it that outcomes match those which are desired.

Social Desirability Bias — This is responding a certain way to be liked by others, including the researcher, which is an example of **friendliness bias** — a participant wanting to agree with the researcher.

There may be a tendency to over-report that which is seen as socially desirable and under-report that which is seen as socially undesirable.

Recency Bias — More weight is put upon that which is recent than on facts that maybe more relevant but are less recent.

Hindsight Bias — "I knew it all along."

Irrational Scalation — Also called **sunk cost fallacy** — So much has been invested into an idea that you cannot just abandon it, so you keep pushing for more investment into it, despite all indications showing that it is a losing proposition.

Knowledge Bias — Choosing what you know rather than what is best or better or even good.

As Christopher J. Pannucci and Edwin G. Wilkins, in the article "Identifying and Avoiding Bias in Research", points out:[1]

> "Bias is not a dichotomous variable. Interpretation of bias cannot be limited to a simple inquisition: is bias present or not? Instead, reviewers of the literature must consider the degree to which bias was prevented by proper study design and implementation. As some degree of bias is nearly always present in a published study, readers must also consider how bias might influence a study's conclusions."[2]

Anyone reading research with a critical eye is called on to be conversant in bias and to be comfortable identifying that bias. Bias exists. Bias does not make a study inaccurate. An informed evaluation of bias helps one to gauge the usefulness of an outcome.

Looking at the various times the term "scientific consensus" has been rolled out over the past decade to silence all debate, it is often apparent that such extraordinary amounts of bias exist so as to make it unable to be deemed scientific in the search for optimal approaches. We are instead left with a great deal of bullying, as can be expected where there is irrational escalation alongside such an influential curse of knowledge.

Any mainstream reporting on one-size-fits-all public health approaches has become so heavily biased as to virtually guarantee that truth will not be reported on.

One may chose to ignore this research, then, waiting for a time in the future when such research may again become usable. "Evidence Based Medicine," has received near cult like fanaticism. In theory it makes a great deal of sense, but it can be taken to pedantic lengths to crowd out both dialogue and dissent, leaving little room for individual outcomes and ridiculing notions as quaint as intuition. Yet certainly, those are important concepts that need consideration alongside evidence. Taken to pedantic lengths, as is now almost always the norm, Evidence Based Medicine feels much more like a form of control rather than a scientific pursuit of the truth. Understandably, it is clear why some would choose to dismiss the entire process of such data heavy control and to rely on faculties that have long worked to get humanity through the trials of life these many years humans have walked the planet.

Alternately, one may choose to engage in the process for keeping such research honest.

Using these powerful tools above, observers can and should poke holes in available research. Identified biases are so effective at that. We are all now consumers of public health research, whether we like it or not. Having such research so present in life and almost always presented in click-worthy headline format is largely a bad thing, but it is the reality we live on and correspondingly not a reality that anyone should be naive about or complacent regarding.

Many research teams have a correspondent with a publicly available email address who has agreed to reply to research questions. A consumer of researcher should feel free to ask questions they find pressing. You must often reach out multiple times if you expect to hear back. If they do not respond after three or four follow-up attempts, carbon copy the whole team. If that does not work, reach out to the department head of the correspondent. Then reach out to all department heads of all authors for the study. If that does not work, reach out to the funding source for the study. Eventually they will respond.

The same can be done to journalists or anyone else who reports upon poorly done research.

Do not bother to do this if it is a passing fancy. There are too many passing fancies and busy researchers will feel incentivized to ignore you. Push firmly, however, against those topics that are important to you and which are dishonestly portrayed, and you may be surprised by how effectively one vocal, committed person can move the needle and help to keep researchers as diligent as possible.

Censoring such poorly compiled news and research is not a useful tool, but being savvy in response to it and realizing its many limitations is very useful.

Reason 51: If You Want To Make A Sacrifice For Society, Make A Sacrifice By Being A Member Of The Control Group

Science likes to use test groups and control groups.

The test group tries something new. The control group tries all else the same with the exception of one specific variable.

When experimenting, researchers seek to use as few resources as possible in experimenting because that experiment could go wrong.

Researchers put as small of a budget, as needed, risk as few lab rats as needed, spend just barely the appropriate amount of time needed.

The whole goal is to, as quickly as possible, determine basic trends.

Until a concept has proven effective, you do not invest any resources beyond what is absolutely needed to arrive at that conclusion. This is exactly why we do research before recommending behaviors in the general population. The very opposite was done in the case of face masks and other one-size-fits-all public health approaches that have been implemented since the Ides of March 2020.

The unmasked are the control group. They are doing a favor for society by staying unmasked. One day, honest researchers will come along and study that control group and be able to identify the crimes that took place due to the mask mandates. They will be able to quantify the harm and prove that no such policy could ever be considered healthy for an individual. This is the test that should have taken place *before* any mask mandate.

All who believe in a pursuit of truth and the effectiveness of the scientific method should welcome that exactly — a robust control group and thorough research.

In sharp contrast, those who seek to hide the folly of this policy and their possible complicity in the crimes of corona communism would prefer that everyone be subject to mandatory masking as well as all other one-size-fits-all public health mandates. Doing so hides their crime and prevents the ability to prove that crime.

You, as an unmasked person, are a living, breathing record of what took place, a record stored in the health of your body, health that can be empirically studied and quantified. Those who remain unmasked, are the members of the control group who can, in the name of science, help to shed light on this sad policy and its ensuing social and medical experiment. You should recognize, as well, the favor you do for society. Unlike any of the touted sacrifices mentioned in media, this is one of the truly virtuous sacrifices to make in 2020, 2021, and beyond. For the good of society, please remain in the control group, and certainly keep your children in the control group. Your decision to remain part of the control group is a great gift to society and to our posterity. Thank you.

Reason 52: The Story Of Vioxx

The ills of 2020 and beyond were a long time coming. Little of what took place was new. In fact, it was more of the same dishonesty from once trusted institutions. The case of Vioxx illustrates this well.

Vioxx was a painkiller introduced in the late 1990's by the American Pharmaceutical giant Merck. It was marketed as an improvement over other prescription painkillers based on a better safety profile and reduced side effects in general. It was approved for the treatment of conditions ranging from rheumatoid arthritis to migraines and quickly became a popular drug around the world. It was later withdrawn from the market due to a large number of deaths associated with its use.

By 2005, virtually every trusted pharmaceutical and medical institution had been proven a total, unrepentant sham, unwilling to engage in the most basic meaningful ethics to save lives, as long as they knew there was across-the-board cooperation. Fifteen years later, no one should be shocked when society-wide, that same behavior occurred from the Ides of March 2020 forward.

The pharmaceutical establishment, medical establishment, doctors, media, government, politicians, and other institutions had long been cooperating to do exactly that. The true shocker should be that anyone in the general public continues to trust such corrupt institutions, even going so far as extending more power to them to rule the lives of average people, despite being proven irredeemably corrupt.

I do not expect you to change the world or to change these institutions, but I do expect you to remove these institutions from positions of influence in your own life. I'm going to use the example of Vioxx to illustrate why you should do exactly that.

On September 30, 2004, Merck announced a worldwide recall of their painkiller Vioxx.

This came a full five years after Merck knew that Vioxx killed people. Millions took it. Billions in profit were earned for Merck. Thousands predictably died who would not have if they would have just kept their previous painkiller, which Merck claimed Vioxx to be safer than.

Not only was this information known, but influence peddlers at Merck got *The New England Journal of Medicine* and the United States Food and Drug Administration to assist in releasing their killer drug and selling it to the public as safe and effective. Silence from these institutions would have been more ethical than their cooperation in this mass murder.

The drama of the story hinges on the hiding of three heart attacks, in order to hide a concerning trend. This made it possible to make a false claim in November 1999 about the heart attack risk related to Vioxx, and to continue to repeat that claim: "While the trends are disconcerting, the number of events are small." This is familiar verbiage to anyone following public health officials as they talk about the one-size-fits-all health mandates: safe and effective is the frontline defense of these mandates. When that defense is pierced "disconcerting but small" is the backup defense.

The lie that a treatment is "safe and effective," always seems to be replaced by the claim that horrifying side effects are "disconcerting but small" in frequency. Ultimately, the truth prevails, but only after many are killed and injured by the treatment. Only those who wrongly put their trust in liars are ever the victim, which carries some poetic justice and a lesson to be cautious around untrustworthy serpents. Trusting a serpent is a fatal mistake in its own.

Those who dare reveal such information publicly are lifesavers, for they speak truth to those who will listen. They are also labelled pariahs and risk career, wealth, and wellbeing. There is a cost to standing against corruption. In all eras there has been a cost. If there were not, corruption would never exist, for the remedy to corruption would come so cheaply.

In their timeline coverage of the events around Vioxx, National Public Radio (NPR) reports: "As of November 1, 1999, 79 patients out of 4,000 taking Vioxx have had serious heart problems or have died, compared with 41 patients taking naproxen."[1]

Taking the experimental Vioxx is nearly twice as dangerous for the heart as taking naproxen. Naproxen is available in generic form. Vioxx was marketed as a safer though more expensive replacement.

It was not safer, but it was more expensive.

The fact that this reporting came from NPR is quite significant. NPR has long been derided for its extreme political bias. Much of its coverage of politicians came with a strong liberal bias. NPR could often be found attacking the enemies of their favorite politicians, while leaving their favorite politicians untouched. At the time of the Vioxx scandal however, NPR was, at least, still doing critical reporting on pharmaceutical companies — a true public service.

This independent coverage by NPR and its critical take on drug companies was recognized as a flaw in the system by the powers that be. No news organization was to exist that behaved this way, let alone a government funded news organization.

By the end of the first year of the Obama Administration, 2009, this matter had been handled and it would theretofore be nearly impossible to find any reporting from NPR that was critical of the pharmaceutical industry. Prior to that, NPR had been a true treasure on pharmaceutical industry coverage. Government media was put in order by the pharmaceutical interests and related interests. The few publically and privately owned media institutions that were unbiased were at that same time put in order as well.

The New York Times was also once such an institution. The medical safety and vaccine safety wing of the Democrat Party had formed and solidified by the 2004 presidential primaries and had been a force to be reckoned with by the 2008 presidential primaries. Such views were surgically removed from friendly media, hardly given a voice in the main stream from 2009 to the present. How this could have happened is not the question as much as the question is "How could we have kept trusting them?"

Once the Vioxx scandal had become too public to ignore, the prominent medical journal, *The Lancet* finally chimed in. *The Lancet* estimated 88,000 had heart attacks and 38,000 died from Vioxx. Other researchers estimate the real numbers were more like 500,000 deaths from Vioxx. It was, more dangerous than naproxen, and even far more dangerous than the commonly used aspirin.

Not only had this drug been the darling of the pharmaceutical industry and the darling of the medical research establishment, doctors loved it too. Twenty-five million Americans received Vioxx prescriptions after being told by their doctors that it was safer than the alternative. Being safer than the alternative was the whole reason for Vioxx's existence. Their patients foolishly believed their doctors' sales pitches.

And the media loved Vioxx. It had an average television advertising budget of $100 million each year. This may explain why, to this day, the American media has remained nearly silent on the topic of Vioxx.

No real inquiry from the media ever took place. No true demand for reform ever took place. Instead, the media obediently told a story of how badly this caught up with Merck in court. That was a total lie

In November 2007, Merck paid a whopping $4.85 billion to settle the personal liability lawsuits of approximately 47,000 plaintiffs and 265 potential class action cases. It was, at the time, believed to be the largest drug settlement ever. Remember even the establishment *Lancet* said 38,000 people died, though not each one of those people went to court seeking recompense. The true death count is far larger than this, but even using that number the details of the settlement are shockingly small. The settlement was not as big of a deal as the media claimed. This did not stop the media from making a huge deal of what a shocker this settlement was and how severe it was.

$4.85 billion divided by 47,000 plaintiffs comes out to $103,191.49 per family before lawyers' fees, expenses, and taxes. Are we really to believe $103,191.49 per person and no jail time is a reasonable resolution for a company that knew for 5 years that they would kill people and did exactly that? Merck may even have ended up ahead. It was making $2 billion per year on Vioxx at the time of the drug recall.

One murder can be enough for cross-border manhunts to occur alongside large media trials with grand public outrage. Multimillion dollar wrongful death suits follow. Yet 38,000 deaths resulting in no jail time, virtually total silence from watchdogs on the particulars of the matter, tiny per death settlement fees, no jail time for a murderer, no reform, no company even put out of business.

Some point out that with the new class of Covid shots, manufacturers are exempt from liability. In the example of Vioxx, pharmaceutical companies were practically exempt from liability already. They went through the world providing inherently dangerous chemicals to people while claiming them to be safer than what the people were already using. They lied to people, telling them that if they switched they would live longer, healthier lives. The exact opposite was true. The people who believed them were cheated out of precious health and life. No one has gone to jail and Merck has had very little financial impact from the mass killing of so many Americans.

The issue at hand here, though, is not three heart attacks, 38,000 additional causes of heart disease or death, 500,000 dead, $4.85 billion, a media that lies to you, doctors that lie to you, a pharmaceutical establishment that lies to you, US Government watchdogs that lie to you. It is not about covering up data to make money. It is not about corruption at *The New England Journal of Medicine* or in the research community as a whole.

Those issues take years to resolve.

The real issue is this: you cannot trust these institutions to put your child first. They do not care about you. They do not care about your family. They do not care about your child. Quit pretending they do. Make them 100% irrelevant in your decision making process.

If you absolutely cannot ignore entities like these, and you must take them into account, perhaps you can garner this lesson from the Vioxx story: you are often far better off doing the exact opposite of what drug makers, the US Government, the media establishment, doctors, and the medical journals advise.

You do not need to change the world. You do not need to change the way your neighbors think. You do not need to move government. All that is nice. But the priority is protecting yourself and your family from these lying sociopaths.

That can be done right now.

That can be done with every decision you make.

Say "No!" to all these nonsense one-size-fits-all public health mandates that they want to push upon you and your family.

I wish this were not the world we lived in. It is.

There should be dozens of widely published conclusive studies about how bad face masks are, widely covered in the media. There should also be total outrage at all levels of government that mask mandates still exist either in the public sector or private sector. Hundreds of public health officials in each state should be put on trial and prevented from ever holding a position of public confidence again.

That is not the time we live in, but we may get there.

The research leaves many questions unanswered about why anyone would be so foolish with such clearly dangerous public health approaches and so tyrannical as to force them upon everyone in society. The rest of this book analyzes the available science to demonstrate that the face masks are not safe for you, your child, or anyone else, and that no person, and certainly no child, should be compelled to wear a face mask.

FACE MASKS ARE NOT SAFE

Reason 53: This List Of Health Concerns That The Political Establishment, The Media Establishment, And The Medical Establishment Will Not Talk About

In the United States, we are used to seeing long pharmaceutical commercials full of exhaustive lists of the harm that could be caused by the medical intervention being pitched in the commercial. Though this list of possible risks and side effects are the norm for almost any medical intervention advertised, the same has not occurred with face masks or other medical interventions said to be safe and effective in preventing the spread of Sars-Cov-2 and the illness known as Covid-19.

When it comes to face masks, the list would look something like this list below, and would require an additional 19 minutes for every 60 second television commercial proclaiming the usefulness of the allegedly safe and effective face mask. Deceitfully, the media establishment calls masks "safe and effective," the political establishment calls masks "safe and effective," and the medical establishment calls masks "safe and effective."

The following is a list of known risks, likely risks, or possible risks caused by wearing a face mask or made worse by wearing a face mask.

This list is not exhaustive, and researchers seemingly daily find evidence of further conditions to add to this list and additional evidence that mask wearing is far worse for the health of a child than previously thought.

Risk To Pregnant Women And Fetuses

1.) Impedes gaseous exchange between mother and fetus,
2.) Too much carbon dioxide in a pregnant mother's blood may lead to too much carbon dioxide in fetal blood,
3.) Exposure to birth defect-causing chemicals and increased risk of giving birth to a child with birth defects,
4.) Significant and irreversible damage to a child's developing brain,
5.) Impaired fetal growth,
6.) Adverse perinatal outcomes in women with chronic respiratory conditions,
7.) Preterm labor, which is regular contractions leading to the opening up of the cervix after week 20 and before week 37 of pregnancy and which may lead to preterm birth,

8.) Pre-eclampsia, which is high blood pressure during pregnancy accompanied by damage to organs,
9.) Respiratory compromise in pregnant women,
10.) Imposes higher workload on pregnant women,
11.) Increased risk of suffocation when worn by a baby,
12.) Virtually every physiological reaction to face masks mentioned on this list below can also occur in a fetus, only it occurs during his most important developmental period of life, likely making the physiological impact much worse,

Breathing And The Lungs

13.) Obstruction of the airway,
14.) Mask-induced increased airway resistance,
15.) Increased breathing resistance,
16.) Increased inhalation resistance,
17.) Increased exhalation resistance,
18.) Breathing problems,
19.) Impeded gas exchange at rest,
20.) Shortness of breath,
21.) Feeling of breathlessness,
22.) Chest discomfort,
23.) Tightness of the chest,
24.) Increased respiratory frequency and depth,
25.) Increased respiratory load,
26.) Increased work of respiratory muscles,
27.) Disturbed respiratory physiology,
28.) Reduced lung function,
29.) Impairments in lung function parameters,
30.) Decreased oxygen intake,
31.) Increased cardiorespiratory stress,
32.) Impairments in cardiopulmonary capacity,
33.) Rebreathing of carbon dioxide,
34.) Increased rebreathing of the body's waste,
35.) Increased inspiratory carbon dioxide levels,
36.) Increased expiratory carbon dioxide levels,
37.) Increased oxygen demand,
38.) Increased oxygen consumption,
39.) Impacted oxygen uptake,
40.) Decreased oxygen saturation,

41.) Increased physiological dead space, which is a larger amount of space in and around the body that does not exchange air and consequently may lead to significant problems as a result,

42.) Reduced gas exchange volume available to the lungs in each breath

43.) Increased maximal inspiratory pressure,

44.) Increased maximal voluntary ventilation,

45.) Impeded gas exchange during exercise,

46.) Increased retention of carbon dioxide in the lungs,

47.) Hyperventilation, which is overly rapid or overly deep breathing,

48.) Decreased ability to compensate for a lack of homeostasis through hyperventilation,

49.) Hypoventilation, which is reduced intake of air into the lungs,

50.) Respiratory distress,

51.) Artificial inducement of COPD-like symptoms, which is chronic obstructive pulmonary disease, a chronic inflammation of the airways, causing restricted airflow,

52.) Oxygen deprivation with effects on the heart, lungs, and brain,

53.) Pneumonia, which is an infection of the airs sacs of the lungs,

54.) Aspiration pneumonia (Pulmonary aspiration is the inhalation of fluid or other substance into the lower lungs. Aspiration pneumonia is the infection and inflammation of air sacs as a result of pulmonary aspiration.),

55.) Passing out during exercise,

56.) Irritation of the respiratory tract,

57.) Airway inflammation,

58.) Foreign bodies in the lungs,

59.) Lung toxicity from inhaled graphene and other particles contained within face masks,

60.) Inhaled mask polypropylene fibers and other fibers contained within face masks,

61.) Sub pleural ground glass opacities due to inhaled mask fibers (While ground glass opacities are indicated in many diseases and conditions, they are hardly as awful as their name would suggest. Their name comes from the hazy look of sandblasted glass. Ground glass opacities (GGO) is merely another way to say "hazy images on an chest x-ray or CT scan." The presence of ground glass opacities indicates increased density in lung tissue.),

62.) Self-contamination,

63.) Clinically relevant fungal, bacterial, and viral infections,

64.) Abscesses in lung tissue,

65.) Increased lower respiratory tract infections caused by the deep seeding of oropharyngeal flora,

66.) Aspergillosis, which is the inhalation of fungal fibers that gather as fungal balls in the lungs,

67.) Inhalation of mold and bacterial colonies living on the surface of masks,

68.) Fibrous thickening of the peribronchiolar interstitium, which is the space around the air sacs of the lungs,

69.) Bronchopulmonary diseases from inhaled synthetic fibers such as:

    1. Asthma,

    2. Alveolitis, which is inflammation of the air sacs of the lungs,

    3. Chronic bronchitis, which is the inflammation of the lining of the bronchial tubes; the bronchial tubes being how air is carried to and from the lungs,

    4. Bronchiectasis, which is abnormal widening of the bronchi or their branches, causing an additional risk of infection,

    5. Spontaneous pneumothorax, which is sudden collapsed lung without any apparent cause,

    6. Chronic pneumonia,

    7. Granulomas, which are masses of tissue produced in response to the presence of an infection or foreign substance,

    8. Pulmonary fibrosis,

    9. Mask induced rhinitis, which is swelling of the mucous membrane of the nose,

70.) Increased disease transmission due to "the nebulizer effect," which is a phenomenon caused by the wearing of mask, in which the mask wearer to pushes more fine particles further out from the mask wearer than a non-mask wearer would,

71.) Pulmonary hypertension, which is abnormally high blood pressure in the blood vessels that support the lungs,

72.) Aggravation of exercise induced asthma,

73.) Bacterial-induced chronic airway inflammation,

74.) Increased risk of severe respiratory failure,

75.) Immotile cilia syndrome caused by humidity and temperature in the upper airway (Cilia is a hair-like structure lining the airways that serves several functions, among that helping to clear the lungs of matter. Immotile cilia lead to disturbance in the clearing of the lungs.),

Heart

76.) Increased heart rate,

77.) Reduced cardiopulmonary capacity,

78.) Lower maximum blood lactation response, which is an indicator of reduced cardiopulmonary capacity,

79.) Mask-induced latent increase in blood gas carbon dioxide levels (toward hypercapnia),

80.) Increase in carbon dioxide retention,

81.) Increased carbon dioxide blood content,

82.) Increased transcutaneous carbon dioxide, which is carbon dioxide levels measured through the skin,

83.) Rapid onset of toxic effects due to the easy uptake of carbon dioxide in the blood and the rapid diffusion into bodily tissue,

84.) Mask-induced latent drop in blood gas oxygen levels (toward hypoxia),

85.) Decreased oxygen availability,

86.) Decreased oxygen saturation of the blood,

87.) Decreased blood oxygen partial pressure,

88.) Hypercapnia, which is abnormally high carbon dioxide in the blood

89.) Including acute (sudden) hypercapnia,

90.) Hypoxia, which is abnormally low oxygen in the blood,

91.) Hypercapnic hypoxemia, which is abnormally low oxygen in the blood at the same time as abnormally high carbon dioxide in the blood,

92.) Increased blood acidity,

93.) Increased lactate concentration,

94.) Increased acidic environment,

95.) Acidosis,

96.) Cardiac overload,

97.) Endothelial dysfunction, which is impaired function of the lining of the blood vessels, an early stage of arteriosclerosis in which the endothelium, the lining of the blood vessels, stops working properly and may cause significant symptoms,

98.) Increased blood pressure,

99.) Increase in systolic blood pressure,

100.) Hypertension, which is abnormally high blood pressure,

101.) Hypotension, which is abnormally low blood pressure,

102.) Vascular damage, which is damage to the arteries and/or veins,

103.) Cardiovascular disease, which is disease of the heart and circulatory system,
104.) Increased heart attack risk,
105.) Increased stroke risk,
106.) Serious arrhythmia, which is an irregular or abnormal rhythm of the heart,
107.) Cardiac dysfunction,
108.) Right or left ventricular dysfunction, which is improper functioning of the portion of the heart that is largely responsible for pumping blood,
109.) Pericarditis, which is swelling or irritation of the saclike tissue around the heart, the pericardium,
110.) Myocardial ischemia, which is reduced blood flow to the heart, preventing the heart muscle from receiving enough oxygen,
111.) Arteriosclerosis, which is the hardening of the arteries,
112.) Coronary heart disease, which is a disease affecting the major blood vessels that supply the heart,
113.) Life threatening staph infections,
114.) Bacteremia, which is bloodstream infection,
115.) Sepsis, which is a condition in which the body's response to an infection damages the body,
116.) Septic arthritis, which is joint trouble caused by the spread of an infection to a joint,
117.) Irreversible fibrosis in heart tissue, which is a change in the heart tissue, leading to impaired performance of the heart,
118.) Subacute bacterial endocarditis, which is an infection of the heart lining and valves that develops over a longer period of time than acute (sudden) bacterial endocarditis,

Kidneys

119.) Reduced renal blood flow,
120.) Reduced renal function,
121.) Reduced glomerular filtration rate, which is the amount of blood that passes through the filters of the kidneys each minute — a reduced rate is an indication of reduced kidney function,
122.) Renal overload,
123.) Generalized nephritis, which is inflammation of the kidneys,
124.) Flares of toxins in the body,

Head

125.) Headaches,

126.) Exacerbation of pre-existing headache disorders,

127.) De novo PPE-associated headaches (PPE is personal protective equipment, such as face masks, N95 respirators, face shields, and other items; de novo, in this specific usage, refers to a headache that did not exist prior to the introduction of PPE and therefore provide a stronger indication that the introduced PPE is a cause of the headache.),

128.) Migraine headaches,

129.) Irritation of cervical nerves in the neck and head by mask straps,

130.) Lightheadedness,

131.) Insomnia,

132.) Drowsiness, which is qualitative neurological deficits,

133.) Dizziness,

134.) Syncope, which is the inability to maintain sufficient blood pressure to allow the brain to properly function, thereby increasing the risk of falling,

135.) Triggers cerebral ischemia, which is the reduction of blood flow to the brain, thereby reducing the amount of oxygen available to brain tissue,

136.) Seizures,

137.) Increased brain volume,

138.) Decrease in cerebrospinal fluid spaces,

139.) Increased intracranial pressure (Generally speaking, as the brain enlarges, pressure on the skull increases.),

140.) Increased vasodilation in the central nervous system,

141.) Increase in cerebral artery flow,

142.) Decreased pulsation of blood vessels in the central nervous system,

143.) Damage to blood vessels that supply the brain,

144.) Decreased cerebral perfusion (Perfusion is the act of pumping blood through the body, cerebral perfusion is the movement of blood — and thereby oxygen — through the tissue of the brain.),

145.) Deterioration of the hippocampus, which is a particularly oxygen-sensitive portion of the brain,

146.) Degeneration of the brain due to reduced oxygen,

147.) Neurodegenerative disease,

148.) Alzheimer's disease,

149.) Meningitis, which is inflammation of the fluid and membranes around the brain and spinal cord,

150.) Autoimmune encephalitis such as basal ganglia encephalitis and pediatric autoimmune neuropsychiatric disorders associated with streptococcal infections, which is also known as PANDAS,

Face

151.) Obstructs flow of blood vessels in the face,
152.) Obstructs flow of lymph in the face,

Skin

153.) Moisture retention,
154.) The sensation of dampness,
155.) The sensation of heat,
156.) Impacted microclimates of the face,
157.) Flushing,
158.) Impacted pH value of skin,
159.) Skin breakdown,
160.) Erythematous, which is the reddening of the skin due to damage of superficial capillaries,
161.) Increased fluid loss through the skin epithelium,
162.) Increased sebum production (Sebum is a Latin word for "grease," and refers to the oil created by the sebaceous glands, specifically on the face, in this example.),
163.) Altered skin flora,
164.) Hypersensitivity to ingredients of industrially manufactured masks,
165.) Impaired skin barrier function,
166.) Increased skin susceptibility to acne and infection,
167.) Redness,
168.) Rash,
169.) Mask associated skin irritation,
170.) Local acne,
171.) Staph infections,
172.) Itching,
173.) Urticaria, which is another word for hives — red, itchy welts on the skin,
174.) Contact dermatitis,
175.) Contact eczema,
176.) Increased disease transmission due to poor hygiene practices around face masks,

Eyes

177.) Impaired field of vision,
178.) Mask-associated ocular irritation,
179.) Increased dry eye symptoms,
180.) The fogging up of glasses,

Ears

181.) The angulation of the outer ear,
182.) Permanently disfigured growth of cartilage of the outer ear,
183.) Auricular chondritis, which is painful inflammation of the cartilage of the ear,
184.) Under-developed auricular cartilage,
185.) Mechanical skin lesions,
186.) Painful lesions of the retro auricular skin (The auricle of the ear is the external portion of the ear; retro auricular skin refers to skin on the back side of the ears or behind the ears.),
187.) Permanent hyperpigmentation (Mask pressure against the skin causes dark marks in the places of pressure as the skin becomes damaged and heals repeatedly.),

Nose

188.) Itching and swelling of mucous membranes, which are the lining of surfaces in the nose and other parts of the body that come in contact with the air and contain cells that produce mucus,
189.) Mucosal irritation of the nose,
190.) Increased nasal secretion,

Mouth

191.) Mouth-breathing,
192.) Mouth dryness,
193.) Reduced saliva,
194.) Oral dysbiosis, which is a harmful imbalance of the microflora of the oral cavity,
195.) Halitosis, which is bad breath,
196.) "Seriously sour breath,"
197.) A newly identified condition known as "mask mouth," in which many of the conditions in this section occur simultaneously, seemingly caused by face mask wearing,
198.) Decaying teeth,
199.) Dental caries, which are more commonly known as cavities,

200.) Mask-induced dental problems,

201.) Receding gum lines,

202.) Gum disease,

203.) Gingivitis, which is inflammation of the gingiva, the lining of the gums around the base of the teeth,

204.) Cheilitis, which is inflammation of the lips,

205.) Angular cheilitis, which is the breaking down of skin at the corners of the mouth,

206.) Cracking and sores at the corner of mouth,

207.) Increased risk of Group A Streptococcus infections,

208.) Candidiasis of the mouth, which is fungal infestation of the mucous membranes with Candida albicans,

209.) Periodontal disease, which is illness of the support structure around the teeth,

210.) Superficial and relatively harmless pathogens in the oral flora are caused to be harmful when they access deeper tissues and the blood

211.) Impaired vocal cord coordination,

212.) Aggravation of facial trauma,

213.) Harm to oral and maxillofacial surgery patients (The maxilla is the upper jaw; oral and maxillofacial surgery is surgery of the mouth, bones of the mouth, and face, and may extended into other portions of the head.),

Communication

214.) Slurred speech,

215.) Acoustic filtering of speech, making speech sound softer, mumbled, muffled, or otherwise harder to hear,

216.) Filter and dull acoustic communication,

217.) Limit facial recognition,

218.) Positive emotions become less recognizable,

219.) Suppression of emotional signals,

220.) Erase positive effects of smiles and laughter,

221.) Increase the likelihood of misunderstanding,

222.) Block emotional signaling,

223.) Disrupt human communication, both verbal and non-verbal,

224.) Negative emotions are amplified,

225.) Reduction of comprehension of outward emotional displays,

226.) Reduction in empathy perception,

227.) Disrupt social interaction,

228.) Disruption of doctor-patient relationship,
229.) Bonding between teachers and learners is reduced,
230.) Interference with pedagogy,
231.) Increased alienation of the deaf and hard of hearing,
232.) Increased stress upon the hearing impaired,
233.) Increased stress upon the mentally impaired,
234.) Reduced social cohesion,
235.) Reduced group cohesion,
236.) Increased stress-related illnesses,
237.) Hinders a baby's acquisition of speech and language,
238.) Increased feelings of isolation,
239.) Social withdrawal,
240.) Increased peer pressure encouraging the wearing of a face mask beyond the recognition of harmful symptoms,
241.) Provokes excessively loud speech,
242.) Triggering new voice disorders,
243.) Increased risk of voice disorder,
244.) Compromise of the pressure gradients required for undisturbed speech,
245.) Increased aerosol production during speech, which leads to increased spread of pathogens,

Immunity

246.) Partial immunosuppression or reduced immune response,
247.) Increased predisposition for viral, fungal, and bacterial illness,
248.) Increased rhinovirus infections,
249.) Increased risk of disease transmission,
250.) Immune-mediated inflammatory disorders, more commonly known as auto-immune diseases, which include rheumatoid arthritis, systemic lupus, Sjorgen's syndrome, along with many others,

Cancer

251.) Promotes the growth, invasion, and spread of cancer,
252.) Poorer survival rates in patients with cancer,
253.) Poorer clinical outcomes,

Body

254.) PPE-associated discomfort,
255.) Mild pain,
256.) Nausea,

257.) Vomiting,

258.) Fatigue,

259.) Vertigo, which is a sensation of whirling and loss of balance,

260.) Exhaustion,

261.) Drowsiness,

262.) Increased stress hormone levels, which include adrenaline, nora-drenaline, and cortisol,

263.) Increased muscle tension,

264.) Impacted working methods,

265.) Malaise with chest pain,

266.) Increased danger of heat stroke,

267.) Increased likelihood that heat will amass in the body,

268.) Increased likelihood that the body will not be able to properly cool itself,

269.) Mask induced thermal stress,

270.) Increased risk of thermal shock,

271.) Increased risk of dehydration,

272.) Impacted homeostasis,

273.) Slowed maximum speed of movement,

274.) Inability to recognize the signs of dehydration,

275.) Psycho-vegetative stress reactions,

276.) Impacted physical workload,

277.) Impacted maximum power output,

278.) Impacted exercise capacity,

279.) Impacted pace of work,

280.) Muscular weakness,

281.) Impact on fast-twitch muscle fiber size,

282.) Muscle damage,

283.) Greater difficulty exercising,

284.) High fever,

285.) Impacted metabolic rate,

286.) Increased leptin release,

287.) Increased harm from caffeinated drinks and other diuretics,

288.) Health deterioration,

289.) Oxidative stress,

290.) Intoxication, which is the poisoning of the body with a toxin, often to the point of impaired physical or mental control,

291.) Increased inflammatory substances such as C reactive protein (An increase of these substances in the body indicates a higher level of inflammation in the body. Inflammation is a swelling or some other immune reaction of the body and indicates a problem.),

292.) Increased cell acidity,

293.) Increased noradrenergic stress response (Involving the hormone norepinephrine also called noradrenaline. This hormone and neurotransmitter mobilizes the body to act and is associated with the fight or flight response and survival adaptation as well as stress in general. It is common for norepinephrine levels to be low when the body is at rest and a person is at ease.),

294.) Increased rate of infection caused by exercising in a face mask,

295.) Increased use of medication,

296.) Toxic shock syndrome,

297.) Atopic predisposition, which is an allergy tendency,

298.) Increased rate of hospitalization,

299.) Sudden death during exercise,

300.) Altered metabolism,

301.) Increased metabolic stress,

302.) Self-induced illness,

303.) Buildup of pathogenic (disease-causing) bacteria,

304.) Epithelial damage, which is damage to the outer layer of cells lining the surface of the body, both internal and external,

305.) Reduced participation,

306.) Increased symptoms of sleep apnea,

307.) Increased rates of sleep apnea,

308.) Autonomic dysfunction,

309.) Increased likelihood of wound infection when worn by a surgeon,

310.) Chronic inflammation,

311.) Accelerated aging process,

312.) Premature mortality,

313.) Diabetes,

314.) Long-term disease relevant consequences,

315.) Mask-Induced Exhaustion Syndrome (MIES),

Thinking

316.) Impaired cognition,

317.) Compromised cognitive performance,

318.) Cognitive impairment, such as thinking impairments and coordination impairments,

319.) Concentration problems,

320.) Decreased IQ,

321.) Reduced motoric abilities,
322.) Impacts caretaker cognition and wellbeing, leading to a higher risk of harm to the individual receiving care,
323.) Decrease in psycho-motoric skills, which include hand-eye coordination, playing an instrument, driving a car, or other actions in which several parts of the body are used in coordination with each other,
324.) Reduced responsiveness,
325.) Impaired thinking,
326.) Suppressed anger,
327.) Increase in psychosomatic illnesses,
328.) Increased feelings of insecurity,
329.) Panic reactions,
330.) Anxiety,
331.) Activation of fight or flight response,
332.) Increased fear,
333.) Mood disturbances,
334.) Disorientation,
335.) Impacted feeling of wellbeing,
336.) Reduced self-determination,
337.) Loss of autonomy,
338.) Feeling of deprivation of freedom,
339.) Self-suppression of own needs and concerns,
340.) An inhibition to habitual actions such as eating, drinking, touching, scratching, and cleaning,
341.) Subconscious, constant distraction,
342.) Reduced attention,
343.) Impacted individual skill,
344.) Psychological impairment,
345.) Failure to recognize hazards,
346.) Mask-induced listlessness,
347.) Avoidable accidents at work,
348.) Impaired operation of automobiles and other machines,
349.) Perception of discomfort,
350.) Increased feelings of discouragement,
351.) Mild depressive feelings,
352.) Depression,
353.) Exacerbation of paranoid schizophrenia symptoms,
354.) Exacerbation of dementia symptoms,
355.) Exacerbation of personality disorder symptoms,

356.) Psychological impact on children,
357.) Developmental impact on children,
358.) Exacerbation of panic attack symptoms,
359.) Exacerbation of panic disorder symptoms,
360.) Inability to recognize a feeling of thirst,
361.) Loss of consciousness,
362.) Concentration disorders,
363.) Trigger sympathetic stress response,
364.) Depressive self-experience,
365.) Lowered health-related self-care,
366.) Effect on neurological diseases,
367.) Narcotic action,
368.) Neurological symptoms,
369.) Confusion,
370.) Increased feelings of numbness,
371.) Syncope in the operating theater,
372.) Reduced quality of medical care when worn by a care provider,
373.) Mistakes and misunderstandings in the operating room,
374.) Impacted postural stability (proprioception),
375.) Altered gait velocity, and
376.) Falls.

PREGNANT MOTHERS,
AND DEVELOPING BABIES

Reason 54: Face Masks Hurt Pregnant Women And Their Babies

Pregnant mothers need to take special care of their bodies, partly because of the burden their own activity places on the baby.

Once considered acceptable, we now know alcohol, cigarettes, and a wide array of drugs, medicines, and supplements can be very harmful to a developing fetus, with impact that can last a lifetime and which can even kill a baby before it reaches full term.

We know very well that what happens to a mother impacts a developing fetus. We also know that the human body can be marvelously robust and can handle many impositions nature throws at a mother.

The face mask is not one of nature's impositions though. The fabric is not natural, nor is the strange reaction to cover the face for months or years at a time natural.

Furthermore, the wearing of a face mask by a pregnant woman, for any reason is simply foolhardy, for we have such an array of information on how it demonstrably harms the mother that it would be unreasonable to expect that it does not also harm a developing fetus.

Should we really need to wait for experiments on fetuses to be conducted before we acknowledge that this is an experiment a healthy mother in the general public should not be engaged in, especially not under the claim that this is safe and effective.

Unknown risk is not acceptable risk when it comes to pregnant mothers, fetuses, and children.

A two-phase controlled clinical study on healthy pregnant women between 27 to 32 weeks gestation in Singapore concluded that:[1]

> "Breathing through N95 mask materials have been shown to impede gaseous exchange and impose an additional workload on the metabolic system of pregnant healthcare workers, and this needs to be taken into consideration in guidelines for respirator use. The benefits of using Nano-material to prevent serious emerging infectious diseases should be weighed against potential respiratory consequences associated with extended N95 respirator usage."

The study authors also point out:

> "Little is known about the effects of N95 masks on the respiratory function of pregnant healthcare workers, who can be subjected to prolonged usage of FFR (Filtering Face-

piece Respirator) because of their vulnerability to complications from influenza, varicella, and other pathogens transmitted via the respiratory tract.[2] It is also known that pregnant women have a significantly greater respiratory burden due to factors such as increased oxygen (O2) demand, increased nasal airway resistance, decreased functional residual capacity due to diaphragmatic splinting; all these contributing to the 'physiologic' dyspnea of pregnancy.[3] There are also robust data linking respiratory compromise and adverse perinatal outcomes in women who have chronic respiratory conditions, from large scale studies on women with conditions such as asthma and obstructive sleep apnea. These outcomes include preterm labor, impaired fetal growth, and pre-eclampsia."[4,5]

Preterm labor "occurs when regular contractions result in the opening of the cervix after week 20 and before week 37 of pregnancy."[6]

Intrauterine growth retardation (IUGR) "may affect up to 10% of pregnancies and results in substantially increased perinatal morbidity and mortality. Although many infants are small on a constitutional basis and not as a result of disease, many others suffer malnutrition from chronic progressive uteroplacental insufficiency. Genetic disease, embryonic infection, and various drug exposures may also result in IUGR."[7]

Preeclampsia is "a pregnancy complication characterized by high blood pressure and signs of damage to another organ system, most often the liver and kidneys. Preeclampsia usually begins after 20 weeks of pregnancy in women whose blood pressure had been normal."[8]

Until proven otherwise, preterm labor, impaired fetal growth, and pre-eclampsia should be considered possible risks of a pregnant woman wearing a face mask.

Reason 55: Face Masks May Cause Mothers To Have Elevated Enough Carbon Dioxide To Prevent Fetuses From Being Able To Clear Their Own Carbon Dioxide

A careful series of gradients exist between mother and baby across the placenta, in order to make life together safe for both of them.

Nature has prepared for many problems that may get in the way of this.

Research indicates nature may not be prepared for mothers in face masks, however.

There was a time when nature was not prepared for hospitals in which surgeons would go from cadaver to mother without washed hands and deliver babies. Many mothers died until doctors got wise to the problem of their filthy hands. Purpuric fever was the result. Many mother needlessly died. Some physicians of the mid-1800's insisted on handwashing to not just prevent purpuric fever but to prevent maternal death by purpuric fever. Most physicians refused to go along with this approach, preferring the status quo belief that gentleman physicians could not be the cause of such a problem. It took years for the medical establishment to address this problem caused by trusted physicians.

There was a time when nature was not prepared for women to supplement their pregnancy with a morning sickness and anti-anxiety "medicine" known as Thalidomide. This morning sickness medicine cause birth defects when taken during pregnancy.[1] Thousands of children who ostensibly would have otherwise been born healthy, were born severely deformed.[1] Starting with the 1957 release of Thalidomide in west Germany which was subsequently licensed in 46 countries.[1] It took years of birth defects before the medical establishment would address this problem. This was a problem partially caused by trusted physicians. These trusted physicians worked in research, in the pharmaceutical industry, in government, and in private practice. Just because they are trained and licensed to practice medicine, widely trusted in society, does not mean that they medical experimentation on you and your family is something you should be prepared to put trust in.

It is no surprise that nature is not always ready for every foolish thing done to mother and child in the process of bringing a child to term and into the world.

In an April 20, 2021 article entitled "Is a Mask That Covers the Mouth and Nose Free from Undesirable Side Effects in Everyday Use and Free of Potential Hazards?"[1] Kai Kisielinski writes:

"As a critical variable, a low blood carbon dioxide level in pregnant women is maintained via an increased respiratory minute volume, stimulated by progesterone.[3] For a pregnant woman and her unborn child, there is a metabolic need for a fetal-maternal carbon dioxide (CO_2) gradient. The mother's blood carbon dioxide level should always be lower than that of the unborn child in order to ensure the diffusion of CO_2 from the fetal blood into the maternal circulation via the placenta.

"Therefore, mask-related phenomena described above, such as the measurable changes in respiratory physiology with increased breathing resistance increased dead space volume and the retention of exhaled carbon dioxide (CO_2) are of importance. If CO_2 is increasingly rebreathed under masks, this manifestation could, even with subliminal carbon dioxide increases, act as a disturbing variable of the fetal-maternal CO_2 gradient increasing over time of exposure and, thus, develop clinical relevance, also with regard to a reduced compensation reserve of the expectant mothers.[3-5]

"In a comparative study, 22 pregnant women wearing N95 masks during 20 minutes of exercise showed significantly higher percutaneous CO_2 values, with average $PtcCO_2$ values of 33.3 mmHg compared to 31.3 mmHg than in 22 pregnant women without masks ($p = 0.04$).[2] The heat sensation of the expectant mothers was also significantly increased with masks, with $p < 0.001$.[2]

"Accordingly, in another intervention study, researchers demonstrated that breathing through an N95 mask (FFP2 equivalent) impeded gas exchange in 20 pregnant women at rest and during exercise, causing additional stress on their metabolic system.[4] Thus, under an N95 mask, 20 pregnant women showed a decrease in oxygen uptake capacity VO_2 of about 14% (statistically significant, $p = 0.013$) and a decrease in carbon dioxide output capacity VCO_2 of about 18% (statistically significant, $p = 0.001$).

"Corresponding significant changes in exhaled oxygen and carbon dioxide equivalents were also documented with increases in exhaled carbon dioxide (FeCO$_2$) (p < 0.001) and decreases in exhaled oxygen (FeO$_2$) (p < 0.001), which were explained by an altered metabolism due to respiratory mask obstruction.[5]

"In experiments with predominantly short mask application times, neither the mothers nor the fetuses showed statistically significant increases in heart rates or changes in respiratory rates and oxygen saturation values. However, the exact effects of prolonged mask use in pregnant women remain unclear overall. Therefore, in pregnant women, extended use of surgical and N95 masks is viewed critically."[4]

For the health of the baby, pregnant women should not be wearing face masks. There is too much uncertainty about the harm and there is no benefit to wearing a face mask.

It took a lot of people suffering, dying, and being laughed at before concerns about purpuric fever or Thalidomide were listened to. There is little difference in the total idiocy around face masks.

A key difference is that the discovery process is going all the more quickly because of internet communication. Additionally, the censorship of the message is much more total among official channels. That challenge is minimal. Stay the course and people of good conscience with wise views will emerge victorious from this battle.

Reason 56: Face Masks On Pregnant Women During Exertion Should Be Avoided To Protect The Unborn Child

Research indicates that the use of a mask for over an hour may be enough to harm a fetus. Also, the use of a mask during exertion for any period of time may be harmful to a fetus.

Kai Kisielinski, in an April 20, 2021 article entitled "Is a Mask That Covers the Mouth and Nose Free from Undesirable Side Effects in Everyday Use and Free of Potential Hazards?"[1] writes:

> "In pregnant women, the use of masks during exertion or at rest over long periods of time is to be regarded as critical as little research has been done on this.[2] If there is clear scientific evidence of increased dead space ventilation with possible accumulation of CO_2 in the mother's blood, the use of masks by pregnant women for more than 1 hour, as well as under physical stress, should be avoided in order to protect the unborn child.[2,3] The hypercapnia-promoting masks could act as a confounder of the fetal/maternal CO_2 gradient in this case."[2-4]

Face masks are so lacking in usefulness, and so dangerous for the fetus, that no pregnant woman, for any reason, nor for any length of time, should wear one.

To do so is entirely negligent.

If there is a pregnant woman in your life who wears a mask, please help her to recognize the harm she is almost certainly doing to her unborn child — IQ damage,[5] physical and mental developmental damage, harm that may last a lifetime. The extent of the harm is unclear and likely far worse than we can imagine.

Life is already complicated enough on a child being brought into the world. Why does a mother need to make it any more difficult?

Her child needs to be fought for. Her child deserves to be fought for. To wear a mask while pregnant is to give up on one's responsibility to give a child the very best that you can.

Not only are pregnant mothers wearing masks when at rest, while lightly active, and while under physical stress — all of which likely cause harm to mother and baby, but there is another time when many mothers are masked. In stark contrast to the recommendations above and with no known benefit to mother or baby, during the greatest and most risky time of physical stress for the mother-child pair, hospitals across the country have made it a requirement that mothers wear masks in the delivery room.

Not only does such a request bring dehumanization at such a tender moment but it senselessly introduces an additional layer of danger. Pregnant mothers should not be masked, children should not be masked, no one should be masked, least of all people in a delivery room.

Reason 57: Face Mask Material May Be Teratogenic — Which Means They May Cause Birth Defect

Much effort is made to protect developing fetuses from chemicals that may harm them. This practice has been dispensed with in the case of face masks. Pregnant mothers need to be aware that the medical community and public health establishment are unlikely to point out these risks.

In an April 20, 2021 article entitled "Is a Mask That Covers the Mouth and Nose Free from Undesirable Side Effects in Everyday Use and Free of Potential Hazards?"[1] Kai Kisielinski writes that toxic chemical used in the manufacturing of face masks may cause birth defects:

> "In addition, it is unclear whether the substances contained in industrially manufactured masks that can be inhaled over longer periods of time (e.g., formaldehyde as an ingredient of the textile and thiram as an ingredient of the ear bands) are teratogenic."[2,3]

There is nothing surprising about this. Toxic chemicals are regularly used all around us. Many of them are unstudied for their effects on the fetus and their ability to cause birth defects.

The legitimate concern that masks add to the toxic load on a mother and child represent another reason not to wear a face mask. This is especially true if you are sensitive to chemicals or if you are one who takes extra precautions to avoid toxic chemicals.

The contents of face masks are not well studied for their teratogenic effects. That is even more the case for cloth face masks, for which there is virtually no study of the harm done by the many chemicals used to create that fabric, to treat that fabric, and to dye that fabric. A great deal of effort goes into studying the toxicity of chemicals on the skin and avoiding overly toxic chemicals in the manufacturing of clothing. These chemicals, however, have not been studied for use in a cloth face mask. Chemicals that are relatively safe on the skin may not be safe to inhale.

Reason 58: Face Masks Are Harmful For Babies

Cot death or SIDS (Sudden Infant Death Syndrome),[1] is a serious concern among children 2 and under, though the first months are most common for such a death to occur. Decades of effort have gone into explaining and preventing this problem of babies who never wake up from their sleep.

There are no magic cut off ages in biology. It is entirely silly to think that a baby at 730 days of age (2-years-old) is unable to wear a face mask, but suddenly at 731 days of age is able to. Biology does not work that way.

Additionally, though this is a greater problem for the young, people of all ages inexplicably never wake from their sleep. The need to view every person as an individual and to handle medical decisions on an individual basis is so very important.

In an article by Nigel Barlow on August 6, 2020, quoting Dr. Rebecca Fletcher:[2]

> "'It is extremely dangerous to cover a baby's mouth and nose and the design of 'cute' baby face coverings that have been brought to our attention look like they would greatly increase the risk of suffocation. I would strongly advise parents not to use any form of face covering for their baby,' said Dr. Rebecca Fletcher, chair of Bury, Rochdale and Oldham Child Death Overview Panel."

No adult should be forcibly masked, no child should be forcibly masked, and certainly, no baby should be masked. This trend of masking babies is a foolhardy reversal on decades of wise practice to leave the air passage of babies unrestricted.

Reason 59: Children Are Far More Vulnerable To Harm From Face Masks Than Adults

Coal miners used to bring canaries into mines with them because canaries were sensitive to noxious fumes that could kill a miner. If the canary died, they knew it was time to get out before the miners were overwhelmed also.

Children are a lot like canaries in the mine. They are the more sensitive version of adults. The impacts of face masks and other one-size-fits-all public health approaches can be seen and felt in children long before adults, if we chose to see them. Unfortunately, most people choose not to see that, which is to the detriment of many a child.

It is additionally, to the detriment of others in society to ignore what is so blatantly happening in front of our very eyes.

These one-size-fits-all health approaches are awful for us. To ignore their impact on children is just as foolhardy as ignoring a fainting canary in front of you: something is amiss.

Kai Kisielinski, in an April 20, 2021 article entitled "Is a Mask That Covers the Mouth and Nose Free from Undesirable Side Effects in Everyday Use and Free of Potential Hazards?"1 writes:

> "Children are particularly vulnerable and may be more likely to receive inappropriate treatment or additional harm. It can be assumed that the potential adverse mask effects described for adults are all the more valid for children (physiological internal, neurological, psychological, psychiatric, dermatological, ear, nose, and throat (ENT), dental, sociological, occupational and social medical, microbiological and epidemiological impairments)."

All negative impacts of face masks should be assumed to be more impactful on children than on adults. This includes breathing restrictions from masks. Breathing restrictions have an even greater ability to cause problems with children. Kisielinski continues:

> "Special attention must be paid to the respiration of children, which represents a critical and vulnerable physiological variable due to higher oxygen demand, increased hypoxia susceptibility of the central nervous system (CNS), lower respiratory reserve, smaller airways with a stronger increase in resistance when the lumen is narrowed. The diving reflex caused by stimulating the nose and upper lip can

cause respiratory arrest to bradycardia in the event of oxygen deficiency."

As Kisielinski points out, rather than being specifically made for the special needs of a child, children are carelessly made to wear adult face masks:

"The masks currently used for children are exclusively adult masks manufactured in smaller geometric dimensions and had neither been specially tested nor approved for this purpose.[2]

"In an experimental British research study, the masks frequently led to feelings of heat ($p < 0.0001$) and breathing problems ($p < 0.03$) in 100 school children between 8 and 11 years of age especially during physical exertion, which is why the protective equipment was taken off by 24% of the children during physical activity.[2] The exclusion criteria for this mask experiment were lung disease, cardiovascular impairment and claustrophobia.[2]

"Scientists from Singapore were able to demonstrate in their level 1b study published in the renowned journal *Nature* that 106 children aged between 7 and 14 years who wore FFP2 masks for only 5 minutes showed an increase in the inspiratory and expiratory CO_2 levels, indicating disturbed respiratory physiology.[3]

"However, a disturbed respiratory physiology in children can have long-term disease-relevant consequences. Slightly elevated CO_2 levels are known to increase heart rate, blood pressure, headache, fatigue and concentration disorders."[4]

Since children are so sensitive to mask use, the following is a short list of reasons cited by Kisielinski why children that children should not wear masks:

"Accordingly, the following conditions were listed as exclusion criteria for mask use:[3] any cardiopulmonary disease including but not limited to: asthma, bronchitis, cystic fibrosis, congenital heart disease, emphysema; any condition that may be aggravated by physical exertion, including but not limited to: exercise-induced asthma; lower respiratory tract infections (pneumonia, bronchitis within the last 2 weeks), anxiety disorders, diabetes, hypertension or epilepsy/attack disorder; any physical disability due to medical, orthopedic or neuromuscular disease; any acute upper respiratory illness or symptomatic rhinitis (nasal obstruction, runny nose or sneezing); any condition with deformity that affects the fit of the mask (e.g., increased facial hair, craniofacial deformities, etc.). It is also important to emphasize the possible effects of masks in neurological diseases, as described earlier."

This expansive and incomplete list by Kisielinski is a far cry from the claim that face masks are safe and effective. Millions of children fall into the category above, of those who face masks are not safe for due to pre-existing health conditions. Additional research points to the likelihood that masks are not safe for anyone in the general public, which includes children. Children, especially, cannot wear a face mask safely.

SOME OF THE HARMFUL COMPONENTS OF FACE MASKS

Reason 60: Graphene In Face Masks
May Pose A Particular Risk

Government always seem to be late to the game when it comes to protecting people. It is ultimately up to the individual to protect one's own health and liberty.

The Canadian Government on April 2, 2021,[1] issued this warning to be particularly careful of face masks containing the nanoparticle graphene.

"Graphene is a novel nanomaterial (materials made of tiny particles) reported to have antiviral and antibacterial properties. Health Canada conducted a preliminary scientific assessment after being made aware that masks containing graphene have been sold with Covid-19 claims and used by adults and children in schools and daycares. Health Canada believes they may also have been distributed for use in healthcare settings. Health Canada's preliminary assessment of available research identified that inhaled graphene particles had some potential to cause early lung toxicity in animals"

That such a warning was issued should trigger red flags that far greater problems with face masks exist. It is not easy to get government to issue such warnings.

The Canadian Government did not just allow unsafe face masks to be used in Canada. That would be forgivable. The Canadian Government *forced* unsafe face masks to be used by Canadians and with great legally imposed consequence to those who would not wear the unsafe masks. For an entire year, this was mandated, despite watchdogs warning of these and other dangers. About such dangers, government remained silent while parroting the line that face masks are "safe and effective."

As of the date of this writing, no such warning has been issued by the US Government. This should be of no surprise to anyone. It is your job to know what is safe for you and for your family. The government has a very long history of not protecting people.

Reason 61: Inhaled Cotton Fibers
Cause Lung Disease

You are constantly inhaling matter into your body. Many features of your respiratory system are protective in keeping that out which does not belong and allowing that in which belongs. These features include: mucus, anti-microbial peptides, nasal turbinates, the glottis, coughs, sneezes, saliva, bacterial competition within the oropharyngeal flora, immunoglobulins, a branching airway, the mucociliary escalatory function, free fatty acids, lysozymes, iron-binding proteins, Immunoglobulin G, surfactants and other components of the alveolar lining, macrophages, polymorphonuclear cells, and lymphocytes.

It is a phenomenal system, but there is a limit to how much the system can be taxed and still continue to work.

A long history of lung diseases occur among those who tax that system and do not recognize early signs of limitation: examples of that include types of pneumoconiosis, such as byssinosis (inhaling unprocessed cotton dust), silicosis (inhaling quartz dust or other silica dust), black lung or coal miners pneumoconiosis (inhaling coal dust), asbestosis (inhaling asbestos dust), farmers lung (inhaling dust or spores from moldy hay), teflon flu or polymer fume fever (inhaling plastic gases), metal fume fever (inhaling metal fumes).

Masks release friable particles. They are able to enter the respiratory system. Wearing a mask appears to overtax the system by introducing friable content into the lungs far beyond the amount that the respiratory system can expel. Additionally, those friable particles are of a character difficult for the body to sufficiently remove.

The consequence of this is lung conditions and lung diseases which are already beginning to appear in the short-term, and which may additionally have unpredictable long-term consequences, perhaps even being irreversible, as many conditions related to foreign matter settling in the lungs tend to be.

In the article "Masks, false safety and real dangers, Part 1: Friable mask particulate and lung vulnerability," Boris Borovoy et al. write:[1]

> "Inhaled cotton fibers have been shown to cause sub pleural ground glass opacities at the surface of the visceral pleura, as well as centrilobular and peribronchovascular interstitial thickening, as well as fibrous thickening of peribronchiolar interstitium. It was found by spectral analysis by infrared

spectrophotometry that the foreign bodies in the lungs had an identical pattern to that of cellulose, which must have come from the inhaled cotton fibers.[2] Cotton and even silk may contribute to COPD in textile workers. Byssinosis is a pulmonary syndrome related to textile work. When textile workers were exposed to organic dusts from textiles in the workplace, both reversible and irreversible pulmonary conditions, such as asthma and COPD developed.[3] It should be remembered that unmasked textile workers would not have such high inspiratory flow as masked individuals."

Even in low inspiratory flow environments, inhaled particles can be harmful. How much more that can be presumed to be true for the high inspiratory flow environment of a face mask. Even a natural fiber, such as cotton, can be harmful to the lungs when inhaled. How much more so for synthetic fiber, such as those of which face masks are made?

We have here another reason face masks should not be worn, especially not by children. We also have another example of how face masks are not likely to be safe for anyone.

Reason 62: Inhaled Synthetic Fibers Cause Lung Disease

It is worth noting that while cotton fibers, which are highly processed, but still of natural derivation, may be problematic, it is also clear that an extensive array of synthetic fibers are of a character and type that are likely to be harmful when inhaled.

This harm again may go far beyond short-term discomfort and may be irreversible harm done to the lungs and body.

In the article "Masks, false safety and real dangers, Part 1: Friable mask particulate and lung vulnerability," Boris Borovoy et al. write:[1]

> "Research on synthetic fibers has shown a correlation between the inhalation of synthetic fibers and various bronchopulmonary diseases, such as asthma, alveolitis, chronic bronchitis, bronchiectasis, fibrosis, spontaneous pneumothorax and chronic pneumonia. Cellular proliferation made up of histiocytes and fibroblasts were found in the lungs of those exposed to synthetic fibers in ambient air. Focal lesions in the lungs showed granulomas and collagen fibers containing both fine dust and long fibers. Some of the lung illnesses from this exposure could be reversed, while others had already proceeded to pulmonary fibrosis."[2]

It is worth noting again — inhaled particles, like those shed by a face mask during normal use, cause reversible and irreversible lung conditions. They can permanently damage the lungs.

This would be less significant if this were a well-researched topic as it relates to face masks.

Instead, masses of people are being masked and thereby experimented on, worst of all children, who are unable to consent to such nonsense, which again, may have permanent, lifelong health consequences for them.

There is a real risk of a constantly masked person with a worn down reused face mask developing irreversible fibrosis of the lungs, an awful disease.

How large that risk is remains unknown, which is unacceptable for a policy mandated on others especially children.

Face masks are ineffective in the prevention of a respiratory virus. If that were not the case, a reasonable person-by-person cost benefit analysis could occur. However, since that is the case and no individual benefit is had by mask wearing, it is unwise to wear a face mask, especially given the unquestionably significant downside risk.

Reason 63: Inhaled Fibers
Cause Pulmonary Fibrosis

Among the many possible diseases cause by inhaled particles, exists a particularly egregious one: pulmonary fibrous.

It is worth noting that inhaled particles lead to fibers in the lungs. We are undertaking a mass experiment in which people are being masked en masse and correspondingly en masse being exposed to an uncommonly high concentration of uncommon, unnatural, friable particles.

No parent should want to include their child in such an experiment. We already have enough evidence to indicate that this experiment, taken long enough, will likely end poorly for those predisposed to pulmonary fibroids.

One problem is that we do not know exactly who those are who are predisposed to pulmonary fibroids. We only know that some people suffer from them and others do not, though they are exposed to similar conditions.

In the article "Masks, false safety and real dangers, Part 1: Friable mask particulate and lung vulnerability," Boris Borovoy et al. write:[1]

> "Pulmonary fibrosis is among the worst diseases that can be suffered or witnessed. It kills exceedingly slowly, by ever-thickening matrix formation, a kind of scar tissue, obstructing the alveoli and reducing their air exchange. The illness worsens slowly over time, and suffocates the victim very gradually. Nothing is available to the sufferer from conventional medicine. Neither medication nor radiation can undo the damage of the fibrous matrix laid down in the lungs' tissue. Similarly, surgery is not available to eliminate the insidious, suffocating mesh that painstakingly takes the life of the unfortunate patient. Neither is any known cure available in the realm of natural or alternative medicine. Neither nutrient, herb, nor any other known treatment can even reduce the fibrogenesis, let alone eliminate it. The 5-year survival rate is only 20%.[2] The only remedy against this scourge is diligent prevention of small and microscopic inhaled foreign bodies.

> "Inhaled particles, particularly nanoparticles, can begin the process of pulmonary fibrosis by forming free radicals such as superoxide anions. The resulting oxidative stress pro-

motes inflammatory responses and surface reactivity.[3] The pathogenesis of idiopathic pulmonary fibrosis begins when Type 2 alveoli are injured and epithelia is not fully healed. Interstitial fibroblasts differentiate into myofibroblasts, which gather in fibrotic foci and form fibers with contractile properties.[4] This is followed by synthesis and deposit of extracellular matrix, which seems to be key in suffocating the air exchange of alveoli."

As Borovoy points out, these tiny artificial particles may cause damage to the body beyond the lungs as well:

"Particles of nanometer to micrometer size have been implicated as causative agents in pulmonary fibrosis.[5] Airborne inhaled nano-size particles are especially dangerous for the lungs, but are small enough to undergo transcytosis across epithelial and endothelial cells to enter blood and lymph, reaching the cardiovascular system, spleen, bone marrow, and have been observed to travel along axons and dendrites of the central nervous system and ganglia, a phenomenon that has been known for decades."[6]

We know that the fibers of face masks are breathed into the body, even reaching deep into the lungs. We know that the body has several ways of dealing with such fibers, the formation of painful and debilitating fibroids being one of them.

We do not know what the long-term impact of the unprecedented mask mandates implemented on and around April 3, 2020 will be, but based on past research with similar inhaled materials, some percentage of the population is likely to experience painful, debilitating fibroids in their respiratory tract.

How many and how badly is a matter that is currently being determined through a massive experiment on the general population. No child deserves such a painful and debilitating sentence and no child deserves to be subject to such experimentation. The only way to protect your child is by refusing to subject your child any longer to such an experiment. The only way to do that is by refusing to let a face mask ever again be placed on your child's face for any reason. That experiment is what you are allowing when you allow your child to be masked.

Reason 64: Prolonged Textile Face Mask Use May Lead To Respiratory Illnesses Like Those Experienced By Textile Workers In The Third World

Mask wearing may cause problems throughout the respiratory system, beyond fibrosis of the lungs.

Kai Kisielinski, in an April 20, 2021 article entitled "Is a Mask That Covers the Mouth and Nose Free from Undesirable Side Effects in Everyday Use and Free of Potential Hazards?" describes this process and consequences further:[1]

> "The WHO sees the integration of individual companies and communities that produce their own fabric masks as a potential social and economic benefit. Due to the global shortage of surgical masks and personal protective equipment, it sees this as a source of income and points out that the reuse of fabric masks can reduce costs and waste and contribute to sustainability."[2]

This effort to institutionalize the unsafe and ineffective mask into existing societal and economic structures is troubling. Rather than acknowledging face masks as unsafe and ineffective and doing away with them, the opposite is being done. The truest way to reduce face mask costs and face mask waste is not to switch to cloth face masks, but to eliminate all face mask mandates and to use the available science to caution people against wearing the unsafe and ineffective face masks.

Kisielinski continues, digging into the toxins contained in the unsafe and ineffective face masks:

> "In addition to the question of certification procedures for such fabric masks, it should also be mentioned that due to the extensive mask obligation, textile (artificial) substances in the form of micro- and nanoparticles, some of which cannot be degraded in the body, are chronically absorbed into the body through inhalation to an unusual extent. In the case of medical masks, disposable polymers such as polypropylene, polyurethane, polyacrylonitrile, polystyrene, polycarbonate, polyethylene and polyester should be mentioned.[3] Ear, nose, and throat (ENT) physicians have already been able to detect such particles in the nasal mucosa

of mask wearers with mucosal reactions in the sense of a foreign body reaction with rhinitis.[4] In the case of community masks, other substances from the textile industry are likely to be added to those mentioned above. The body will try to absorb these substances through macrophages and scavenger cells in the respiratory tract and alveoli as part of a foreign body reaction, whereby toxin release and corresponding local and generalized reactions may occur in an unsuccessful attempt to break them down.[5] Extensive respiratory protection in permanent long-term use (24/7), at least from a theoretical point of view, also potentially carries the risk of leading to a mask-related pulmonary[6] or even generalized disorder, as is already known from textile workers chronically exposed to organic dusts in the Third World (byssinosis)."[5]

It has long been understood that third world textile workers have grown ill as a result of their exposure to fibers in their workspace. The same used to take place in developed nations. Similar fibers from face masks end up in the lungs of those who wear them. That is guaranteed to be harmful to some wearers. How harmful that is and how many are harmed has not yet been determined.

Even if face mask wearing were discontinued today, in fifteen or twenty years, we would finally begin to see the long-term effects of what happened when so many people inhaled so many fibers from face masks deep into their respiratory tract for a two year period of time.

Every time you put on a face mask, you make yourself a lab rat in that experiment. Every time you put your child in a face mask, you make your child one of Dr. Fauci's beagle puppies in this experiment. We do not know how many will be harmed in this experiment. Some are certain to be. How little you value your child's wellbeing and your role of trust as a parent if you are allowing your child to be a subject in such a nonsensical experiment. We already know face masks are not safe and are not effective.

No further testing needs to be done. The data is all there for those who are willing to have a look. Your child deserves better than to be a subject in an experiment.

Reason 65: Your Child Inhales Dangerous Chlorine Compounds While Wearing A Face Mask

Many toxic substances are inhaled when someone wears a mask. As the Association of American Physicians and Surgeons points out:[1]

> "The Hamburg Environmental Institute (July 2020) warned of the inhalation of chlorine compounds in polyester masks as well as problems in connection with face mask disposal."[2]

Even worse is likely to be contained in a face mask. If the face mask is made from a random piece of cloth, that is even more likely to be the case.

If everyone wore the same type of mask, from the same manufacturers, made according to identical material and standards, we would have a way to identify the risks associated with inhaling chemicals contained within the mask and given off by the masks.

However, under the preposterous public health recommendations of "make a mask of any design, out of any material, and wear it constantly as your moral duty," we cannot even begin to quantify the array of toxic chemicals inhaled.

There is no certification of this process. There is little recognition that any danger could possibly exist, which is the first step to certifying the safety of face mask manufacturing.

Quite to the contrary, watchdogs from public health to medical boards to industry groups continue to parrot the line that face masks are safe and effective. That behavior is entirely preposterous since the exact same piece of material worn as a piece of clothing on the body could be deemed entirely unsafe for the skin and dangerous to manufacture. That same item made into a face mask is given no such consideration. This is yet another reason you should not wear a face mask and your children should not either.

Reason 66: Exhaled Air Contains Over 250 Substances Meant To Be Removed From Your Body And Not Breathed Back In

Not only is the air inside the face mask full of harmful chemicals because of the material the face mask is made of, the air inside the face mask is full of harmful waste chemicals coming out of your body, concentrated in the space behind the mask and breathed back into your body.

In an April 20, 2021 article entitled "Is a Mask That Covers the Mouth and Nose Free from Undesirable Side Effects in Everyday Use and Free of Potential Hazards?" Kai Kisielinski writes:[1]

> "In view of the increased dead space volume, the long-term and increased accumulation and rebreathing of other respiratory air components apart from CO_2 is also unexplained, both in children and in old and sick people. Exhaled air contains over 250 substances, including irritant or toxic gases such as nitrogen oxides (NO), hydrogen sulfide (H_2S), isoprene and acetone."[2]

You may ask, "So what? Does that do anything?" The answer is yes. Kisielinski continues:

> "For nitrogen oxides[3] and hydrogen sulfide,[4] pathological effects relevant to disease have been described in environmental medicine even at a low but chronic exposure.[3-5] Among the volatile organic compounds in exhaled air, acetone and isoprene dominate in terms of quantity, but allyl methyl sulfide, propionic acid and ethanol (some of bacterial origin) should also be mentioned."[6]

But it does not just stop there. We know that individually, the rebreathing of these waste products of your body, independent of other waste products, are harmful. We have no idea how they react with each other though. There has been little need of this study, because researchers of the past had a hard time envisioning how government would conclude it wise to mask all people, or how a population would conclude it wise to acquiesce to such outlandish, ineffective, and unsafe orders.

We have no idea how the chemical waste components interact with other components, to harm he who is foolish enough to rebreathe his own waste, much like a dog takes to his own vomit. Kisielinski concludes:

179

"Whether such substances also react chemically with each other underneath masks and in the dead space volume created by masks, and with the mask tissue itself, and in what quantities these and possible reaction products are rebreathed, has not yet been clarified. In addition to the blood gas changes described above (O_2 drop and CO_2 rise), these effects could also play a role with regard to undesirable mask effects. Further research is needed here and is of particular interest in the case of prolonged and ubiquitous use of masks."

Kisielinski points out that more research is needed here to answer some of these questions. The wrong way to conduct that research is on the general population, least of all on children.

Perhaps you want to give yourself as a lab rat for the benefit of science and will agree to wear a face mask. Research subjects need to be fully informed of the research taking place and possible risks. That is not taking place in the population-wide mask research not being done. To the contrary, the population is being told a lie that the unsafe and ineffective face masks are safe and effective.

No informed consent is possible when a person is being lied to and told that the hundreds of known side effects of face mask wearing do not exist. What we are seeing take place — massive, uninformed experimentation on a population, children included — is patently wrong.

BACTERIA, FUNGI, AND VIRUSES ON THE SURFACE OF FACE MASKS

Reason 67: Eighty-Two Bacterial Colonies And Four Mold Colonies Found On A Child's Face Mask After Eight Hours

Is one child's mask the be all and end all of the story?

No. Absolutely not. It is anecdotal evidence and anecdotal evidence is the start of a story that continues through more thorough research — research that should be done BEFORE recommending masking. One child's mask shows this much — you are not being told the whole story.

As the Association of American Physicians and Surgeons points out:[1]

> "Recent study (in German) cultured 82 bacterial colonies and 4 mold (fungoid) colonies from a child's mask after 8 hours of wear."

The face mask turns into a harmful biohazard when worn. We know it is not helpful to wear. Far from being helpful, the fact that it turns into a biohazard that we are expected to allow our children to breathe through is harmful and wrongheaded.

Reason 68: Face Masks Are Breeding Grounds For Bacteria In A Way Our Unmasked Faces Are Not

The skin is covered in bacteria. The face is covered in bacteria. The respiratory system is full of bacteria. The body generally manages that fine. It is all very normal and healthy. The bacteria is not the problem. Introduce a mask, though, and it forms a breeding ground for bacteria that we pass air through. Our bodies, then, have an unfamiliar bacterial burden to deal with and have no defenses on the face mask with which to deal with them.

If I handed you a petri dish of lab grown bacteria that is known to be harmful to humans, would you walk around with it in front of your face all day? Of course not. Would you smear it on a face mask each morning and breathe through that face mask, filling your lungs with those pathogens? Of course not.

Yet that is what we do while wearing a face mask. Boris Borovoy et al. write in "Microbial challenges from masks:"[1]

> "Bacteria are on average ten times the size of viruses, particularly coronaviruses, and have less penetration through masks.[2] Therefore, at least part of the re-circulated flow of bacteria in aerosolized and droplet exhalation does not escape the vicinity of the oral and nasal environment. Bacteria and other microbes are not only retained in this space, but masks themselves are warm, moist repositories of these microbes.

> "Laboratory testing of used masks from 20 train commuters revealed that 11 of the 20 masks tested contained over 100,000 bacterial colonies. Molds and yeasts were also found. Three of the masks contained more than one million bacterial colonies.[3] Because such particles have been cultured from masks, they are expected to remain fully available to the airways while a mask is worn."

"Fully available to the airways," means while wearing a face mask, you are constantly reintroducing harmful bacteria into your body that your body does not want or know how to handle. Borovoy continues:

> "The outside surfaces of surgical masks were found to have high levels of the following microbes, even in hospitals,

more concentrated on the outside of masks than in the environment.[4] Staphylococcus species (57%) and Pseudomonas species (38%) were predominant among bacteria, and Penicillium species (39%) and Aspergillus species. (31%) were the predominant fungi. These correlated with the same bacteria and fungi found in samples of the ambient air where the masks were worn."[5]

Exhaling aerosolized bacteria in normal conditions tends to disable them quickly because their aerosol carrier dries up. In the damp environment of a mask, however, that does not happen. Borovoy continues:

"The mechanism of pathology originating from masks is likely as follows: Microbe-carrying droplets, trapped in masks, stay damp while the mask is worn, whereas without a mask, exhaled droplets and aerosol are known to dry quickly. In the continually damp environment of the mask, bacteria start to proliferate, are re-inhaled and then transferred throughout the body, as discussed below."

Masks are breeding grounds for bacteria in a way our unmasked faces are not. Do not wear them. Stop immediately. Definitely do not let your child wear them.

Reason 69: Bacteria On Masks Are Not Benign And Have Been Proven To Be Very Harmful

If the bacteria contained on masks were not harmful, the growth of bacteria on face masks might be no big deal. Unfortunately, that is not the case.

The bacteria on face masks are not benign, but quite harmful. Everyone walking around in a face mask is breeding colonies of very harmful bacteria on their face, inhaling them into their bodies in higher than normal quantities, and exhaling them into the air around them in higher than normal quantities.

Some call that harmful behavior normal and healthy and beneficial.

Their normal breath poses virtually no harm to you. Their breath *through* their mask, however, may be very harmful to you.

Stay away from them.

What they are doing is very strange.

They are turning themselves into a walking biohazard that they otherwise would not have been in the absence of a face mask.

To demonstrate the harmful colonies formed by mask wearing, Boris Borovoy points to a long used form of mask in the general population, a CPAP (Continuous Positive Airway Pressure machine) commonly worn to treat sleep apnea:[1]

> "CPAP has been used for decades, but universal masking is very new. We know that wearing the CPAP mask has led to life-threatening Legionella pneumonia as well as Streptococcus infections.[2] This disproves the hypothesis that microbial growth on masks is always benign."

This is a perfect example, that disproves the idea that face mask bacteria is harmless.

The difference between a CPAP and a face mask, however is that a CPAP is worn in a bedroom, in a relatively isolated environment. A face mask is worn in public, and spreads its foul and unnatural collection of pathogens through a population unprepared for such a foul and unnatural collection of pathogens being spread in such quantities. The wearing of a face mask is the artificial creation of a biohazard for others in a way that a CPAP is not.

Yet the official narrative around face masks is very different. Borovoy continues about why pathogenic bacteria collected on a face mask is harmful for the mask wearer, from the mouth down to the lungs:

"Aspiration pneumonia is a consequence of oral bacteria aspirated into the lungs. The teeth and gums are reservoirs for respiratory pathogens.[3,4] Oral dysbiosis is a disordered ecosystem of commensal as well as pathogenic bacteria in the mouth. Dental caries and periodontal disease are common results of such dysbiosis. One dental practice estimates that 50% of their patients are suffering from mask-induced dental problems, including decaying teeth, receding gum lines and 'seriously sour breath.'[5] The dentists theorize that these new oral infections are mostly caused by the tendency for people to mouth-breathe while wearing a mask, which is not consistent with the evolution of the form and functionality of the airways of humans or any other species.

"The oral flora is known to comprise over 700 bacterial species, inhabiting the epithelial debris, nutrients and oral secretions in the oral environment. Streptococci, lactobacilli and staphylococci are among the most common of these bacteria. Together, they comprise the biofilm that coats the surfaces of the oral cavity. Clearly, the bacteria benefit from the host, but the host may also benefit from the bacteria and contribute to our immunity by the production of secretory antibodies against new pathogens. The commensal relationship of oral flora with the host is generally benign and stable, unless the same bacteria achieve access to deeper tissues and blood. A number of serious and life-threatening diseases result when this happens.

"Bacteria that live in the mouth and upper respiratory tract may be aspirated and cause infection in the lungs. We know that mask-wearers have greater inspiratory flow than non-mask wearers.[6] This is presumably due to the hypoxic condition of mask obstruction to the airways. As a result, microbes may be more likely to be aspirated while wearing a mask than not wearing one.

"Damage to the airways results from bacterial colonization. When bacteria localize to the site(s) of infections in the respiratory tract and induce local airway inflammation, epithelial damage results. Such damage only requires bacterial colonization of the airways to begin this process, and to progress to bacterial-induced chronic airway inflammation.[7] This process begins with resident bacteria in oral secretions being aspirated and then adhering to the respiratory epithelium. These stimulate cytokine production and inflammation."[8]

Researchers realize that a dirty mouth may lead to disease of the lungs, which is why special care is taken to keep the mouths of at risk hospital patients clean. Borovoy continues:

"In fact, the very same periodontopathic bacteria are involved in the pathogenesis of respiratory diseases. These may be some of the diseases implicated in Covid-19.[9] Conversely, oral hygiene measures have correlated with improved outcomes in pneumonia patients[10] and those generally with respiratory tract infections,[11] as well as other lung diseases, such as COPD."[12]

An additional worry is a pathogenic synergy of microbes that may be more likely to occur in a moist mask, devoid of defenses against such pathogens, defenses which exist in the body. Borovoy continues:

"Infections do not only take hold from one species of pathogenic microbes. A pathogenic synergy can result in the flourishing of a particular pathogen. This was found to be the case with Aggregatibacter actinomycetemcomitans together with Streptococcus gordonii, both of which are commonly found in the mouth and in its abscesses.[13] With the concentration and culturing of microbes on the surface of a mask, is this pathogenic synergy made more likely while wearing a mask?"

It does not just stop there with bacterial infection. Additional harm is done that points to pathogenic synergy for mask wearers that makes them more prone to non-bacterial disease as well. Borovoy even goes as far as to conclude:

"Cloth mask wearers had significantly higher influenza-like illness when compared to unmasked."[14]

Jingy Xiao's review of randomized controlled trials in the CDC peer review journal of epidemiology *Emerging Infectious Diseases*, unequivocally shows masks do not help to prevent the spread of a respiratory virus.[15] Here, Borovoy is making an argument for how and why masks, in fact, increase the risk of influenza.

We know that face masks do not work, so there is no downside to not wearing a face mask. However, there is a downside to wearing a mask, since masks are covered in harmful bacteria and wearing a face mask helps that pathogenic bacteria and other pathogenic microorganisms access deeper tissues in the body, thereby putting the wearer at greater risk of harm.

Reason 70: Face Mask Wearing Causes Harmful Bacteria To Proliferate In An Environment Outside The Protection Of The Many Pathogen-Defenses The Body Has

The body can defend itself from pathogens. The body cannot defend a face mask from pathogens. The face mask provides an ideal environment for the growth of pathogens outside of the body's defenses. As it is worn over the nose and mouth, and air is filtered through it, the face mask also provides an ideal delivery mechanism for concentrated colonies of pathogens to be brought into the body. Because inspiratory flow is greater in a face mask, a face mask is ideal for bringing these pathogens deep into the lungs. Since expiratory flow is greater in a face mask, the face mask is also ideal for propelling those pathogens further into the environment around the mask wearer. This increased expiratory flow is due, in part, to wearers speaking more loudly and more forcefully, producing what is known as "the nebulizer effect."

Kai Kisielinski, in an April 20, 2021 article entitled "Is a Mask That Covers the Mouth and Nose Free from Undesirable Side Effects in Everyday Use and Free of Potential Hazards?" writes about the growth of pathogens on a face mask, outside of the body's defenses:[1]

> "Masks cause retention of moisture.[2] Poor filtration performance and incorrect use of surgical masks and community masks, as well as their frequent reuse, imply an increased risk of infection.[3-5] The warm and humid environment created by and in masks without the presence of protective mechanisms such as antibodies, the complement system, defense cells and pathogen-inhibiting and on a mucous membrane paves the way for unimpeded growth and, thus, an ideal growth and breeding ground for various pathogens such as bacteria and fungi[6] and also allows viruses to accumulate.[7] The warm and humid mask microclimate favors the accumulation of various germs on and underneath the masks,[8] and the germ density is measurably proportional to the length of time the mask is worn. After only 2 hours of wearing the mask, the pathogen density increases almost tenfold in experimental observation studies."[7,9]

There are various vectors by which masks can become contaminated. Kisielinski continues:

> "From a microbiological and epidemiological point of view, masks in everyday use pose a risk of contamination. This can occur as foreign contamination but also as self-contamination. On the one hand, germs are sucked in or attach themselves to the masks through convection currents. On the other hand, potential infectious agents from the nasopharynx accumulate excessively on both the outside and inside of the mask during breathing.[6,10] This is compounded by contact with contaminated hands. Since masks are constantly penetrated by germ-containing breath and the pathogen reproduction rate is higher outside mucous membranes, potential infectious pathogens accumulate excessively on the outside and inside of masks. On and in the masks, there are quite serious, potentially disease-causing bacteria and fungi such as E. coli (54% of all germs detected), Staphylococcus aureus (25% of all germs detected), Candida (6%), Klebsiella (5%), Enterococci (4%), Pseudomonads (3%), Enterobacter (2%) and Micrococcus (1%) even detectable in large quantities."[6]

Like Boris Borovoy, Kisielinski also concludes the face masks do not harbor purely benign microbes, but many strains of harmful microbes:

> "In another microbiological study, the bacterium Staphylococcus aureus (57% of all bacteria detected) and the fungus Aspergillus (31% of all fungi detected) were found to be the dominant germs on 230 surgical masks examined.[8]

> "After more than six hours of use, the following viruses were found in descending order on 148 masks worn by medical personnel: adenovirus, bocavirus, respiratory syncytial virus and influenza viruses."[7]

Kisielinski also points to masks as a perfect breeding ground for such pathogens:

> "From this aspect, it is also problematic that moisture distributes these potential pathogens in the form of tiny droplets via capillary action on and in the mask, whereby further proliferation in the sense of self- and foreign contamination by the aerosols can then occur internally and externally

with every breath.[11] In this regard, it is also known from the literature that masks are responsible for a proportionally disproportionate production of fine particles in the environment and, surprisingly, much more so than in people without masks."[12]

Kisielinski takes it further, getting into the topic of the nebulizer effect. Not only is your unnatural, dirty mask on your face harmful to you, your unnatural, dirty mask on you face is harmful to me:

"It was shown that all mask-wearing subjects released significantly more smaller particles of size 0.3–0.5 μm into the air than mask-less people, both when breathing, speaking and coughing (fabric, surgical, N95 masks, measured with the Aerodynamic Particle Sizer, APS, TS, model 3329).[12] The increase in the detection of rhinoviruses in the sentinel studies of the German RKI from 2020[13] could be a further indication of this phenomenon, as masks were consistently used by the general population in public spaces in that year."

Naturally, every person should be allowed to make his own health decisions.

If your dirty face mask is shown by research to harm me, however, and not wearing a face mask is parroted mindlessly by the media as harmful to all others, then what is the right solution?

The best solution is to leave others alone and to stay away from those who will not allow you to be left alone. Barring that, the more natural solution is the preferable solution.

Interventions are contrary to nature and lead inevitably to a cascade of interventions as it becomes clear that unintended consequences arise. The best solution is, therefore, to avoid intervention as much as possible and to defer to nature.

The very problem with the face mask, the very reason for this book, is the unwillingness of the public health community to trust that the body can do just fine in the face of Covid-19 and other respiratory ailments without these one-size-fits-all interventions.

The deeper we get into these cascades of interventions around Covid, the clearer it is becoming that we are creating more unintended consequences.

This is the nature of going down paths that diverge from nature while pretending that man has all the solutions.

If one or two people choose to experiment on themselves, that is one thing. If one or two billion children are forced to be experimented on, that is an entirely different level of moral and ethical violation.

Looking back on 2020 and 2021, the body, just as it was created, could have handled Covid-19 just fine and with far less harm to society than has occurred as a result of the interventions of 2020 and 2021.

Public health officials who participated must be culled from all positions of trust and never again allowed such power.

Reason 71: The Build Up Of Fungi And Bacteria In Face Masks

Breathing, coughing and sneezing into a mask creates a buildup of fungi, bacteria, viruses, and a host of other particles that emanate from the body's excretions.

Wearing a moist pouch full of visible and invisible bodily excretions around all day is foul and would never be allowed in any other circumstance.

Appropriately, the face mask is pejoratively referred to as a "face diaper."

Reason 72: Face Masks Cause Sore Throats

Not only are face masks not effective at preventing a person from getting sick from a respiratory virus, but face masks also cause sore throats. Dr. Armando Meza, an infectious disease specialist in Texas, reports:

> "Humidity will let bacteria continue to grow inside the mask so if you were growing bacteria in that area and you were breathing that inside, you can potentially get an infection, especially strep or any other bacteria that can cause infection." [1]

The body has potent anti-pathogen defenses that keep each of us alive every day. These defenses are not made to protect a person who straps a moist sack full of strep onto his face. Doing so artificially undermines the body's pathogen defenses and leads to sore throats and other infections of the respiratory tract.

This harm done by the wearing of an unsafe and ineffective face mask is another reason neither you nor your child should wear a face mask.

Have you ever said to yourself, "I need strep-throat more often?" Have you ever said to yourself, "My family needs strep-throat more often?" If you have not, then no one in your family should be wearing a face mask.

Reason 73: Face Masked People May Be At Greater Risk For Fungal Infections Of Lungs Than Unmasked

The wearing of a face mask is not only ineffective at preventing the spread of a respiratory virus, but wearing a face mask adds to the risk of fungal infections of the lungs. Boris Borovoy et al. write in "Microbial challenges from masks:"[1]

"Aspergillosis is an infection of the lungs by the spores of the Aspergillus fumigatus fungus. These spores are ubiquitous in the environment, indoors and outdoors, and are usually harmless. There are many environmental sources of Aspergillus. Decaying leaves and compost in the outdoors around trees and plants, as well as indoors in bathrooms are common locations of Aspergillus. These spores may be inhaled by those with weakened immune systems and can be a cause or a result of bronchiectasis.[2] This is a chronic airway infection syndrome, and as indicated above, a risk from inhaled fibers. Fungal fibers may be inhaled and accumulate as fungal balls known as aspergillomas. At its worst, Aspergillosis can proceed to systemic infection, with consequences to the brain, heart and kidneys. Invasive aspergillosis spreads rapidly and may be fatal."

Fungi may produce chemicals that suppress the immune system. Borovoy writes:

"Aspergillus as well as candida also produce gliotoxins, which are immunosuppressive toxins that in turn enable proliferation of candida. The mechanism of immunosuppression appears to be by alteration of the structure and function of PMN neutrophils."[3]

These problems of fungal infection are made even worse by mask wearing, as Borovoy writes:

"It is possible that a warm moist environment, such as a mask worn outdoors or in bathrooms may pick up and harbor fungal spores as well as particulate and/or loose fibers. This is normally not a concern for a healthy person or an unmasked person. When mold spores are inhaled by a healthy person, immune system cells surround and destroy them. Masks provide an alternative environment whereby mold and fungi are held and trapped beyond typical airborne levels. When maintained over the airways, this can create a risk for the mask-wearer. Simply, if the masks retain fungal spores, these may be dislodged with inhalation."

In addition to bacterial and viral infections, elevated risk of fungal infection is an additional reason not to wear a face mask.

Reason 74: Mayo Clinic: Face Mask Wearing Is Leading To An Increase In Staph Infections, As Can Be Expected As They Help Bacteria Access Deeper Quarters Of The Body

Oral bacteria accessing deep tissue in the body can lead to harmful infections. Boris Borovoy et al write in "Microbial challenges from masks:"[1]

"When oral bacteria gain access to blood and deep tissues, they may cause pneumonia, abscesses in lung tissue, subacute bacterial endocarditis, sepsis and meningitis.[2] It is important to consider that endocarditis can be a lifelong infection. Strep pyogenes bacteria has been observed for decades to cause irreversible fibrosis in heart tissue long after the bacteria were no longer found.[3] This bacteria is known by many as 'flesh eating strep.' Former Streptococcus infections that had seemingly resolved a long time ago may still be positive in an Antistreptolysin O test. For years afterward, flares of toxins can be released in the body at times of stress or secondary infection and cause debilitating symptoms."

Additional diseases may be caused by oral bacteria reaching deep tissue. Borovoy writes:

"Additionally Type 2 diabetes, hypertension, and cardiovascular diseases have been the result of oral bacteria gaining access to deeper tissue.[4] These are among the diseases reported as co-morbidities associated with an increased risk of death attributed to Covid-19. COPD[5] and in this enormous study, cancer can also result simply from the access of oral bacteria to deeper tissue.[6]

"Immune-mediated inflammatory disorders, commonly known as auto-immune diseases are correlated with oral dysbiosis. We know that transient bacteria from an oral infection or a dental procedure can gain access to the blood for systemic circulation. Those bacteria can produce toxins that trigger tissue damage or other pathological changes. These molecules may react with antibodies that produce large complexes, which are associated with acute and chronic inflammatory changes.[7,8] Such auto-immune diseases as rheumatoid arthritis, systemic lupus erythematosus and Sjogren's syndrome all have features of oral dysbiosis."[9]

Brain tissue can even be reached by such infections. Borovoy writes:

"Autoimmune encephalitis occurs when microbes access brain tissue, triggering neurological or psychiatric symptoms. This complex of diseases include basal ganglia encephalitis, and can be triggered by bacterial, viral and fungal infections. Some of the most pernicious of this group of diseases is pediatric autoimmune neuropsychiatric disorders associated with streptococcal infections (PANDAS). Group A Streptococcus (GAS) is a very common illness, and the most common bacterial infectious agent of sore throat, 'strep throat,' and is one of the microbial agents involved in PANDAS. GAS causes one million to 2.6 million cases of strep throat each year.[10]

"Repeated infections in the nasal cavity can lead to Th1 and Th17 lymphocytes in the surrounding nasal tissue. These are pro-inflammatory and target host cells in a misdirected immune response. The Th17 cells travel into the brain along the olfactory nerves, through the cribriform plate from the nose or throat or palate and into the brain. These in turn stimulate cytokines, which then stimulate microglia. The endothelial cells in the blood brain barrier are broken down by damaging both the tight junctions in the endothelium, and by increasing transcytosis of auto-antibodies that are circulating in the blood to access the brain. This mechanism has been shown to lead to the abrupt onset of neurological and psychiatric symptoms associated with the PANDAS diagnosis."[11]

Borovoy cites the Mayo Clinic, tying mask wearing to a new prevalence of deadly infections:

"Our nasal passages are colonized by Staphylococcus bacteria, among other organisms. Under typical circumstances, these pose no threat to the individual; however, Mayo Clinic has warned, (although this statement has now been erased from their site.) 'A growing number of otherwise healthy people are developing life-threatening staph infections because of mask wearing:'"[12]

A convincing explanation for why this sensible, early warning has been removed from the Mayo Clinic website has not been provided. How many have suffered from life-threatening infections as a result of the removal of such a warning? Who removed this warning? Can that person ever be allowed in a position of public trust again? These are questions that will one day need to be answered.

Mask wearing may cause these infections to be more likely because of their ability to colonize oral bacteria outside the body's defenses, but close enough to impact the body by forming part of the respiratory "dead space." As Borovoy points out:

"One of the risks of mask wearing is that masks maintain bacteria in greater numbers and for a longer period of time. This increases the risk of those bacteria entering the respiratory system and/or blood stream through micro wounds."

Borovoy lists some of these conditions:

"The following are some of the diseases and conditions that may result. Bacteremia is a condition in which bacteria can travel to internal organs, muscle, bone and prosthetic devices. Toxic shock syndrome is a condition in which some strains of Staphylococcus produce toxins that create high fever, nausea, vomiting and other symptoms. Septic arthritis occurs when staph bacteria infect the joints, which may result in pain, swelling and fever.

"The risk of pericarditis caused by staphylococcus has been known since at least 1945.[13] This life-threatening disease has been treated with prolonged antibiotic therapy and aggressive drainage of the pericardium,[14] and, in severe cases, surgical resection of the pericardium.[15] Purulent pericarditis is the most serious consequence of bacterial pericarditis, and is always fatal if untreated. Even in treated patients the mortality rate is 40%.[16]

"Streptococcus is a commensal organism of the oral mucosa, and is the most common infective agent causing endocarditis.[17] It is not so unusual for oral Streptococci to gain access to the bloodstream, and oral Streptococci comprise more than half of colonies cultured from blood following dental procedures. 'Oral streptococcal bacteremia is frequently associated with the development of septic shock and death.'"[18]

Borovoy demonstrates a long-term concern for deeper tissue infection by oral bacteria:

> "Cardiovascular and rheumatological outcomes from mask-wearing are unlikely to be realized in the United States for at least several months due to the recentness of mask wearing; although we can learn from the history of prevalence of cardiovascular disease many years after the 1918-1919 forced masking pandemic described previously. These are enormous concerns on the horizon for future public health considerations."

While Borovoy predicts a several month lag time as possible, in discovering these newfound symptoms and conditions resulting from face mask wearing, the lag time may be significantly longer.

In a free and open environment for scientific discussion, Borovoy's prediction would be sensible. However, in the heavily censorious environment we are in, in which a lack of public discourse and a lack of scientific debate exists on this topic, the usual channels are not able to effectively work. Accordingly, the scientific method is unable to be applied as easily in the absence of robust research and debate.

That only further illustrates the need for brave sentinels such as Borovoy. Deep tissue infection from oral bacteria represents another reason not to wear a face mask.

BONDING, LEARNING,
AND THE DEVELOPING MIND

Reason 75: Face Masks Harm
A Child's Developing Mind

Theory abounds on the topic of how a child's mind develops. Researchers do not know exactly how a child's mind develops, but researchers have useful metrics to explore that realm of possibility, and conversely to observe harm and stress placed upon a child that puts a distracting burden upon the developing mind.

Masks appear to harm developing children as they experience neurological symptoms far above baseline. Though it should not require a study to tell us so, we are likely to one day see that the impositions from March 2020 onward were a repeated onslaught against the developing mind of a child.

In the article "Review of scientific reports of harms caused by face masks," from December 2020, Silke Schwarz writes:[1]

> "Background: Narratives about complaints in children and adolescents caused by wearing a mask are accumulating. There is, to date, no registry for side effects of masks.

> "Methods: At the University of Witten/Herdecke an online registry has been set up where parents, doctors, pedagogues and others can enter their observations. On October, 20, 2020, 363 doctors were asked to make entries and to make parents and teachers aware of the registry.

> "Results: By October, 26, 2020 the registry had been used by 20,353 people. In this publication we report the results from the parents, who entered data on a total of 25,930 children. The average wearing time of the mask was 270 minutes per day. Impairments caused by wearing the mask were reported by 68% of the parents. These included irritability (60%), headache (53%), difficulty concentrating (50%), less happiness (49%), reluctance to go to school/kindergarten (44%), malaise (42%) impaired learning (38%) and drowsiness or fatigue (37%)."

More than two-thirds of parents reported visible impairment in their child from wearing a mask. This begs a question. How many more children experienced difficulty from the mask, but their parents did not notice or were unwilling to notice?

Through more careful observation, we may one day realize that number is near 100% of children who have cognitive effects from mask wearing.

Reason 76: Face Masks Affect
A Person's Ability To Think Clearly

With the cognitive effects caused by mask wearing, it can be no surprise that clear thinking is impeded by mask wearing.

Kai Kisielinski, in an April 20, 2021 article entitled "Is a Mask That Covers the Mouth and Nose Free from Undesirable Side Effects in Everyday Use and Free of Potential Hazards?" writes:[1]

> "The sum of the disturbances and discomforts that can be caused by a mask also contributes to distraction (see also psychological impairment). These, in conjunction with a decrease in psycho-motoric skills, reduced responsiveness and overall impaired cognitive performance (all of which are pathophysiological effects of wearing a mask) [2-7] can lead to a failure to recognize hazards and, thus, to accidents or avoidable errors at work.[2,8,9] Of particular note here are mask-induced listlessness ($p < 0.05$), impaired thinking ($p < 0.05$) and concentration problems ($p < 0.02$) as measured by a Likert scale (1–5).[3] Accordingly, occupational health regulations take action against such scenarios. The German Industrial Accident Insurance (DGUV) has precise and extensive regulations for respiratory protective equipment where they document the limitation of wearing time, levels of work intensity and defined instruction obligation."[10]

This is a very broad set of impacts on the thought process that should not be taken lightly. No child should be masked until the magnitude of this impact is better understood and quantified.

Reason 77: Face Masks Cause Degeneration Of Brains Because Of Lack Of Oxygen

The brain needs oxygen. In a very short amount of time, the brain degenerates with a lack of oxygen. It is not a matter of if this happens, it is a matter of what point it happens at.

The question then is "How much face mask wearing does it take to cause degeneration of the brain?"

We do not know the answer to that. The topic is not well studied. This is a question that needed answering *before* the mass masking of children, not a year later. All masking of children should cease until this question is sufficiently answered.

Vernon Coleman writes in the article: "Masks And Mask Wearing: 100 Facts You Must Know," January 11, 2021,[1] about the work of a doctor who he so effectively summarizes, from a YouTube video that has now been taken down:

> "Dr. Margarite Griesz-Brisson MD PhD is a leading European neurologist and neurophysiologist. In October 2020, she warned that rebreathing our exhaled air, because of wearing masks, will create oxygen deficiency and an excess of carbon dioxide in the body. 'We know,' she said, 'that the human brain is very sensitive to oxygen deprivation. There are nerve cells in the hippocampus that cannot last longer than three minutes without oxygen.'"

The brain has warning signs associated with this problem. To continue quoting Coleman:

> "Dr. Griesz-Brisson pointed out that the acute warning symptoms of oxygen deprivation are headaches, drowsiness, dizziness, difficulty in concentration and slowing down of reaction times. The real danger is, however, that when the oxygen deprivation becomes chronic, the symptoms disappear because the body gets used to them."

While those warning signs go away, the damage does not, as Coleman states:

> "However, efficiency remains impaired and the damage to the brain continues. 'We know that neurodegenerative disease takes years to decades to develop. If today you forget your phone number, the breakdown in your brain would

have already started two or three decades ago.' Dr. Griesz-Brisson explains that while the mask wearer thinks that they are becoming accustomed to re-breathing exhaled air, the problems within the brain are growing as the oxygen deprivation continues."

The brain does not recover from this when face mask wearing stops. Coleman continues:

"She also points out that brain cells which die, because of a shortage of oxygen, will never be replaced. They are gone forever. She goes on to argue that everyone is entitled to claim exemption from mask wearing because oxygen deprivation is so dangerous — and masks do not work."

This is especially harmful to children. Coleman continues:

"Finally, Dr. Griesz-Brisson points out that children and teenagers must never wear masks, partly because they have extremely active and adaptive immune systems but also because their brains are especially active and vulnerable. The more active an organ is the more oxygen it needs. And so the damage to children's brains is huge and irreversible. She warns that dementia is going to increase in ten years, and the younger generation will not be able to reach their potential because of the mask wearing. Oxygen deprivation adversely affects the heart and the lungs but it also damages the brain.

"And the damage will be permanent. 'My conclusion has to be that no one has the right to force us to deprive our bodies of oxygen for absolutely no good reason. Depriving individuals of oxygen is a crime perpetrated by those demanding that we wear masks. Those who let it happen and those who collaborate are also guilty. And those who wear masks in situations where they are not legally required are operating in a criminal activity.' Inevitably, Dr. Griesz-Brisson's interview was removed from YouTube as part of the global suppression of medical information."

The long-term neurological harm perpetrated on children forced to wear masks, truly is a crime. No child should be compelled to participate in it. No parent should allow their child to be exposed to even to a second of mandated masking.

Reason 78: Face Mask Wearing Causes Reduced Attention And Slower Speed In Athletes

When trying to determine the effects of masks on a child's cognition, we can look to other areas of life that are easier to measure, in order to see if impacts on cognition should even be a concern.

There are theories that wearing "training masks" intended to mimic altitude training, may benefit athletes. This theory has been used to glibly dismiss the growing body of evidence around the harm done to children by exercising in a face mask. Effectively, people arguing from this point of view claim that face masks help strengthen a child's body.

The body of available evidence shows that face masks should not be worn during exercise. There is physiological evidence against the wearing a face mask during exercise, and impacts on cognition are a concern, as can be seen from studies done on elite athletes. Evidence shows face masks are harmful, and training masks may be harmful as well.

In an April 20, 2021 article entitled "Is a Mask That Covers the Mouth and Nose Free from Undesirable Side Effects in Everyday Use and Free of Potential Hazards?"[1] Kai Kisielinski writes that training masks do not have proven performance enhancing benefit:

> "According to the literature, performance-enhancing effects of masks regarding cardiovascular optimization and improvement of oxygen uptake capacity cannot be proven.

> "For example, in an experimental reference study (12 subjects per group), the training mask that supposedly mimics altitude training (ETM: elevation training mask) only had training effects on the respiratory muscles. However, mask wearers showed significantly lower oxygen saturation values ($SpO2\%$) during exercise ($SpO2$ of 94% for mask wearers versus 96% for mask-less, $p < 0.05$),[2] which can be explained by an increased dead space volume and increased resistance during breathing. The measured oxygen saturation values were significantly lower than the normal values in the group of mask wearers, which indicates a clinical relevance.

> "The proven adaptation effect of the respiratory muscles in healthy athletes[2] clearly suggests that masks have a disrup-

tive effect on respiratory physiology. In another intervention study on mask use in weightlifters, researchers documented statistically significant effects of reduced attention (questionnaire recording, Likert scale) and a slowed maximum speed of movement detectable by means of sensors (both significant at $p < 0.001$), leading the researchers to conclude that mask use in sport is not without risks. As a secondary finding, they also detected a significant decrease in oxygen saturation SpO2 when performing special weight-lifting exercises ('back squats') in the mask group after only 1 minute of exercise compared to the mask-free group ($p < 0.001$)."[3]

While wearing a face mask is harmful to elite athletes, this may be even more harmful to those who are untrained or sick. As Kisielinski points out:

"The proven tendency of the masks to shift the chemical parameter oxygen saturation SpO2 in a pathological direction (lower limit value 95%) may well have clinical relevance in untrained or sick individuals. Sports medicine confirmed an increase in carbon dioxide (CO_2) retention, with an elevation in CO_2 partial pressure in the blood with larger respiratory dead space volumes."[4]

Further evidence from studies of the impact of masks on one's ability to exercise, indicates harm on children, the elderly, and the pre-diseased. Kisielinski continues:

"In fact, dead space-induced CO_2 retention while wearing a mask during exercise was also experimentally proven. The effects of a short aerobic exercise under N95 masks were tested on 16 healthy volunteers. A significantly increased end-expiratory partial pressure of carbon dioxide ($PETCO_2$) with plus 8 mmHg ($p < 0.001$) was found.[5] The increase in blood carbon dioxide (CO_2) in the mask wearers under maximum load was plus 14% CO_2 for surgical masks and plus 23% CO_2 for N95 masks, an effect that may well have clinical relevance in the pre-diseased, elderly and children, as these values strongly approached the pathological range."[5]

Recognizing the harm that can be done, even to the high end of elite athletes, by face masks, adds to the body of evidence on why neither children nor anyone else should be encouraged to wear a face mask, let alone forced into one.

FACE MASKS DISRUPT COMMUNICATION

Reason 79: Face Masks Are Disruptive To Basic Human Communication

Each of the chapters in this book constitute a reason not to put a face mask on a child.

This is one of many chapters in this book that should not need to be written. It should be enough to say about this or many other chapters "Because masks quite obviously cause harm X, they should never be worn by children, nor worn by anyone around children."

Masks hinder human communication, even down to the most basic level and should therefore not be worn.

Kai Kisielinski, in an April 20, 2021 article entitled "Is a Mask That Covers the Mouth and Nose Free from Undesirable Side Effects in Everyday Use and Free of Potential Hazards?" writes:[1]

"Experts point out that masks disrupt the basics of human communication (verbal and nonverbal). The limited facial recognition caused by masks leads to a suppression of emotional signals. Masks, therefore, disrupt social interaction, erasing the positive effect of smiles and laughter but at the same time greatly increasing the likelihood of misunderstandings because negative emotions are also less evident under masks."[2]

This same decrease in empathy harms the doctor patient relationship, as Kisielinski demonstrates:

"A decrease in empathy perception through mask use with disruption of the doctor-patient relationship has already been scientifically proven on the basis of a randomized study (statistically significant, with $p = 0.04$).[3] In this study, the Consultation Empathy Care Measury, the Patient Enablement Instrument (PEI) Score and a Satisfaction Rating Scale were assessed in 1030 patients. The 516 doctors, who wore masks throughout, conveyed reduced empathy towards the patients and, thus, nullified the positive health promoting effects of a dynamic relationship. These results demonstrate a disruption of interpersonal interaction and relationship dynamics caused by masks."

The WHO even recognizes how fundamentally important communication is, especially for children and how it must be weighed when anyone considers placing a mask on a child. This question had hardly been weighed prior to the masking mandates of April 3, 2020:

> "The WHO guidance on the use of masks in children in the community, published in August 2020, points out that the benefits of mask use in children must be weighed up against the potential harms, including social and communicational concerns."[4]

Quite naturally, other experts are concerned. Kisielinski adds:

> "Fears that widespread pandemic measures will lead to dysfunctional social life with degraded social, cultural and psychological interactions have also been expressed by other experts."[2,5-7]

Face masks being so disruptive to basic human communication, provides yet another reason for face masks never to be worn by children and never to be worn around children.

Do your child a favor and insist that anyone he speaks to have no mask on when that person interacts with your child. Such drastic refusal of anyone in a mask may not be exactly what the world wants of you, but it is exactly what your child needs of you.

Reason 80: We All Read Lips

The mother of a child who reads lips, wrote me elaborating on how we all read lips:

> *Dear Mr. Stevo*
>
> *As a mother of vaccine injured deaf and autistic adult son, I am intimately familiar with the subject.*
>
> *But I can also assure you — most people hear with their eyes!*
>
> *Especially children — they cannot learn language properly if they do not watch articulation and facial expression.*
>
> *Do you remember The West Wing? I understood pretty much everything, but I know many Americans, native English speakers, who have a hard time understanding the dialogues because Aaron Sorkin loves "walking while talking."*
>
> *Face diapers are monuments of insanity, and those who do not understand the maskholes are not always kidding. That is the reason you should always face the hard of hearing person when speaking to him/her. This is also the reason for mistakes and misunderstandings in the operating room, and no amount of acoustical treatment could remedy this problem.*
>
> *In some states, there are exemptions from mask wearing requirements for people who communicate with the deaf and hard of hearing.*
>
> *But it is a real tragedy that so many people comply, and I commend you for your continuous attention to the matter.*
>
> *Best regards*
>
> *Irena Stepanova*

While this may not need stating to many observant parents, this mother states the case so well of how we all use lip reading to communicate.

When a room grows loud, it is normal for people to stare at lips. When a person speaks a different native language than you, it is normal for you to look at that person's lips to understand better. The normal communication of life, once taken for granted, has become so difficult, as everything from food orders to car orders are now flubbed purely because of a face mask being involved in the exchange.

This is another reason masks should be worn by no one.

How arrogant of public health officials to suggest a 10 cent polypropylene mask from Wuhan could improve upon millennia of strategies for continued human existence and that only through a mandate would anyone want to wear this allegedly helpful device.

Reason 81: Babies And Children Especially Read Lips

It is normal for babies and children to want to read lips. To mask them is abnormal and to mask the lips they are trying to read is even more abnormal.

In the article "Review of scientific reports of harms caused by face masks," David Lewkowicz, writes:[1]

> "We discovered that babies begin lip-reading at around 8 months of age. ... Crucially, once lip-reading emerges in infancy, it becomes the default mode of speech processing whenever comprehension is difficult. ...

> "Overall, the research to date demonstrates that the visible articulations that babies normally see when others are talking play a key role in their acquisition of communication skills. Research also shows that babies who lip-read more have better language skills when they are older. If so, this suggests that masks probably hinder babies' acquisition of speech and language."

No one should be in a mask — not babies, not children, and definitely not anyone allowed to interact with them.

Reason 82: Face Masks Act
As An Acoustic Filter

Not only do masks prevent lip reading, they act as an acoustic filter, effectively causing everyone to sound as if they are mumbling.

Kai Kisielinski, in an April 20, 2021 article entitled "Is a Mask That Covers the Mouth and Nose Free from Undesirable Side Effects in Everyday Use and Free of Potential Hazards?" writes:[1]

> "The results of a Chilean study with healthcare workers show that masks act like an acoustic filter and provoke excessively loud speech. This causes a voice disorder.[2] The increased volume of speech also contributes to increased aerosol production by the mask wearer."[3]

All well raised children in the United States learn to look a person in the eyes while shaking hands, to smile, to speak up, and to speak clearly.

Masking undoes this upbringing on how to be friendly, approachable, and generally successful in how you present yourself to another.

In these ways, and so many other ways, mask wearing helps set a truly low cultural standard.

Reason 83: Face Masks Cause Further Harm To The Mentally Impaired And Hearing Impaired

Masks separate those who have average and above average ability to communicate for their age group. They really cause harm to those with impairments communicating.

Kai Kisielinski, in an April 20, 2021 article entitled "Is a Mask That Covers the Mouth and Nose Free from Undesirable Side Effects in Everyday Use and Free of Potential Hazards?" writes:[1]

> "The disruption of non-verbal communication due to the loss of facial expression recognition under the mask can increase feelings of insecurity, discouragement and numbness as well as isolation, which can be extremely stressful for the mentally and hearing-impaired."[2]

No one with communicational impairments should be forced into a mask or have a mask worn around them, but also, no one is perfect at communicating.

We all have our impairments. To prevent additional communicational problems, no one should be forced to wear a mask or forced to communicate with anyone in a mask.

The cultural norm right now is to encourage everyone to be masked. The better cultural norm, a cultural norm interested in the wellbeing of the people involved, a cultural norm based on the science of how harmful mandatory masking is, should be a cultural norm in which no one is masked, and in which people who are masked are looked at negatively.

To mask is anti-social.

Reason 84: Face Masks Reduce The Ability For A Child To Bond And Reduce The Ability For A Child To Learn

From a young age, American children are taught to look others in the eye, to smile, and to give a good handshake. It sends signals to the other person that you are a capable person worthy of his time many similarly expressive traditions are taught.

Important social bonds are formed in these first seconds of interaction as rapport is developed, largely on a non-verbal level, overwhelmingly reliant on the face and its cues.

Suddenly, we have done away with that and suggested the face is so irrelevant, social bonds are so irrelevant, that all must be masked without so much as a societal conversation about the harm done to a child when a face is masked.

I am here to start that conversation and mean to win it with your help.

In the article "Review of scientific reports of harms caused by face masks," Manfred Spitzer, writes:[1]

> "Covering the lower half of the face reduces the ability to communicate, interpret, and mimic the expressions of those with whom we interact. Positive emotions become less recognizable, and negative emotions are amplified. Emotional mimicry, contagion, and emotionality in general are reduced and (thereby) bonding between teachers and learners, group cohesion, and learning — of which emotions are a major driver. Face masks block emotional signaling between teachers and students:"

Children should not be masked, and no one in the presence of children should be masked.

Reason 85: Face Masks Harm Relationships

Face masks harm relationships.

In a face mask ...
The smile is gone.
Trust is reduced.
Fear is encouraged, instead of smiling at a stranger.
People look down more.
People are more likely to turn away.
People are less likely to connect.
People mumble more.
People interact less.

Masks perpetuate this fear-driven narrative that everyone from best friend, to child, to your own mother, is a walking biohazard who could end your life.

That is simply not the perspective that has gotten us to this point in human history and through many disease outbreaks of the past.

You cannot logically burn down a culture in the name of protecting oneself from a virus by using things that do not even work to protect you from a virus.

Yet, that is what so many are actively doing. Is it logical? No.

Do they care about your logic? Probably not.

Draw a firm line. Do this by identifying your boundaries, communicating your boundaries, and defending your boundaries. Logic has its limits.

Quit asking for permission. Just be the leader of your home and protect.

Reason 86: Face To Face Contact Is Reduced When Children Wear Masks

People are already unlikely to look one another in the eye.

Screens have replaced so much natural, human communication.

Masks are a natural extension for a society disinterested in recognizing our humanness, disinterested in recognizing the importance of face to face communication.

To put on a mask makes you a part of that trend of dehumanizing another and showing an unwillingness to look him in the face.

Refusing the mask, refusing the mask be worn in your presence, insisting on normal human face to face interaction, places you in opposition to that toxic trend.

For your own wellbeing, for the wellbeing of your family, stand in opposition to that trend.

Reason 87: Face Masks Block Emotional Signaling Between Students And Teachers, Students And Parents, Students And Students, And Between Students And All Other Humans

So much emotion is communicated through the face, and so much of the face is blocked by a face mask.

Denis Rancourt of the Ontario Civil Liberties Association writes:[1]

"In sum, recognition of, and response to, the outward emotional displays of one's peers' faces is a critical and necessary component of social interaction in schools. It helps pupils and teachers to modify their behavior in order to align with social communication and behavioral norms. When these emotional displays are inhibited by face masks, our ability to communicate effectively with one another is reduced and we are primarily left with mimicking negative (frown) emotions. All of this happens primarily outside of conscious awareness, and hence, is hard to be consciously controlled or even corrected. Since emotions are a major driver of group cohesion, the decreased emotionality, and decreased positive emotionality in particular, may interfere with smooth classroom action. Given the fact that the very process of learning is facilitated by emotions (this is their main raison d'être), face masks are likely to cause some interference with pedagogy."[2]

Given the harm done to a child by both the child wearing a mask and by others wearing a mask around that child, masks should not be worn by children or around children. Some would say it is a person's option to wear a mask or not. That is an awful approach. No parent should tolerate that anti-social, harmful behavior around a child.

Parents protect their children from all manner of harm. That is just their duty and they willingly accept how to make that happen. Some parents sadly treat the harm of a face mask differently than other harms. Generally speaking though, parents who understand the harm that face masks cause a child do not need to be educated on how to stop that harm. They just figure out a way.

They figure out a way to keep this and all other age inappropriate harm away from their child. That is part of being a parent.

Just like all other forms of sociopathy, there is no age at which the harm of wearing a face mask becomes age appropriate.

Reason 88: Both Face Masks And Face Shields Cause Fear In Children

What is happening is not normal. Children get that. Doctors' offices are already uncomfortable enough environments for children. They are also an environment in which problems with face masks can be measured.

In an April 20, 2021 article entitled "Is a Mask That Covers the Mouth and Nose Free from Undesirable Side Effects in Everyday Use and Free of Potential Hazards?" Kai Kisielinski writes:[1]

> "Both masks and face shields caused fear in 46% of children (37 out of 80) in a scientific study. If children are given the choice of whether the doctor examining them should wear a mask they reject this in 49% of the cases. Along with their parents, the children prefer the practitioner to wear a face visor (statistically significant with $p < 0.0001$)."[2]

Stand in favor of empathy. Stand in favor of understanding another without them having to say a word. Faces are practically made for that. Stand in favor of that human communication that so enriches us and bonds us.

Refuse the face mask.

Do not allow it on your child, and do not allow it in your child's presence.

Masks must come to be regarded as a supremely anti-human, sociopathic, divisive, and harmful tool. Anyone who would wear one is sending a signal about their comfort to do harm to another.

Toxic attitudes toward humanity must be done away with as well.

It is worth noting that it is not just the face mask, it is the face visor too. Many children intuitively understand how weird this universal face masking all is. They may not have the words to describe it, but so many children can sense the wrongness of it.

Children prefer a face visor over a face mask and prefer a human face over either.

We can expect similar results in non-clinical settings and can add both face masks and face shields causing fear in children as a reason that no one should be masked or shielded in the presence of children.

Of course, there are some children who feel fear in the absence of a face mask — parents, school, screen time, and society have filled them with the same irrational psychosis that *The New England Journal of Med-*

icine has described as "a reflexive reaction to anxiety."[3] Parents can intervene and stem that cycle of fear related to face masks and other one-size-fits-all health mandates.

It is a parent's duty to protect a child from the psychosis of the world, not to magnify it.

Negligent parenting is no reason to mask children, thereby normalizing the wrongheadedness of the negligence. To the contrary, the root cause: the negligent parenting, should be addressed. Masking children or anyone around children is unsafe, ineffective, experimental, and must be immediately stopped.

Reason 89: Face Masks Are Particularly Harmful On A Person's Wellbeing

So much communicational harm is done by face masks, so much biological harm as well. Knowing that, how can we possibly expect anyone to feel good in a face mask?

There appears to be a correlation between temperature increase under the mask and wellbeing of the individual wearing the mask, possibly based on the masks impact on numerous body systems.

Kai Kisielinski, in an April 20, 2021 article entitled "Is a Mask That Covers the Mouth and Nose Free from Undesirable Side Effects in Everyday Use and Free of Potential Hazards?" writes:[1]

> "[There is] a significant temperature increase of 1.9 °C on average (to over 34.5 °C) in the mask-covered facial area (p < 0.05).[2] Due to the relatively larger representation in the sensitive cerebral cortex (homunculus), the temperature sensation in the face is more decisive for the feeling of wellbeing than other body regions.[3,4] The perception of discomfort when wearing a mask can, thus, be intensified. Interestingly, in our analysis, we found a combined occurrence of the physical variable temperature rise under the mask and the symptom respiratory impairment in seven of eight studies concerned, with a mutual significantly measured occurrence in 88%. We also detected a combined occurrence of significantly measured temperature rise under the mask and significantly measured fatigue in 50% of the relevant primary studies. These clustered associations of temperature rise with symptoms of respiratory impairment and fatigue suggest a clinical relevance of the detected temperature rise under masks. In the worst case scenario, the effects mentioned can reinforce each other and lead to decompensation, especially in the presence of COPD, heart failure and respiratory insufficiency."

Wanting your child and those around you to be supported, secure, and to have a general sense of wellbeing, we must deny anyone the ability to mask them or anyone else.

Reason 90: Face Masks Help You Raise A Sociopath

It is unclear why there is increased difficulty in society for face to face communication, but anti-social behavior, as traditionally defined, is on the rise. Discomfort in face to face communication among people of all ages is one of many telling signs of this increase in anti-social behavior.

What is clear, is that a face mask reduces social cohesion between those who are masked, doing harm to the masked and unmasked alike.

Masks create difficulty bonding, learning, empathizing, and communicating. These are the trends of society and key features that distinguish a sociopath from a healthy person.

As previously pointed out, Denis Rancourt of the Ontario Civil Liberties Association writes:[1]

> "Covering the lower half of the face reduces the ability to communicate, interpret, and mimic the expressions of those with whom we interact. Positive emotions become less recognizable, and negative emotions are amplified. Emotional mimicry, contagion, and emotionality in general are reduced and (thereby) bonding between teachers and learners, group cohesion, and learning — of which emotions are a major driver."[2]

Masking is the exact behavior and produces the exact outcome that should not be wanted by anyone seeking to raise a healthy child. A healthy child is one with both a healthy body and healthy mind.

Will every child who wears a mask become a sociopath? Of course not.

Do we really need to wait 20 years to find out how many do?

All one-size-fits-all health approaches, whether they be voluntary or mandatory must be stopped now — masking being one among many.

Reason 91: Face Mask Peer Pressure Is So Great That Mask Wearing Is Encouraged Far Beyond The Point Of Harm To The Mask Wearer

Is wearing a face mask ideal?

No.

Is wearing a face mask effective?

No.

Is using a face mask safe?

No.

Recognizing all that, it should be clear that no face masks should ever be worn by anyone in the general public, either voluntarily or mandated: that is the ideal.

If one is to wear a face mask, it is worth noting that pressure to fit in, to be like others, to be part of the group, can be so extreme that it can cause one to ignore the very real signs of something being amiss in one's body. Long before those signs appear, something is amiss. Such is the nature of what scientists describe as "sub-threshold stimuli." People are harmed by toxins before the threshold for conscious detection is reached.

Kai Kisielinski, in an April 20, 2021 article entitled "Is a Mask That Covers the Mouth and Nose Free from Undesirable Side Effects in Everyday Use and Free of Potential Hazards?" writes:[1]

> "From a doctor's viewpoint, it may also be difficult to advise children and adults who, due to social pressure (to wear a mask) and the desire to feel they belong, suppress their own needs and concerns until the effects of masks have a noticeable negative impact on their health.[2] Nevertheless, the use of masks should be stopped immediately at the latest when shortness of breath, dizziness or vertigo occur.[3,4] From this aspect, it seems sensible for decision makers and authorities to provide information, to define instruction obligations and offer appropriate training for employers, teachers and other persons who have a supervisory or caregiving duty. Knowledge about first aid measures could also be refreshed and expanded accordingly in this regard."

The risk of peer pressure encouraging the wearing of face masks beyond the point of safety, is so potent that it is best to entirely eliminate the possibility of peer pressure by drawing a firm boundary. Never wear a face mask again for any reason. Never let your child be masked again for any reason.

By taking that approach, all peer pressure risk of wearing a face mask past the point of harm is confidently eliminated.

HARM TO THE HEAD

Reason 92: Face Masks Are Long Known To Cause Headaches

Masks cause headaches and a host of other side effects in those who wear them. Researchers have known that a long time.

In an April 20, 2021 article entitled "Is a Mask That Covers the Mouth and Nose Free from Undesirable Side Effects in Everyday Use and Free of Potential Hazards?"[1] for *International Journal of Environmental Research and Public Health*, Kai Kisielinski writes:

> "Initial headaches ($p < 0.05$) were experienced by up to 82% of 158, 21–35 year-old mask wearers in another study of N95 respiratory protection with one third (34%) experiencing headaches up to four times daily. Participants wore the mask for 18.3 days over a 30-day period with a mean of 5.9 hours per day."[2]

In this study 87% of participants had headaches and 34% had headaches four times each day. How could we force that on a person without expecting it to affect them, their cognition, and the quality of their work.

N-95 masks are not the same as surgical masks. The surgical mask results are troubling as well. Kisielinski points out a majority of surgical mask wearers suffer headaches as well:

> "Significantly increased headache ($p < 0.05$) could be observed not only for N95 but also for surgical masks in participants of another observational study of healthcare workers.[3]

> "In another study, the researchers classified 306 users with an average age of 43 years and wearing different types of masks, of whom 51% had an initial headache as a specific symptom related exclusively to increased surgical and N95 mask use (1 to 4 hours, $p = 0.008$)."[4]

What is going on that causes headaches? Kisielinski continues:

> "Researchers from Singapore were able to demonstrate in a trial involving 154 healthy N95 health service mask wearers that a significant increase in mask-induced blood carbon dioxide levels (measured by end-expiratory partial pressure of carbon dioxide $PETCO_2$) and a measurably greater vasodilatation with an increase in cerebral artery flow in the cere-

bri media resulted. This was associated with headaches in the trial group (p < 0.001).[5]

"According to the researchers, the aforementioned changes also contribute to headaches during the prolonged use of masks with a shift towards hypoxia and hypercapnia. Furthermore, stress and mechanical factors such as the irritation of cervical nerves in the neck and head area caused by the tight mask straps pressuring the nerve strands also contribute to headaches.[2]

"In the analysis of the primary studies, we were able to detect an association between the N95 mask and headaches. In six out of 10 studies, the significant headache appeared in conjunction with the N95 mask (60% of all studies)."

A majority of people report headaches in a mask. The impact to the person reaches far beyond a headache.

No one should be masked, least of all our children. No one performing a procedure on another should be masked, least of all those performing a procedure on a child.

No one in a mask should be around your child because of the communicational problems, but also because of the medical harm that could be done if that person is treating your child.

Reason 93: Face Masks Trigger Migraines

A portion of the population regularly suffers from headaches, some quite severe.

Face masks appear to exacerbate those headaches.

In the August 20, 2020 article "Review of scientific reports of harms caused by face masks," Dina Karvounides writes:[1]

> "Many common triggers such as dehydration, fasting, sleep problems, and stressors were discussed above. Here we highlight [computer] screen use and mask wearing as potential additional school-related triggers. ... Pressure created by the mask or its straps against various contact points on the face or scalp could trigger headache"

Migraine headaches are a subset of headaches, often more disabling and impactful upon cognition. For a face mask to both cause a migraine and to be safe to the wearer is not possible.

Reason 94: Face Masks Are So Bad For You That The Vast Majority Of Healthy People Get Headaches From Wearing Them

It is worth noting that headaches in face masks are not suffered just among the sick. They are suffered among the healthy too. How much more harmful of an impact, then, can be expected among the sick, children, and the elderly.

"Well, *I* do not get a headache from wearing a face mask," some may say. That indicates, for some that others have no reason to complain. However, absence of evidence is not evidence of absence. Keep wearing a face mask if you find it the right fit for you. One day you will likely come to regret that decision. Do not, however, force a face mask upon others.

Face masks should not be forced on others, no should other types of Personal Protective Equipment (PPE).

According to Jonathan J.Y. Ong, in the article "Headaches Associated With Personal Protective Equipment – A Cross-Sectional Study Among Frontline Healthcare Workers During Covid-19:"[1]

> "Most healthcare workers develop de novo PPE-associated headaches or exacerbation of their pre-existing headache disorders."

Breaking those numbers down further, study authors observed:

> "A total of 158 healthcare workers participated in the study. Majority [126/158 (77.8%)] were aged 21-35 years. Participants included nurses [102/158 (64.6%)], doctors [51/158 (32.3%)], and paramedical staff [5/158 (3.2%)]. Pre-existing primary headache diagnosis was present in about a third [46/158 (29.1%)] of respondents. Those based at the emergency department had higher average daily duration of combined PPE exposure compared to those working in isolation wards [7.0 (SD 2.2) vs 5.2 (SD 2.4) hours, P < .0001] or medical ICU [7.0 (SD 2.2) vs 2.2 (SD 0.41) hours, P < .0001]. Out of 158 respondents, 128 (81.0%) respondents developed de novo PPE-associated headaches. A pre-existing primary headache diagnosis (OR = 4.20, 95% CI 1.48-15.40; P = .030) and combined PPE usage for >4 hours per day (OR 3.91, 95% CI 1.35-11.31; P = .012) were independently associated with de novo PPE-associated

headaches. Since Covid-19 outbreak, 42/46 (91.3%) of respondents with pre-existing headache diagnosis either 'agreed' or 'strongly agreed' that the increased PPE usage had affected the control of their background headaches, which affected their level of work performance."

Many are harmed by face mask policies — both the wearer and those around the wearer are harmed. Face masks should not be forced upon anyone. They should instead be widely ridiculed in society.

The truth is, they are not "forced" on anyone. There are numerous ways around wearing a face mask and around having a face mask worn in front of you. You can skip to the end of the book or sign up at www.RealStevo.com to learn some of the techniques that work so well. What it really comes down to, though, is resolving to never wear a face mask again. It is also about figuring out how to live as unimpeded as possible while others slowly open their eyes to how nonsensical face mask policies are and themselves work up the courage to also resolve to never again wear a face mask.

Reason 95: Face Mask Wearing Causes Neurological Harm And Cognitive Impairment

A headache is so much more than a pain in the head. It is a symptom. It often indicates more severe problems.

Kai Kisielinski, in an April 20, 2021 article entitled "Is a Mask That Covers the Mouth and Nose Free from Undesirable Side Effects in Everyday Use and Free of Potential Hazards?"[1] for *International Journal of Environmental Research and Public Health*, writes:

> "In a scientific evaluation of syncope in the operating theater, 36 of 77 affected persons (47%) were associated with wearing a mask.[2] However, other factors could not be ruled out as contributory causes."

The author of the paper continue:

> "Physicians from New York studied the effects of wearing masks of the surgical-type mask and N95 among medical personnel in a sample of 343 participants (surveyed using standardized, anonymized questionnaires). Wearing the masks caused detectable physical adverse effects such as impaired cognition (24% of wearers) and headaches in 71.4% of the participants. Of these, 28% persisted and required medication. Headache occurred in 15.2% under 1 hour of wear, in 30.6% after 1 hour of wear and in 29.7% after 3 hours of wear. Thus, the effect intensified with increasing wearing time.[3]

> "Confusion, disorientation and even drowsiness (Likert scale questionnaire) and reduced motoric abilities (measured with a linear position transducer) with reduced reactivity and overall impaired performance (measured with the Roberge Subjective Symptoms during-Work Scale) as a result of mask use have also been documented in other studies.[3-8]

> "The scientists explain these neurological impairments with a mask-induced latent drop in blood gas oxygen levels O2 (towards hypoxia) or a latent increase in blood gas carbon dioxide levels CO_2 (towards hypercapnia).[8] In view of the scientific data, this connection also appears to be indisputable.[9-12]

"In a mask experiment from 2020, significant impaired thinking (p < 0.03) and impaired concentration (p < 0.02) were found for all mask types used (fabric, surgical and N95 masks) after only 100 minutes of wearing the mask.[6] The thought disorders correlated significantly with a drop in oxygen saturation (p < 0.001) during mask use."

To see a headache as a problem that can be handled with an aspirin ignores the root cause and the other symptoms likely to accompany a headache. A headache is a sign that something is wrong and needs addressing.

Because some in medicine are so myopic as to ignore the root cause of a problem, face masks are seen as some as "No big deal," and "Nothing a little aspirin cannot fix."

They harm the wearer.

They should not be worn.

Reason 96: Face Masks Make Headaches Worse And May Make Other Neurological Pathologies Such As Aneurysms And Tumors Worse

Beyond a headache, are additional neurological pathologies that may be made worse by a face mask.

Kai Kisielinski, in an April 20, 2021 article entitled "Is a Mask That Covers the Mouth and Nose Free from Undesirable Side Effects in Everyday Use and Free of Potential Hazards?" writes that more mask use leads to more headaches and other symptoms:[1]

> "In patients with headaches, a worsening of symptoms can be expected with prolonged mask use.[2-5] As a result of the increase in blood carbon dioxide (CO_2) when the mask is used, vasodilatation occurs in the central nervous system and the pulsation of the blood vessels decreases.[2] In this connection, it is also interesting to note radiological experiments that demonstrate an increase in brain volume under subthreshold, but still within normal limits of CO_2 increase in the blood by means of structural MRI. The blood carbon dioxide increase was produced in seven subjects via rebreathing with resulting median carbon dioxide concentration of 42 mmHg and an interquartile range of 39.44 mmHg, corresponding to only a subthreshold increase given the normal values of 32–45 mmHg. In the experiment, there was a significant increase in brain parenchymal volume measurable under increased arterial CO_2 levels ($p < 0.02$), with a concomitant decrease in CSF spaces ($p < 0.04$), entirely in accordance with the Monroe–Kelly doctrine, according to which the total volume within the skull always remains the same. The authors interpreted the increase in brain volume as an expression of an increase in blood volume due to a CO_2 increase-induced dilation of the cerebral vessels.[6] The consequences of such equally subthreshold carbon dioxide (CO_2) increases even under masks[7-13] are unclear for people with pathological changes inside the skull (aneurysms, tumors, etc.) with associated vascular changes[2] and brain volume shifts[6] especially due to longer exposure while wearing a mask, but could be of

great relevance due to the blood gas-related volume shifts that take place."

This research is by no means conclusive. It opens a door through which further researchers may choose to step. What is clear is that many aspects of face mask harm have not been well researched and are certainly not well understood. Face masks are, therefore, unable to be considered safe, least of all on your child.

Reason 97: What They Are Doing To Your Children Makes Your Children Stupider And Gives Your Children Learning Disabilities

We have each met stupid people. They could have been helped by a few extra IQ points.

Maybe that person had lead in his drinking water as a child, maybe his mother drank fluoridated water while he was in utero, maybe his mother smoked crack, maybe he was dropped on his head as a baby, or maybe genetically that is just how he was born.

Whatever the case, he has had a little bit of a harder life because he has gone through life with fewer intellectual resources.

Knowing that, what parent could possible want to sentence a child to a lower IQ? Certainly not me.

A Brown University study,[1] still awaiting peer review, says what so many observant parents and so many chapters of this book say: face masks, lockdowns, and social distancing appear to make kids a lot stupider, costing a child 21 IQ points, dropping them from a 100 point medium IQ to a 79 point medium IQ in this longitudinal study of 600 children.

Do I consider a single, not yet peer reviewed study to be the gospel truth? Certainly not. I think the premise is solid though, next to parental intuition, millennia of human experience, and the other several hundred pieces of research cited in this book.

Mask your child and your child will be stupider. Let others wear masks around your child and your child will be stupider. Socially distance and lockdown your child and your child will be stupider.

Do I know which of those components are worse than others? Not really, nor can I see how that is relevant at this point in time. If you love your kids, turn off the TV, quit believing the narrative, and get them back to normal as quickly as possible.

Treat the 2019-2020 Covid-19 season as the minor flu season that it was. Eventually, everyone else will catch up with you. If you participated in any of this, you can never give your child back the lost development you denied him over the past year, but you can prevent him from having to endure this psychosis for even one more moment.

HARM TO THE MIND

Reason 98: The Powerful Impact Of Despair

In 2017, for the first time since 1963, the life expectancy of Americans declined two years in a row. *The British Medical Journal* looked into a broader cause behind the decline: despair.[1]

Grace Donnelly in the article, "Here's why life expectancy in the US dropped again this year," published in *Fortune* on February 9, 2018, writes:[2]

> "Life expectancy in the US dropped for the second year in a row, according to the CDC's National Center for Health Statistics.

> "The new average life expectancy for Americans is 78.7 years, which puts the US behind other developed nations and 1.5 years lower than the Organisation for Economic Cooperation and Development (OECD) average life expectancy[3] of 80.3. The OECD is a group of developed countries[4] that includes Canada, Germany, Mexico, France, Japan, and the U.K.

> "A new study published in the BMJ journal[5] looked into a broader cause behind the decline: despair.

> "'We are seeing an alarming increase in deaths from substance abuse and despair,' said Steven Woolf, an associate professor of emergency medicine at Virginia Commonwealth University and co-author of the report.[6]

> "He added that the amount of the decrease in life expectancy is actually less alarming than the fact that addiction and a decline in the emotional wellbeing of Americans have been significant enough to drag down the country's average length of life.

> "The research points to the opioid epidemic, backing up a CDC report from last year[7] that linked the drop directly to a 21% increase in overdose deaths from the year before and cited a 137% increase in opioid-related deaths between 2000 and 2014.

> "The increase in deaths caused by drugs and alcohol, particularly among white Americans, is 'unclear, complex, and not explained by opioids alone,' according to Woolf.[8]

"On average, 115 people in the US die each day[9] from an opioid overdose, and six Americans per day are dying from alcohol abuse – the highest rate in 35 years,[10] according to federal data.

"The report also highlights a rise in the suicide rate, which increased 24% between 1999 and 2014,[11] as well as health conditions from diabetes to HIV/AIDS that are negatively impacting the lives of Americans.

"The authors of the study point out that the solutions to problems politicians recognize as detrimental to the quality of life in the US are often rejected[12] when it comes down to policy making, and it is American citizens who feel the impact of inaction.

"'The consequences are dire: not only more deaths and illness but also escalating healthcare costs, a sicker workforce, and a less competitive economy,' the authors wrote.[13] 'Future generations may pay the greatest price.'"

The impact of despair on those who wear a face mask must not be overlooked. By 2018, despair was seen as a leading factor in earlier death. Combined with the vast system of house arrest known as "lockdowns," school closures, event closures, venue closures, business closures, and general destabilization of daily life, face masks have been another painful, alienating factor in a society that was already having a hard time managing the significant despair felt by so many.

If these methods worked to protect people, perhaps we would have a reason to debate this topic, but we have been fooled. These methods do not work and were known not to work. The unsafe and ineffective face mask is just another intervention on a long list of interventions that have brought harm to people. Despair was already at a crisis state in America, the West, and the developed world. The days since the Ides of March 2020 have added to that.

While this trend precedes Covid-19, the powerful trend should not be ignored in understanding Covid-19. The general public, societal, and governmental leadership who are already caught in a great decline.

A healthy and free society would never have accepted the strange and senseless public health precautions of 2020 and beyond. No one who perceives their daily activity as vitally valuable to others would have accepted the declaration that they were now "non-essential."

Many signs point to you and I being in the midst of a society in collapse, with few realizing that is taking place.

This book and much of my other writing is on that topic. As minor as the face mask may be to some, it is a powerful symbol to you and others that you participate fully in the trend of society or that you stand resolutely against it.

Reason 99: Face Masks Are Psychologically Harmful For You

Beyond cognition, there is additional harm done to the mind and personal wellbeing by how face masks psychologically harm an individual: both the one wearing a face mask and individuals around a masked person, whether they be verbally interacting with the masked person or not.

Baruch Vainshelboim writes in "Face masks in the Covid-19 era: A health hypothesis:"[1]

> "Psychologically, wearing face mask fundamentally has negative effects on the wearer and the nearby person. Basic human-to-human connectivity through face expression is compromised and self-identity is somewhat eliminated.[2-4] These dehumanizing movements partially delete the uniqueness and individuality of person who wearing the face mask as well as the connected person.[4] Social connections and relationships are basic human needs, which innately inherited in all people, whereas reduced human-to-human connections are associated with poor mental and physical health."[5,6]

Vainshelboim ties face masks into a greater trend in so-called "social" technology, isolating people:

> "Despite escalation in technology and globalization that would presumably foster social connections, scientific findings show that people are becoming increasingly more socially isolated, and the prevalence of loneliness is increasing in last few decades.[5,7] Poor social connections are closely related to isolation and loneliness, considered significant health related risk factors."[5-8]

The social isolation and the sense of loneliness may even be lethal. Vainshelboim correlates social isolation with mortality:

> "A meta-analysis of 91 studies of about 400,000 people showed a 13% increased morality risk among people with low compare to high contact frequency.[8] Another meta-analysis of 148 prospective studies (308,849 participants) found that poor social relationships was associated with 50% increased mortality risk. People who were socially isolated or fell lonely had 45% and 40% increased mortality

risk, respectively. These findings were consistent across ages, sex, initial health status, cause of death and follow-up periods.[7] Importantly, the increased risk for mortality was found comparable to smoking and exceeding well-established risk factors such as obesity and physical inactivity.[7] An umbrella review of 40 systematic reviews including 10 meta-analyses demonstrated that compromised social relationships were associated with increased risk of all-cause mortality, depression, anxiety suicide, cancer and overall physical illness."[6]

Vainshelboim is not saying anything new here. He is saying what we already knew — a person who is perpetually isolated and lonely, has a lower quality of life and shorter life. Many intuitively realize that deep down. What Vainshelboim does is to tie this to masks as well, practically thumping every reader on the head and saying "PAY ATTENTION, YOU KNOW THIS ALREADY. WHAT YOU ARE DOING IS STUPID."

Vainshelboim goes beyond the harmful effects of loneliness and isolation on the individual and also digs into the effects of added physical stress on the body and mind:

"As described earlier, wearing face masks causing hypoxic and hypercapnic state that constantly challenges the normal homeostasis, and activates 'fight or flight' stress response, an important survival mechanism in the human body.[9-11] The acute stress response includes activation of nervous, endocrine, cardiovascular, and the immune systems.[2,12-14] These include activation of the limbic part of the brain, release stress hormones (adrenalin, neuro-adrenalin and cortisol), changes in blood flow distribution (vasodilation of peripheral blood vessels and vasoconstriction of visceral blood vessels) and activation of the immune system response (secretion of macrophages and natural killer cells)."[2,3]

That describes the harm on the wearer. Vainshelboim goes further, illustrating how the act of seeing someone else in a face mask causes psychological and physical harm to another as well.

"Encountering people who wearing face masks activates innate stress-fear emotion, which is fundamental to all humans in danger or life threating situations, such as death or unknown, unpredictable outcome. While acute stress response (seconds to minutes) is adaptive reaction to challenges and part of the survival mechanism, chronic and prolonged state of stress-fear is maladaptive and has detrimental effects on physical and mental health. The repeatedly or continuously activated stress-fear response causes the body to operate on survival mode, having sustained increase in blood pressure, pro-inflammatory state and immunosuppression."[2,3]

It is impossible to read Vainshelboim and continue to say that face masks do no harm. Another reason not to wear them, not to allow your children in them, and not to allow anyone around you or your children in them is that they do grievous psychological harm.

Reason 100: Face Mask Wearing Is Linked To Substantial Psychological Side Effects

Mask wearing is harmful on the mental health of those wearing them and likely harmful on the mental health of those surrounded by people wearing them.

Kai Kisielinski authored an April 20, 2021 article entitled "Is a Mask That Covers the Mouth and Nose Free from Undesirable Side Effects in Everyday Use and Free of Potential Hazards?"[1] Kisielinski describes senses of loss, deprivation, and interference stemming from mask wearing, along with impaired performance, impaired decision making, and change in behavior:

> "The mask also causes an impaired field of vision (especially affecting the ground and obstacles on the ground) and also presents an inhibition to habitual actions such as eating, drinking, touching, scratching and cleaning the otherwise uncovered part of the face, which is consciously and subconsciously perceived as a permanent disturbance, obstruction and restriction[2] Wearing masks, thus, entails a feeling of deprivation of freedom and loss of autonomy and self-determination, which can lead to suppressed anger and subconscious constant distraction, especially as the wearing of masks is mostly dictated and ordered by others.[3,4] These perceived interferences of integrity, self-determination and autonomy, coupled with discomfort, often contribute to substantial distraction and may ultimately be combined with the physiologically mask-related decline in psycho motoric abilities, reduced responsiveness and an overall impaired cognitive performance.

> "It leads to misjudging situations as well as delayed, incorrect and inappropriate behavior and a decline in the effectiveness of the mask wearer."[2,5-8]

When something is amiss with the head and face, ones wellbeing can be easily affected. Kisielinski continues:

> "The use of masks for several hours often causes further detectable adverse effects such as headaches, local acne, mask-associated skin irritation, itching, sensations of heat and dampness, impairments and discomfort predominantly affecting the head and face.[2,4,5,9-13] However, the head and

face are significant for wellbeing due to their large representation in the sensitive cerebral cortex (homunculus)."[2]

Fear and insecurity can be caused by mask wearing — in children, as well as in adults. Kisielinski points this out:

"According to a questionnaire survey, masks also frequently cause anxiety and psychovegetative stress reactions in children – as well as in adults — with an increase in psychosomatic and stress-related illnesses and depressive self-experience, reduced participation, social withdrawal and lowered health-related self-care.[14] Over 50% of the mask wearers studied had at least mild depressive feelings.[14]

Not only do the masks themselves induce fear and other psychological and physiological harm, but the media coverage and commentary from medical and public health professionals on the topic add to the fear. As Kisielinski writes here, this fear-inducing behavior creates "a social dynamic that seems partly unfounded from a medical and scientific point of view:"

"Additional fear-inducing and often exaggerated media coverage can further intensify this. A recent retrospective analysis of the general media in the context of the 2014 Ebola epidemic showed a scientific truth content of only 38% of all publicly published information.[15] Researchers classified a total of 28% of the information as provocative and polarizing and 42% as exaggerating risks. In addition, 72% of the media content aimed to stir up health-related negative feelings. The feeling of fear, combined with insecurity and the primal human need to belong,[16] causes a social dynamic that seems partly unfounded from a medical and scientific point of view."

This is not entirely lost on public health officials either, that the mask is so tied to one's psychological wellbeing and sense of belonging. That detail is used to pressure compliance. As Kisielinski shows:

"The mask, which originally served purely hygienic purpose, has been transformed into a symbol of conformity and pseudo-solidarity. The WHO, for example, lists the advantages of the use of masks by healthy people in public to include a potentially reduced stigmatization of mask wearers, a sense of contribution to preventing the spread of the virus and a reminder to comply with other measures."[17]

Here, a mere tip of the iceberg is shown by the wearing of a face mask. The psychological harm is poorly understood and is likely considerable.

Reason 101: Face Mask Wearing Leads To Panic Attacks And Exacerbates Significant Other Psychiatric Conditions

Panic attacks and other psychiatric conditions can be triggered by face masks.

Kai Kisielinski wrote an April 20, 2021 article entitled "Is a Mask That Covers the Mouth and Nose Free from Undesirable Side Effects in Everyday Use and Free of Potential Hazards?" Panic attacks are understandably a problem exacerbated by face masks, both psychologically and physically. Kisielinski writes:[1]

> "Masks can cause increased rebreathing with an accumulation of carbon dioxide in the wearer due to increased dead space volume,[2-5] with often statistically significant measurable elevated blood carbon dioxide (CO_2) levels in sufferers.[6-18] However, changes that lead to hypercapnia are known to trigger panic attacks.[19,20] This makes the significantly measurable increase in CO_2 caused by wearing a mask clinically relevant."

Relatively minor changes in carbon dioxide in the body can trigger panic attacks. As Kisielinski points out:

> "Interestingly, breath provocation tests by inhaling CO_2 are used to differentiate anxiety states in panic disorders and premenstrual dysphoria from other psychiatric clinical pictures. Here, absolute concentrations of 5% CO_2 already suffice to trigger panic reactions within 15–16 minutes.[19] The normal exhaled air content of CO_2 is about 4%.

> "It is obvious from experimental studies on masked subjects that concentration changes in the respiratory gases in the above-mentioned range with values above 4% could occur during rebreathing with prolonged mask use.[4,13]

> "The activation of the locus coeruleus by CO_2 is used to generate panic reactions via respiratory gases.[20,21] This is because the locus coeruleus is an important part of the system of vegetative noradrenergic neurons, a control center in the brainstem, which reacts to an appropriate stimulus and changes in the gas concentrations in the blood by releasing the stress hormone noradrenaline."[20]

Further psychiatric harm can be triggered from the same physical circumstances described here. Kisielinski writes:

"From the physiological, neurological and psychological side effects and dangers described above (Sections 3.1, 3.3 and 3.4), additional problems can be derived for the use of masks in psychiatric cases. People undergoing treatment for dementia, paranoid schizophrenia, personality disorders with anxiety and panic attacks, but also panic disorders with claustrophobic components, are difficult to reconcile with a mask requirement, because even small increases in CO_2 can cause and intensify panic attacks."[19-22]

Furthermore, this can be very difficult on dementia patients and others who have no concept of what a Covid-19 protection measure is. Kisielinski writes:

"According to a psychiatric study, patients with moderate to severe dementia have no understanding of Covid-19 protection measures and have to be persuaded to wear masks constantly.[23]

"According to a comparative study, patients with schizophrenia have a lower acceptance of mask-wearing (54.9% agreement) than ordinary practice patients (61.6%).[24] The extent to which mask-wearing can lead to an exacerbation of schizophrenia symptoms has not yet been researched in detail.

"When wearing masks, confusion, impaired thinking, disorientation (standardized recording via special rating and Likert scales, $p < 0.05$) and in some cases a decrease in maximum speed and reaction time (measured with the linear-position transducer, $p < 0.05$) were observed.[9,25-30] Psychotropic drugs reduce psycho-motoric functions in psychiatric patients. This can become clinically relevant especially with regard to the further reduced ability to react and the additional increased susceptibility to accidents of such patients when wearing masks."

The CDC even recognizes this problem in their own guidelines, but downplays the seriousness of how many are affected. Kisielinski writes:

"In order to avoid an unintentional CO_2-triggered anesthesia,[28] fixed and medically sedated patients, without the possibility of continuous monitoring, should not be masked according to the criteria of the Centers for Disease Control and Prevention, USA (CDC). This is because of the possible CO_2 retention described above, as there is a risk of unconsciousness, aspiration and asphyxia."[2,3,5,27,31,32]

The healthy and the sick alike are harmed by mask wearing, providing yet another example of why face masks should not be worn by the general public — least of all by your child.

Reason 102: Face Masks Cause Unstudied Psychological Harm To Children

Based on our knowledge of psychology to date, face masks likely have tremendous psychological impacts upon children and upon the population as a whole.

This topic has been very lightly studied, a shocking detail given the tremendous amount of research in child psychology often touted as being so necessary for the wellbeing of children.

Major researchers in child psychology have been surprisingly quiet and obedient in what has been a travesty visited upon children.

You will forever know who in child psychology is worth reading and who is not worth the time to even consider based on whether or not they were vocal about the need for research on face masks in 2020 and beyond.

As Denis Rancourt points out in "Review of scientific reports of harms caused by face masks:"[1]

> "One research focus area that appears to be entirely lacking, in examining the harms of masks, is the broad psychological (and therefore social) impact of mandatory masking policies applied to the general population."

Denis Rancourt continues:

> "There can be little doubt that forced masking of the general population has a significant potential to deteriorate the three fundamental psychological needs of the individual: autonomy, competence, and relatedness. This harm to individuals and the societal implications have not been studied. The impact may be gargantuan.

> "Only infants and school children have so far been considered using the perspective of psychological and developmental impact (as described below).

> "The 11 August 2020 Commentary of Scheid et al. is not helpful, because it incorrectly disregards physiological impacts and examines psychology solely from the perspective of mask compliance.[2]

> "When considering whether a world of masked adults and children, at a crucial period in a baby's or child's life, can have long-term detrimental psychological and development

impact, I propose that the following hierarchical sequence of thought experiments is useful:

- "Would babies and children entirely raised by mechanical robots be adversely affected?
- "Would babies and children entirely raised by masked adults, and themselves forced to be masked beyond two years of age, be adversely affected?
- "What periods, durations and circumstances of masking, distancing and shielding could have long-term psychological or developmental negative consequences?"

Did they use that platform to stand in defense of children? Did they stay silent? In those two simple questions, so much about the character of a person in that position can be answered.

We all can be grateful too the brave researchers cited in this book who stuck their necks out to stand up for children and adults alike in the face of bad science and tyrannical masking orders.

Ultimately, however, it comes down to your ability to say "No!" in your own life and to never wear a face mask again and to never mask your child again — no matter what the penalty is. Once you know the truth about how harmful masks are, it becomes hard to justify doing otherwise.

EXERCISE IN FACE MASKS HARMS BOTH THE HEALTHY AND SICK

Reason 103: CDC And WHO Advise Against Wearing Face Masks During Exercise

Face masks can be dangerous to exercise in, which is why exercising in them is not recommended. Wearing masks can be dangerous if light activity and this is especially true during vigorous activity.

Kai Kisielinski, in an April 20, 2021 article entitled "Is a Mask That Covers the Mouth and Nose Free from Undesirable Side Effects in Everyday Use and Free of Potential Hazards?" writes:[1]

> "These facts are an indication that the use of masks also triggers the effects described above leading to hypoxia and hypercapnia in sports. Accordingly, the WHO and Centers for Disease Control and Prevention (CDC) advise against wearing masks during physical exercise."[2,3]

The CDC tackles this topic in an article entitled "Guidance for Wearing Masks:"[4]

> "People should not wear masks while engaged in activities that may cause the mask to become wet, like when swimming at the beach or pool.
>
> "People who are engaged in high intensity activities, like running, may not be able to wear a mask if it causes difficulty breathing."

This guidance was updated on April 19, 2021:

> "Masks should always be used in public settings, but if you are unable to wear a mask because of difficulty breathing during high intensity activities, choose a location with greater ventilation and air exchange (for instance, outdoors versus indoors) and where you can keep at least 6 feet of distance from others during the activity. If such a location is not available, opt for low-intensity activities such as walking or yoga that allow for mask wearing.
>
> "If you are able to wear a mask, remove your mask if it gets moist from sweat and replace it with a clean mask.
>
> "Opt for an activity that does not require using mouth guards or helmets. Wearing a mask with these types of protective equipment is not safe if it makes it hard to breathe.

"Supervise children who are wearing a mask while playing sports."

The World Health Organization (WHO) tackles it in a May 5, 2021 article entitled "Coronavirus disease (Covid-19) advice for the public: Myth busters," saying:

"FACT: People should NOT wear masks while exercising.

"People should NOT wear masks when exercising, as masks may reduce the ability to breathe comfortably.

"Sweat can make the mask become wet more quickly which makes it difficult to breathe and promotes the growth of microorganisms. The important preventive measure during exercise is to maintain physical distance of at least one meter from others."

No one should be exercising in a face mask. Though they use couched language, even the CDC and the WHO say that masks should not be worn during exercise.

Reason 104: Face Masks Are Dangerous When Worn During Exercise

Oxygen and carbon dioxide levels are drastically affected by mask wearing.

Kai Kisielinski, in an April 20, 2021 article entitled "Is a Mask That Covers the Mouth and Nose Free from Undesirable Side Effects in Everyday Use and Free of Potential Hazards?" writes:[1]

> "In an interesting endurance study with eight middle-aged subjects (19–66), the gas content for O_2 and CO_2 under the masks was determined before and after exercise. Even at rest, the oxygen availability under the masks was 13% lower than without the masks and the carbon dioxide (CO_2) concentration was 30 times higher. Under stress (Ruffier test), the oxygen concentration (% O_2) below the mask dropped significantly by a further 3.7%, while the carbon dioxide concentration (% CO_2) increased significantly by a further 20% (statistically significant with $p < 0.001$). Correspondingly, the oxygen saturation of the blood (SpO_2) of the test persons also decreased significantly from 97.6 to 92.1% ($p < 0.02$).[2]

> "The drop in the oxygen saturation value (SpO_2) to 92%, clearly below the normal limit of 95%, is to be classified as clinically relevant and detrimental to health."

This is another reason no one should be exercising in a face mask — doing so may be "clinically relevant and detrimental to health."

Reason 105: Exercising In
A Face Mask Will Hurt You

Exercising in a face mask harms the body beyond short-term carbon dioxide and oxygen levels.

In the *Medical Hypotheses* journal, "Exercise with face mask; Are we handling a devil's sword? — A physiological hypothesis," Baskaran Chandrasekaran and Shifra Fernandes write:[1]

> "Exercising with face masks may reduce available oxygen and increase air trapping preventing substantial carbon dioxide exchange. The hypercapnic hypoxia may potentially increase acidic environment, cardiac overload, anaerobic metabolism and renal overload, which may substantially aggravate the underlying pathology of established chronic diseases."

Face masks are already harmful to the wearer. They appear to be made more harmful by exercise. No one, especially not a child, should be exercising in a face mask.

This is true no matter how insistent someone else is that such masks be worn. Pushy behavior from those who wish to sweep a topic under the rug does not make a truth any less true.

Reason 106: Exercising With A Face Mask May *Increase* Infection Rates

Not only is a face mask not helpful in preventing the spread of a respiratory virus, exercising in a face mask may actually *increase* infection rates.

In the *Medical Hypotheses* article, "Exercise with face mask; Are we handling a devil's sword? — A physiological hypothesis," Baskaran Chandrasekaran and Shifra Fernandes write:[1]

> "Though, moderate exercise, in the long run, is found to increase natural killer cell count and downregulate inflammatory factors such as tumor necrosis factors, acute bouts of vigorous exercise over a while may influence these changes negatively. Exercising with face masks induces an acidic environment, and thus mobility of hypoxic natural killer cells to the target cells would be affected, aggravating the chances of infection during the pandemic. A further change in humidity and temperature in the upper airway causes immotile cilia syndrome predisposing individuals to lower respiratory tract infections by deep seeding of oropharyngeal flora"[2]

Here we have another reason face masks should not be worn — not at rest and not during physical exertion, not by you and not by your child. Doing so may increase your risk of infection.

Reason 107: Even Activity As Simple As Walking Is Made Measurably Harder By A Face Mask, Even Among Healthy People

Exercise and other heavy physical exertion is made harder in a face mask, but so is light activity such as walking. This is measurably true, even if some people dismiss this fact as "no big deal."

Kai Kisielinski authored an April 20, 2021 article entitled "Is a Mask That Covers the Mouth and Nose Free from Undesirable Side Effects in Everyday Use and Free of Potential Hazards?" In it Kisielinski writes:[1]

"As early as 2012, an experiment showed that walking in the 20 masked subjects compared to the identical activity without masks significantly increased heart rates (average +9.4 beats per minute, $p < 0.001$) and breathing rates ($p < 0.02$). These physiological changes were accompanied by transcutaneous significantly measurable increased transcutaneous carbon dioxide ($PtcCO_2$) levels ($p < 0.0006$) as well as respiratory difficulties in the mask wearers compared to the control group.[2]

"In a recent experimental comparative study from 2020, 12 healthy volunteers under surgical masks as well as under N95 masks experienced measurable impairments in the measured lung function parameters as well as cardiopulmonary capacity (lower maximum blood lactate response) during moderate to heavy physical exertion compared to exertion without masks ($p < 0.001$).[3] The mask-induced increased airway resistance led to increased respiratory work with increased oxygen consumption and demand, both of the respiratory muscles and the heart. Breathing was significantly impeded ($p < 0.001$) and participants reported mild pain. The scientists concluded from their results that the cardiac compensation of the pulmonary, mask-induced restrictions, which still functioned in healthy people, was probably no longer possible in patients with reduced cardiac output."[3]

Light activity is harder in cloth masks as well. Kisielinski writes:

"In another recent study, researchers tested fabric masks (community masks), surgical masks and FFP2/N95 masks

268

in 26 healthy people during exercise on a cycle ergometer. All masks also showed a measurable carbon dioxide (CO_2) retention ($PtcCO_2$) (statistically significant with $p < 0.001$) and, for N95 masks, a decrease in the oxygen saturation value SpO_2 (statistically significant at 75 and 100 W with $p < 0.02$ and $p < 0.005$, respectively). The clinical relevance of these changes was shown in an increase in breathing frequency with fabric masks ($p < 0.04$) as well as in the occurrence of the previously described mask specific complaints such as a feeling of heat, shortness of breath and headaches. The stress perception was recorded on a Borg scale from 1 to 20. During physical exertion under an N95 mask, the group with masks showed a significant increase in the feeling of exhaustion compared to the group without with 14.6 versus 11.9 on the scale of 20. During the exposure, 14 of the 24 subjects wearing masks complained of shortness of breath (58%), four of headaches and two of a feeling of heat. Most of the complaints concerned FFP2 masks (72%)"

With even basic activity like walking made harder with a face mask, we have yet another example of why not to put on a face mask, and why not to put a face mask on your child.

Reason 108: Exercising In
A Face Mask Harms The Sick

Healthy people may not always notice the stress on the body of wearing a face mask. Sick individuals may be more likely to notice the stress and may even have underlying conditions aggravated.

In the *Medical Hypotheses* article, "Exercise with face mask; Are we handling a devil's sword? — A physiological hypothesis," Baskaran Chandrasekaran and Shifra Fernandes write:[1]

> "Increased cardiorespiratory stress. The reduced availability of O_2 and CO_2 would increase the heart rate and blood pressure exponentially even at low workloads. This physiological alteration may increase aortic pressure and left ventricular pressures, leading to an upsurge of cardiac overload and coronary demand.[2] Further increased respiratory load against the 'valve breathing,' leads to increased respiratory muscle load and pulmonary artery pressure, in turn, adding to the cardiac overload. These changes may be subtle in healthy individuals during exercise. Still, in persons with established chronic illness, these changes may aggravate the underlying pathophysiology, leading to hospitalization or increased use of medication."

It is worth noting that exercise mimics other types of physiological stress. Face masks are, therefore, not just harmful during exercise, but any physiological stress.

The harm of face mask wearing on the healthy and sick alike during time of exercise and other physiological stress is another reason not to wear a face mask or put one on a child.

Reason 109: N95 Wearing Hurts The Sick

The harm done to a dialysis patient by the wearing of an N95 respirator is significant and can be lethal to some who are critically ill. As the Association of American Physicians and Surgeons write:[1]

> "A 2004 observational study of end stage renal disease patients during dialysis for 4 hours, 39 patients, mean age, 57 years. 70% had decreased PaO2 (from 100 to 92); 19% had hypoxemia (PaO2 <70); all patients had increased respiratory rate 16 to 18; chest discomfort (3 baseline patients to 11 patients); respiratory distress (1 baseline patient to 17 patients)."[2,3]

This data comes from a study entitled "The physiological impact of wearing an N95 mask during hemodialysis as a precaution against SARS in patients with end-stage renal disease."

N95 masks can be life threatening to some who are critically ill. The AAPS report continues:

> "Stanford engineers discovered that N95 masks cause a reduction in O2 intake so significant that it can be life threatening to someone [with] lung disease or respiratory distress.

> "Stanford engineers estimated that N95 masks cause a 5% to 20% reduction in O2 intake. This can cause dizziness and lightheadedness. This can be life-threatening for someone with lung disease or with respiratory distress."[4]

Face mask wearing is harmful for the healthy and sick. N95 wearing is even more harmful for the healthy and sick. Not only should a face mask never be forced onto your child, an N95 mask should not either.

Reason 110: Simple Activity Is Made Measurably Harder By Mask Wearing In Unwell People

Much evidence exists on the harmfulness of N95 masks on both the healthy and infirm.

Kai Kisielinski, in an April 20, 2021 article entitled "Is a Mask That Covers the Mouth and Nose Free from Undesirable Side Effects in Everyday Use and Free of Potential Hazards?" writes:[1]

> "In an observational study of ten 20 to 50 year-old nurses wearing N95 masks during their shift work, side effects such as breathing difficulties ("I cannot breathe"), feelings of exhaustion, headache ($p < 0.001$), drowsiness ($p < 0.001$) and a decrease in oxygen saturation SpO2 ($p < 0.05$) as well as an increase in heart rate ($p < 0.001$) were statistically significant in association with an increase in obesity (BMI).[2] The occurrence of symptoms under masks was also associated with older age (statistically significant correlation of fatigue and drowsiness with $p < 0.01$ each, nausea with $p < 0.05$, an increase in blood pressure with $p < 0.01$, headache with $p < 0.05$, breathing difficulties with $p < 0.001$)."[2]

N95 masks are hard on patients with COPD as well. Kisielinski writes:

> "In an intervention study involving 97 patients with advanced chronic obstructive pulmonary disease (COPD) the respiratory rate, oxygen saturation and exhaled carbon dioxide equivalents (capnometry) changed unfavorably and significantly after the use of N95 masks (FFP2 equivalent) with an initial 10-minute rest and subsequent 6-minute walking. Seven patients discontinued the experiment due to serious complaints with a decrease in the oxygen saturation value SpO2 and a pathological carbon dioxide (CO_2) retention as well as increased end-expiratory partial pressure of carbon dioxide ($PETCO_2$).[3] In two patients, the $PETCO_2$ exceeded the normal limits and reached values of >50 mmHg. An FEV1 < 30% and a modified Medical Research Council (mMRC) Dyspnea Scale Score of $\geq$3, both indicators of advanced COPD, correlated with mask intolerance overall in this study.

"The most common symptom under mask was breathless-ness at 86%. In the dropouts of the study, dizziness (57%) and headaches were also often recorded. In the mask-tolerant COPD patients, significant increases in heart rate, respiratory rate and end-expiratory carbon dioxide partial pressure $PETCO_2$ could be objectified even at rest, after on-ly 10 minutes of mask-wearing ($p < 0.001$), accompanied by a decrease in oxygen saturation SpO_2 ($p < 0.001$).[3] The results of this study with an evidence level IIa are indicative for COPD mask wearers."

Not just N95 respirators, face masks are also harmful to COPD suffer-ers. Kisielinski writes:

"In another retrospective comparative study on COPD and surgical masks, examiners were able to demonstrate statisti-cally an increase in arterial partial pressure of carbon diox-ide ($PaCO_2$) of approximately +8 mmHg ($p < 0.005$) and a concomitant mask-related increase in systolic blood pres-sure of +11 mmHg ($p < 0.02$).[4] This increase is relevant in hypertensive patients, but also in healthy people with bor-derline blood pressure values as pathological value range triggered by mask-wearing can be induced. In 39 hemodial-ysis patients with end-stage renal disease, a type N95 mask (FFP2 equivalent) caused a significant drop in blood oxy-gen partial pressure (PaO2) in 70% of patients at rest (on hemodialysis) within only 4 hours ($p = 0.006$). Despite a compensatory increased respiratory rate ($p < 0.001$), ma-laise with chest pain occurred ($p < 0.001$) and even resulted in hypoxemia (drop in oxygen below the normal limit) in 19% of the subjects.[5]

"The researchers concluded from their findings that elderly or patients with reduced cardiopulmonary function have a higher risk of developing a severe respiratory failure while wearing a mask.[5]

"In a review paper on the risks and benefits of masks worn during the Covid-19 crisis, other authors provide an equally critical assessment of mandatory mask use for pa-tients with pneumonia, both with and without Covid-19 pneumonia disease."[6]

Both N95 respirators and face masks are dangerous to the critically ill. Face masks are not safe and effective. Face masks are unsafe to the healthy and especially to the critically ill.

Reason 111: The Overweight, Those With COPD, Lung Disease, Cardiac Disease, Pregnant Women, And Stroke Patients Must Be Particularly Cautious Around Face Masks

There is a narrative that the sick should wear face masks for their safety. That is not accurate. The sick are more vulnerable to external threats to their bodies — face masks included.

The healthy need to be cautious around face masks, because of the serious harm that can be done by wearing a face mask. Those who are ill need to be even more cautious.

In an April 20, 2021 article entitled "Is a Mask That Covers the Mouth and Nose Free from Undesirable Side Effects in Everyday Use and Free of Potential Hazards?"[1] Kai Kisielinski identifies an important set of details lost in the 2020 and 2021 frenzy to mask everyone:

> "Elderly, high-risk patients with lung disease, cardiac patients, pregnant women or stroke patients are advised to consult a physician to discuss the safety of an N95 mask as their lung volume or cardiopulmonary performance may be reduced.[2] A correlation between age and the occurrence of the aforementioned symptoms while wearing a mask has been statistically proven.[3] Patients with reduced cardiopulmonary function are at increased risk of developing serious respiratory failure with mask use according to the referenced literature.[4] Without the possibility of continuous medical monitoring, it can be concluded that they should not wear masks without close monitoring. The American Asthma and Allergy Society has already advised caution in the use of masks with regard to the Covid-19 pandemic for people with moderate and severe lung disease.[5] Since the severely overweight, sleep apnea patients and overlap-COPD sufferers are known to be prone to hypercapnia, they also represent a risk group for serious adverse health effects under extensive mask use.[6] This is because the potential of masks to produce CO_2 retention may not only have a disruptive effect on the blood gases and respiratory physiology of sufferers, but may also lead to further serious adverse health effects in the long-term. Interestingly, in an animal experiment an increase in CO_2 with hypercapnia

leads to contraction of smooth airway muscles with constriction of bronchi.[7] This effect could explain the observed pulmonary decompensations of patients with lung disease under masks."[2,4]

Nine groups of people are here mentioned, constituting large percentages of society, yet the narrative persist that masks are mandatory, safe, and effective. To the savvy person none of these are true. In fact, masks are optional, unsafe, and ineffective.

Reason 112: Japanese Government Warns Face Masks May Cause Heatstroke

The Japanese government advises people not to wear masks outdoors specifically because of the risk of the body overheating in a face mask and being unable to regulate as well. Have you ever heard anyone in the United States government or media make such a claim? If not, you may want to ask yourself why they have not, and what that says about them. You may also want to ask that of them, but most importantly you should take this chapter to heart and seek to protect you and your loved ones from face masks, face mask mandates, and other awful advice given by authority figures that the public is assured can be trusted.

In the article "Japan gov't asks people to take off masks outdoors to avoid heatstroke, keep 2m apart," dated May 27, 2020, Mayumi Nobuta writes:

"TOKYO — The Japanese environment and health ministries on May 26 released a guide calling on people to keep their masks off outside to avoid heatstroke in hot, humid weather, while keeping at least 2 meters from others to lessen the chance of infection with the novel coronavirus.

"According to the Ministry of Environment, the danger of heatstroke increases when wearing a mask as the heart and respiratory rates rise and that puts stress on the body. The guide also recommends people control indoor humidity with ventilation fans or opening windows, and to hydrate frequently." [1]

Face masks make it easy to get heatstroke. Face masks also make it harder for a wearer to recognize the feeling of being thirsty. In the May 19, 2020 article "Wearing masks in summer can lead to heatstroke; Japan doctors urge self-hydration," Shinji Kurokawa writes:

"A group of doctors aiming to reduce the number of heatstroke patients is currently spreading awareness about the hidden stages of dehydration leading to severe symptoms, before the arrival of summer. The group points out the danger of wearing a mask in summer, such as 'Heat is more likely to amass inside the body,' and 'As the inside of the mask becomes damper and more humid, you are less likely to feel signs of thirst.' The doctors warn that people may become dehydrated without being aware of it, leading to higher risks of heatstroke.

"The doctor group also calls for people to drink more water than usual as a preventative measure. They advise against taking drinks containing caffeine to stay hydrated, as caffeine is a diuretic, increasing urinary output. In addition, the group stresses the importance of regularly doing light indoor exercises or other forms of exercise during this relatively cool season, in order to practice sweating and developing a body that can lower its temperature by perspiring.

"Masuji Hattori, a pediatrician at Hyogo College of Medicine and head of the group, commented, 'Heatstroke patients being sent to hospitals in ambulances risk placing an increased burden on the medical field already strained over the novel coronavirus. Heatstroke is an illness that can be totally avoided if proper precautions are taken. We would like for each individual to make serious efforts to take such measures.'" [2]

If wearing a face mask helps heat to amass inside the body and causes people not to be able to feel thirst, one sensible and simple measure that can be taken to prevent a heatstroke is to not wear a face mask.

Reason 113: Face Mask Fatalities In Kids

In the May 8, 2020 article "After Multiple Deaths, Officials Call for No Masks in Gym Class" for *Sixth Tone,* Zhang Wanqing writes:[1]

"Several education bureaus in China are rethinking Covid-19 control policies after three students died running in masks at school, *The Beijing News* reported Friday.

"Bureaus in the eastern city of Xiamen, the southern province of Hainan, and the central city of Changsha have issued notices that either discourage schools from requiring students to wear masks during gym class or prohibit the facial accessories during exercise outright.

"'In light of the recent sudden deaths of students due to running in masks ... students should stay at least 1 meter apart and not wear masks during physical education (PE) class,' Hainan's education bureau said.

"In late April, just after many schools across China reopened following months of closure due to the Covid-19 pandemic, a student from a middle school in Zhoukou, a city in the central Henan province, died after running in PE class while wearing a mask.

"'The death certificate issued by the hospital said 'sudden death,' Li Jian, the father of the deceased child, told domestic publication *Health Times*. 'I still did not understand the cause of the sudden death, but I suspected it was from running in a mask...It was sunny that afternoon, the temperature was about 20 degrees Celsius (68 degrees Fahrenheit). How could it be comfortable to run in a mask?'

"The same month, two more students died under similar circumstances in the cities of Wenzhou and Changsha."

A similar situation took place in Japan. In a May 28, 2021 article "Fifth-grader in Osaka dies after outdoor PE class, may have been wearing mask," Masaki Takahashi writes:[2]

"OSAKA — A fifth-grader at a municipal elementary school in the city of Takatsuki, Osaka Prefecture, collapsed during a February physical education class and later died in hospital, it has been learned.

"It is possible the student was wearing a mask for corona-virus prevention at the time. Although the Takatsuki Municipal Board of Education said there is no known causal relationship between the mask and the child's death, it urged all its elementary and junior high schools to thoroughly take care of students' health.

"According to the city education board, the child suddenly collapsed while running on school grounds outside at around 9:05 a.m. on Feb. 18. The teacher in charge and others took them to the school nurse's office and called an ambulance. The child was taken to hospital, but died shortly after. It is believed the child was wearing a mask before they started running, but when the teacher rushed to the scene, the child's mask was hanging over their chin.

"The city education board's guidelines do not require students to wear masks during PE, but allow students to if they wish. The board says the class was conducted in accordance with the guidelines."

These are public health problems with justifiable cause for concern. Millions of children in the United States were masked at play after the Ides of March 2020 and continue to be. Do parents not deserve a fully transparent conversation on the three deaths mentioned above? The media will not allow that, social media will not allow that, public health officials will not allow that.

Instead, we are left with a situation in which events, such as these occurring in the United States, and they almost certainly have, are quietly swepted under the rug. We are told that there is nothing to see here and to move along.

Obediently, some people do. You and I do not have to be that type of person. Rather than commiting to obey illegitimate authority, we can commit to a search for the truth.

Reason 114: Exercise With Face Masks Can Be Lethal

There have been reports of sudden cardiac death while exercising in a face mask.

Did face masks cause the death?

Did face masks trigger the death?

Are deaths while exercising totally unrelated to a face mask?

These questions should have been answered before a single of our precious children were told to compete in a mask, made to take gym class in a mask, or forced to go through even one minute of the day in a mask.

Whether it be a high school long distance runner or an obese, middle-aged maskhole winded from climbing his structure up to the sidewalk over a 6 inch curb, the effort it takes to breathe through a face mask while one's heart rate is elevated is readily apparent.

Face masks simply should not be worn by those exerting effort.

Reason 115: Face Mask Wearing Has The Opposite Effect Of The Health-Promoting Deep Breathing Encouraged In Prayer, Meditation, And Holistic Healing

So much importance is placed on taking a deep breath. Air is so important to us that we cannot live minutes without it. People make careers out of helping others breathe better. Whether it be pray, meditating, or holistic healing — the necessity of deep breathing is recognized. Even in allopathic medicine, this is recognized to a degree.

Putting on a face mask is the exact opposite of all that. It creates resistance to that. It creates obstruction to that. It is entirely counter to so much of what we know is important about breathing.

In an April 20, 2021 article entitled "Is a Mask That Covers the Mouth and Nose Free from Undesirable Side Effects in Everyday Use and Free of Potential Hazards?"[1] Kai Kisielinski writes:

> "Additionally important is the connection of breathing with the influence on other bodily functions,[2,3] including the psyche with the generation of positive emotions and drive.[4] The latest findings from neuro-psychobiological research indicate that respiration is not only a function regulated by physical variables to control them (feedback mechanism), but rather independently influences higher-level brain centers and, thus, also helps to shape psychological and other bodily functions and reactions.[4-6]

> "Since masks impede the wearer's breathing and accelerate it, they work completely against the principles of health-promoting breathing[2,3] used in holistic medicine and yoga. According to recent research, undisturbed breathing is essential for happiness and healthy drive,[5,7] but masks work against this."

Mask wearing is contrary to so many good principles around breathing. This is another of the many examples of how face masks are harmful to you and should not be worn — not by you and certainly not by your child.

SURGEONS, HEALTH WORKERS, DRIVERS, AND CONFLICTED DOCTORS

Reason 116: Surgical Face Masks Were Made For Surgery And Might Not Even Work For That

Some people play know-it-all and say "Surgical masks are only supposed to be used by surgeons in surgery, not by the general public."

The evidence agrees, surgical masks should not be used by the general public, least of all children.

However, in speaking this truth, some people perpetuate a lie that surgical masks make sense even among surgeons.

It is likely they do not.

Surgical masks may not even work in a surgical setting. They may even make that setting more dangerous for a patient.

Consequently, a lesson we can take from this is that it is good to only say things that you know to be true. Something I know to be true is that face masks are unsafe for children and ineffective at preventing the spread of a respiratory virus.

A 2015 Cochrane Library review entitled "Disposable surgical face masks for preventing surgical wound infection in clean surgery"[1] determined:

"That wearing a face mask during surgery neither increases nor decreases the number of wound infections occurring after surgery. We conclude that there is no clear evidence that wearing disposable face masks affects the likelihood of wound infections developing after surgery."

Those authors write:

"Surgeons and nurses performing clean surgery wear disposable face masks. The purpose of face masks is thought to be two-fold: to prevent the passage of germs from the surgeon's nose and mouth into the patient's wound and to protect the surgeon's face from sprays and splashes from the patient. Face masks are thought to make wound infections after surgery less likely. However, incorrectly worn masks may increase the likelihood of the wound getting contaminated with germs. We wanted to discover whether wearing a face mask during surgery makes infections of the wound more likely after the operation."

Far from the use of face masks being proven safe and effective, even in the surgical suite — their intended and traditional use — review authors conclude:

> "More research in this field is needed before making further conclusions about the use of face masks in surgery."

After decades of face mask wearing by surgeons, the practice is still unable to be shown to be anything but tradition and superstition. Face mask wearing, even among surgeons, is simply not based in data or evidence.

Far from relying on the scientific method to dispassionately prove or disprove a claim, the wearing of face masks is more scientism, an appeal to authority, the most popular logical fallacy of 2020.

Reason 117: Face Masks Cause Medical Care To Be Worse For Children

Prior to Covid-19, masked doctors routinely removed their face masks when talking to a patient, because they realized that they were able to connect better with a patient, and it allowed a patient to feel more comfortable. A doctor unable to connect with a patient is a doctor unable to help that patient feel confident in a treatment.

Just like the rest of us, a child is not really a passive participant in his healthcare. A child, like any patient, needs a measure of confidence in the process taking place.

Being masked and seeing others masked generates fear, creates disconnect, and raises anxiety. Bonding is reduced and trust as well.

A child, at the mercy of adults to make a decision, deserves the ability to bond and find a sense of confidence in the adults around him. I do not mean in the saccharine television drama depiction of children developing bonds because of sweet quality moments. Such moments are largely lies.

Connectedness is diminished behind a face mask, both for the wearer and those looking at him. Bedside manner is done away with. The importance of seeing your own expressions effortlessly mirrored in the face of one who agrees with you is done away with. The most basic aspects of natural empathy between patient and doctor are done away with.

Not only should your child not be masked, his healthcare provider needs to not be masked.

Reason 118: Surgeons, Doctors, And Other Medical Staff In Face Masks May Be More Likely To Harm Patients

Harm to patients caused by medical care, or iatrogenic harm, is believed by some to be the third leading cause of death in the United States.[1] The Hippocratic Oath, the foundation of medical ethics insists medical professionals "do no harm." While the Hippocratic Oath is not taken by all doctors and is considered dated by some, it still forms the foundation of medical ethics dating back at least twenty-five hundred years.

There are many stressors upon practitioners in the medical system that make it more likely that an individual patient will suffer harm.

Additional stressors are not needed and especially with such specious evidence supporting their efficacy. Face masks are such a stressor. Before further masking of personnel in hospitals is continued, the risk-benefit profile must be updated with an honest conversation.

Until that is done, I will not be treated by a medical professional in a mask and I encourage the same high standard for you and your family.

As Maximos Fountzas writes in the article "Personal protective equipment against Covid-19: Vital for surgeons, harmful for patients?:"[2]

"Either in the case of a second lockdown or not, the safety of Personal Protective Equipment (PPE) use against Covid-19 for surgeons should be investigated. All parts of PPE increase surgeon's body temperature and sweating, leading to an impairment of surgeon's comfort, especially during prolonged and complicated surgical procedures. As mentioned above, PPE seems to be associated with important side effects, like dermatoses and headaches for healthcare workers. The PPE-associated discomfort and side effects during surgery may increase surgeons' anxiety and fatigue while performing difficult operations."

Are we to lie to ourselves and pretend that surgeons are some type of superhuman exempt from the same cognitive decline of mask wearing measured in others in the population? To do so would be foolish. Are we to pretend doctors, nurses, and other personnel do not experience the same cognitive decline while wearing a face mask?

A long history of medical research exists around the topic of keeping surgeons at the top of their game in order to create a safe environment for patients. Many of the same principles apply to other professionals in order to keep them at the top of their game for the wellbeing of the individual patient.

Universal masking must come to an immediate end, especially in hospitals, until further research has been conducted to properly assess the risk and benefit of this practice on the outcome of individual patients.

Reason 119: The Nebulizer Effect

An additional harm caused by having masks worn around your children is the nebulizer effect. A nebulizer is "a device used to reduce a liquid medication to extremely fine cloudlike particles; useful in delivering medication to deeper parts of the respiratory tract."[1]

Mask wearing has the tendency to create smaller exhaled particles and for louder speech to increase the production of fine particles, much like a nebulizer — pushing more, smaller particles further out into the air than a non-mask wearer.

Kai Kisielinski, in an April 20, 2021 article entitled "Is a Mask That Covers the Mouth and Nose Free from Undesirable Side Effects in Everyday Use and Free of Potential Hazards?" writes:[2]

> "Masks, when used by the general public, are considered by scientists to pose a risk of infection because the standardized hygiene rules of hospitals cannot be followed by the general public.[3] On top of that, mask wearers (surgical, N95, fabric masks) exhale relatively smaller particles (size 0.3 to 0.5 μm) than mask-less people and the louder speech under masks further amplifies this increased fine aerosol production by the mask wearer (nebulizer effect)."[4]

Like so much of the actual science, this too, is in total contradiction to everything we are being told is true about masks.

Of course, if you realize the importance of a healthy body, rather than living in fear of a germ, it is irrelevant whether a particle is aerosolized near or far, big or small.

This is simply an additional detail that further illustrates the ineffectiveness of mandatory masking. It is one more detail that has been swept under the rug in order to fit a deceitful narrative about the unsafe, ineffective, and experimental practice of mandatory masking.

Reason 120: Face Masks Impair Cognition Among Healthcare Workers

Masks cause impaired cognition in all of humans. While the medical community may see themselves as superhuman, they are mere humans and suffer from the same harmful effects of face mask as the rest of us.

As Denis Rancourt points out in "Review of scientific reports of harms caused by face masks:"[1]

> "A total of 343 healthcare professionals on the Covid-19 front lines participated in this study [New York City]. 314 respondents reported adverse effects from prolonged mask use with headaches being the most common complaint (n = 245). Skin breakdown was experienced by 175 respondents, and acne was reported in 182 respondents. Impaired cognition was reported in 81 respondents...Some respondents experienced resolved side effects once masks were removed, while others required physical or medical intervention."[2]

Rancourt continues:

> "Prolonged use of N95 and surgical masks by healthcare professionals during Covid-19 has caused adverse effects such as headaches, rash, acne, skin breakdown, and impaired cognition in the majority of those surveyed. ..."

If you ask this, you risk getting banned in 2020 and beyond: "Is it really so silly an idea to ask aloud whether face masks on medical professionals are harmful for children and other patients?"

Given the evidence that healthcare workers are, in fact, cognitively affected, more than questions are warranted: for the wellbeing of the child, no one should be wearing a mask around a child.

Reason 121: Face Masks On Medical Workers Hurt Kids

There is a constant worry about how face masks are needed to protect others from the possible spread of a virus. That is a debunked theory.

A more pressing worry should be, "How does wearing a face mask lead to the wearer *harming* others?"

In high pressure medical settings, caretaker error is fairly common and vigilance by patient and family is needed to help caretakers do the best work possible for the patient.

Unfortunately, the mass masking of caretakers measurably impacts caretaker cognition and wellbeing, which correspondingly makes the wearing of face masks harmful to their patients.

In a study of 343 healthcare professionals on the Covid-19 frontlines in New York City, 314 respondents reported adverse events from pro-longed mask use. According to the authors of that study:"[1]

> "Impaired cognition was reported in 81 respondents. ...
> Some respondents experienced resolved side effects once
> masks were removed, while others required physical or
> medical intervention."

Some may feel virtuous when in a face mask, but given the fact that we know masks do not work, do we really want our children treated by people wearing a device that creates "impaired cognition" in nearly a quarter of respondents?

I desire to have clear thinking medical personnel treating my family, and you should too.

A flaw of this study is that it relies on frontline workers to self-report their cognitive impairment. This does not capture those who suffer impaired cognition and do not report it. Nor does it capture those who suffer impaired cognition but do not notice it.

Regardless of the backlash that may be felt, parents need to stand up to this madness of mask wearing by all hospital personnel. Parents should not want their children treated by anyone but the most capable.

In the name of virtue signally, and compliance, we are disadvantaging our children by saddling the medical community with a burden that causes cognitive impairment in nearly a quarter of frontline workers and likely far more.

A study from Singapore[2] identifies impaired work performance among healthcare workers with a history of headaches who wore Personal Protective Equipment (PPE) such as face masks for more than four hours per day, affecting the work performance of 9 out of 10 with headaches and 42 out of a 158 participants (27%).

> "Since Covid-19 outbreak, 42/46 (91.3%) of respondents with pre-existing headache diagnosis either 'agreed' or 'strongly agreed' that the increased PPE usage had affected the control of their background headaches, which affected their level of work performance."

Surgery too becomes more dangerous with the use of face masks and other PPE. Instead of simply having the difficulty of the operating equipment to deal with and the challenge of the human body, the virtue signaling of face masks gives surgeons another challenge.

> "The PPE-associated discomfort and side effects during surgery may increase surgeons' anxiety and fatigue while performing difficult operations."

Like every aspect mentioned in this chapter, this may be a consequence of mask wearing that a surgeon is aware of or is not aware of. That does not change the level of impact on ability, and it is not affected by any number of physicians paraded through the media to claim that any technology at any moment is "safe and effective," face masks included, and that those cautioning safety on this strange new trend of virtue signaling are "over-reacting."

Your child deserves the best medical care. **DO NOT LET SOMEONE IN A MASK TREAT YOUR CHILD. DOING SO IS NEGLIGENT.**

Reason 122: Face Masks Do Not Bring About Greater "Health" As Defined By The World Health Organization

When we look at the Covid-19 precautions of 2020 and beyond, and we step back and ask ourselves, "What is the purpose of all of this?" ideally the answer is, "To ensure greater health and wellbeing."

We know that wearing a face mask does not achieve greater wellbeing, it harms both the wearer and the non-wearer. Nor does it bring health as defined by the WHO.

Kai Kisielinski, in an April 20, 2021 article entitled "Is a Mask That Covers the Mouth and Nose Free from Undesirable Side Effects in Everyday Use and Free of Potential Hazards?" writes:[1]

> "The WHO definition of health: 'health is a state of complete physical, mental and social wellbeing and not merely the absence of disease or infirmity.'"[2]

Face masks produce the opposite of health, as defined by the WHO. That is another good reason that no one should be made to, recommended to, or encouraged to wear one — least of all your child.

Reason 123: Reminder: The World Health Organization Even Says Face Masks May Be Dangerous To Your Child

The World Health Organization goes further and says a face mask may be dangerous for your child:[1]

"The likely disadvantages of the use of mask by healthy people in the general public include:

- potential increased risk of self-contamination due to the manipulation of a face mask and subsequently touching eyes with contaminated hands;
- potential self-contamination that can occur if non-medical masks are not changed when wet or soiled. This can create favorable conditions for microorganism to amplify;
- potential headache and/or breathing difficulties, depending on type of mask used;
- potential development of facial skin lesions, irritant dermatitis or worsening acne, when used frequently for long hours;
- difficulty with communicating clearly;
- potential discomfort;
- a false sense of security, leading to potentially lower adherence to other critical preventive measures such as physical distancing and hand hygiene;
- poor compliance with mask wearing, in particular by young children;
- waste management issues; improper mask disposal leading to increased litter in public places, risk of contamination to street cleaners and environment hazard;
- difficulty communicating for deaf persons who rely on lip reading;
- disadvantages for or difficulty wearing them, especially for children, developmentally challenged persons, those with mental illness, elderly persons with cognitive impairment, those with asthma or chronic respiratory or breathing problems, those who have

had facial trauma or recent oral maxillofacial surgery,
and those living in hot and humid environments."

These details have all been covered in the pages of this book. It is good to see official bodies that agree with the thesis of this book: Face masks hurt kids. Why exactly the media is painting a very different narrative is unclear. To merely cite official organs can be enough to get one deplatformed in the current era. Censors of course censor the truth. A lie is pointless to censor.

Reason 124: No One Even Uses A Face Mask Correctly

To return to the importance of not lying to a child, not lying to yourself, not lying to anyone, and just being an honorable person — hardly anyone even uses a mask correctly.

Mask studies are done in ideal laboratory conditions and in real world medical settings with trained personnel using controlled methods of proper masking.

A mask in some lady's purse, or some guy's pocket, or dangling from a rearview mirror for six months is not that.

The face mask narrative is all a big lie that you can no longer involve yourself or your children in.

Exclude yourself from the charade. It is that simple.

In a study on the correct use of face masks, The Association of American Physicians and Surgeons points out in:[1]

> "Overall, data were collected from 714 men and women. Of all ages, only 90 participants (12.6%) passed the visual mask fit test. About 75% performed strap placement incorrectly, 61% left a 'visible gap between the mask and skin,' and about 60% did not tighten the nose-clip."[2]

Face masks are not used correctly. We should not pretend that they are. Even when used correctly, they do not work. They are neither safe to the wearer, nor are they affective at preventing the transmission of a respiratory virus.

Reason 125: Experiments Are Often In "Ideal" Settings And Therefore Carry A Bias

Even if experiments showed face masks to be safe and effective, which they do not. L. A. Morris writes in the *HSE Contract research report No. 27/1991* article, "Dead Space and inhaled carbon dioxide levels in respiratory protective equipment:"

> "A further point to consider is that much of the exposure data derives from experiments on healthy male subjects, usually military personnel.[2] Such data must be applied with caution to an industrial population where there may be a wider spread of physical capabilities."[3]

Little has changed. Many studies carry the same bias of using healthy test subjects rather than a typical distribution of a normal population. Children have not been well represented in such studies.

Furthermore, masking is done in ideal conditions, often with medically trained staff.

Real world, non-hospital settings differ, as anyone who has seen a mask pulled from a pocket or purse can attest. Studies are done on masks that are sterile, applied with proper and consistent procedure, with sterile hands. No such implementation of protocol exists in the real world. This is further indication that masks are anything but safe and effective. That is the case in studies and is the case in real world settings. Masks are unsafe and ineffective when used by the general population, as has taken place throughout this period of mask mandates.

This is yet another reason why mandates must be brought to an end.

Reason 126: Face Masks Are Visibly Misused

Masks do not work and are misused. Kai Kisielinski, in an April 20, 2021 article entitled "Is a Mask That Covers the Mouth and Nose Free from Undesirable Side Effects in Everyday Use and Free of Potential Hazards?" writes:[1]

"Originally born out of the useful knowledge of protecting wounds from surgeons' breath and predominantly bacterial droplet contamination,[2-4] the mask has been visibly misused with largely incorrect popular everyday use, particularly in Asia in recent years.[5] Significantly, the sociologist Beck described the mask as a cosmetic of risk as early as 1992.[6] Unfortunately, the mask is inherent in a vicious circle: strictly speaking, it only protects symbolically and at the same time represents the fear of infection. This phenomenon is reinforced by the collective fear mongering, which is constantly nurtured by main stream media.[7]

"Nowadays, the mask represents a kind of psychological support for the general population during the virus pandemic, promising them additional anxiety-reduced freedom of movement. The recommendation to use masks in the sense of 'source control' not out of self-protection but out of 'altruism'[8] is also very popular with the regulators as well as the population of many countries. The WHO's recommendation of the mask in the current pandemic is not only a purely infectiological approach, but is also clear on the possible advantages for healthy people in the general public. In particular, a reduced potential stigmatization of mask wearers, the feeling of a contribution made to preventing the spread of the virus, as well as the reminder to adhere to other measures are mentioned.[9]

"It should not go unmentioned that very recent data suggest that the detection of Sars-Cov-2 infection does not seem to be directly related to popular mask use. The groups examined in a retrospective comparative study (infected with Sars-Cov-2 and not infected) did not differ in their habit of using masks: approximately 70% of the subjects in both groups always wore masks and another 14.4% of them frequently.[10] In a Danish prospective study on mask-wearing carried out on about 6000 participants and published in 2020, scientists found no statistically significant difference in the rates of Sars-Cov-2 infection when comparing the group of 3030 mask wearers with the 2994 maskless participants in the study (p = 0.38)."[11]

To pretend a misused face mask can work when a properly worn face mask does not work is nonsense. Do not involve yourself or your own in such a lie.

Reason 127: Mandating Face Mask Wearing Is Unethical

Health is not the only question related to masking. It is not a matter of utility. It is the fact that no one can be forced into a mask or any other medical intervention against their will. This is a long standing concept of international law.

Kai Kisielinski, in an April 20, 2021 article entitled "Is a Mask That Covers the Mouth and Nose Free from Undesirable Side Effects in Everyday Use and Free of Potential Hazards?" writes:[1]

> "In addition to protecting the health of their patients, doctors should also base their actions on the guiding principle of the 1948 Geneva Declaration, as revised in 2017. According to this, every doctor vows to put the health and dignity of his patient first and, even under threat, not to use his medical knowledge to violate human rights and civil liberties.[2] Within the framework of these findings, we, therefore, propagate an explicitly medically judicious, legally compliant action in consideration of scientific factual reality[3-11] against a predominantly assumption-led claim to a general effectiveness of masks, always taking into account possible unwanted individual effects for the patient and mask wearer concerned, entirely in accordance with the principles of evidence-based medicine and the ethical guidelines of a physician."

Forced mask wearing is unethical. No one should be forced into wearing a face mask.

Reason 128: Some Doctors Are Conflicted And Unable To Properly Represent Their Patients' Interests

Doctors are being asked to represent the interests of their patients in this matter, but cannot because they have conflicts of interest, conflicts of conscience, and conflicts of politics that have nothing to do with a patient and his or her wellbeing.

A patient's wellbeing is the primary thing that a patient's doctor should be concerned with.

Kai Kisielinski, in an April 20, 2021 article entitled "Is a Mask That Covers the Mouth and Nose Free from Undesirable Side Effects in Everyday Use and Free of Potential Hazards?" writes:[1]

"Among the medical profession and scientists, the users and observers of medical devices, there have been simultaneous calls for a more nuanced approach.[2-4] While there has been a controversial scientific discussion worldwide about the benefits and risks of masks in public spaces, they became the new social appearance in everyday life in many countries at the same time.

"Although there seems to be a consensus among the decision makers who have introduced mandatory masks that medical exemptions are warranted, it is ultimately the responsibility of individual clinicians to weigh up when to recommend exemption from mandatory masks. Physicians are in a conflict of interest concerning this matter. On the one hand, doctors have a leading role in supporting the authorities in the fight against a pandemic. On the other hand, doctors must, in accordance with the medical ethos, protect the interests, welfare and rights of their patient's third parties with the necessary care and in accordance with the recognized state of medical knowledge.[5-7]

"A careful risk–benefit analysis is becoming increasingly relevant for patients and their practitioners regarding the potential long-term effects of masks. The lack of knowledge of legal legitimacy on the one hand and of the medical scientific facts on the other is a reason for uncertainty among clinically active colleagues."

This conflict of interest, so prevalent among doctors, is a great reason to fire any doctor who will not allow you or your children into his office unmasked. He is putting his interest first. Not yours. A good doctor has no business behaving that way.

Reason 129: Face Masks While Driving Are A Hazard To Your Children

As can be expected, impaired cognition from face masks is not only harmful to children in medical settings, it is harmful to children and all people in other settings as well. As passengers or pedestrians, a driver wearing a face mask is a hazard to your child.[1,2]

On April 23, 2020 a New Jersey Driver got into a car accident because of a face mask. Robert Gearty reported for *Fox News* in an article titled "NJ police say 'excessive wearing' of coronavirus mask contributed to driver passing out, crashing car:"[3]

> "A New Jersey woman who crashed her car into a power pole may have passed out after wearing an N95 coronavirus mask behind the wheel for several hours, police said.

> "The woman was taken to a local hospital with a complaint of pain after Thursday's accident on a two-lane road, the Lincoln Park Police Department said. 'The crash is believed to have resulted from the driver wearing an N95 mask for several hours and subsequently passing out behind the wheel due to insufficient oxygen intake/excessive carbon dioxide intake,' the department said on Facebook Friday.

> "The department offered further explanation in a subsequent post, noting the 'overwhelming response' to its original statement.

> "'It was stated in the original post that we 'believed' the excessive wearing of an N95 mask was a contributing factor to this accident,' the department said. 'While we do not know this with 100% certainty, we do know that the driver had been wearing an N95 mask inside the vehicle for several hours and ultimately passed out while operating the vehicle.'

> "Police added, 'We also know that nothing was uncovered at the accident scene that would suggest that the driver was under the influence of drugs or alcohol. All this being said, it is certainly possible that some other medical reason could have contributed to the driver passing out.'"

You should not drive your children with a mask on. You should not let others drive your children with a mask on. You should not want others on the road driving with a mask on. Doing so presents an unnecessary and unreasonable risk to others on the road, akin to driving while texting, driving while drowsy, and drunk driving. Allowing masked drivers near your children is negligent.

Do we really need 20 years of conclusive studies and thousands of people harmed and killed before we accept what so many of us intuitively know to be true?

Masks impair cognition and should not be worn when cognition is important, which is really all the time, but especially around children, when operating machinery, or doing any work that affects others.

DOUBLE MASKS, CLOTH MASKS, FACE SHIELDS

Reason 130: The Face Mask Mandate Was Issued Without A Single Scientific Paper Cited In Support Of Cloth Face Masks Providing Respiratory Protection

Throughout Covid, we have been expected to listen to talking heads and slick marketing campaigns rather than data, science, or wisdom. It has been a lot of scientism, and not much of the scientific method.

The Association of American Physicians and Surgeons points out:[1]

> "Covid-19 is as politically-charged as it is infectious. Early in the Covid-19 pandemic, the WHO, the CDC and NIH's Dr. Anthony Fauci discouraged wearing masks as not useful for non-healthcare workers. Now they recommend wearing cloth face coverings in public settings where other social distancing measures are hard to do (e.g., grocery stores and pharmacies). The recommendation was published without a single scientific paper or other information provided to support that cloth masks actually provide any respiratory protection."

"Where is the evidence for any of this?" is a question that should be used any time an expert wants you to change your behavior. If an expert wants you to lockdown your society, mask your kids, and volunteer to have your lives and livelihoods declared non-essential, there is not a good enough set of evidence that should get you to acquiesce.

They have no evidence. Do not wear the mask. Do not mask your child. It is time to end this and to go back to all the good evidence-based parts of daily life that you loved before the world lost its mind and started taking even a single dictate by a public health bureaucrat seriously.

Reason 131: Wearing Cloth Face Masks Leads To More Flu-Like Illness Than Wearing No Face Mask, Causing Exactly The Opposite Outcome That Mandatory Masking Is Supposed To Prevent

Face masks are bad for you in so many ways, and they do not work to prevent the spread of a respiratory virus. Cloth masks are so much worse for you. According to one study, in a cloth mask you have a 13 times higher rate of contracting an influenza-like illness by wearing a cloth face mask. Baruch Vainshelboim writes in "Face masks in the Covid-19 era: A health hypothesis:"[1]

> "With respect to cloth face mask, a Randomized Control Trial (RCT) using four weeks follow up compared the effect of cloth face mask to medical masks and to no masks on the incidence of clinical respiratory illness, influenza-like illness and laboratory-confirmed respiratory virus infections among 1607 participants from 14 hospitals.[2] The results showed that there were no difference between wearing cloth masks, medical masks and no masks for incidence of clinical respiratory illness and laboratory-confirmed respiratory virus infections. However, a large harmful effect with more than 13 times higher risk [Relative Risk = 13.25 95% CI (1.74 to 100.97) was observed for influenza-like illness among those who were wearing cloth masks.[2] The study concluded that cloth masks have significant health and safety issues including moisture retention, reuse, poor filtration and increased risk for infection, providing recommendation against the use of cloth masks."[2]

The same study showed ineffective medical masks were penetrated by 44% of particles, whereas *really* ineffective cloth masks were permeated by 97% of particles.

Regardless of this difference, we know when we turn to randomized control trials, that face masks simply do not work to prevent the spread of a respiratory virus.

Do not wear face masks and definitely do not wear cloth masks.

Reason 132: Cloth Face Masks Are Awful

Cloth masks are harmful for you, likely worse than other types of masks. Cloth masks are ineffective, likely more so than other types of masks. Cloth masks carry disease, likely worse than other types of masks.

Much is said in favor of cloth masks, but many significant questions remain. How often should one change them? How often should one wash them? What should one make them out of? What design should one use? I would love to see the data on any of that. The data simply does not exist. The data about cloth masks is that wearing one is far worse than wearing nothing at all.

People who make up tall tales about reality and present them as fact are called liars.

Though there are lots of liars in the face mask debate and others trying to push unsafe, ineffective, and non-consensual one-size-fits-all approaches on others, the idea that someone's crusty, reusable, cloth mask is saving society is among the most ridiculous claims being made.

In 2015, *The British Medical Journal* published a paper entitled, "A Cluster Randomized Trial of Cloth Masks Compared with Medical Masks in Healthcare Workers."[1] The paper was written by nine authors from the University of New South Wales, the University of Sydney, the National Institute of Hygiene and Epidemiology in Vietnam and the Beijing Centers for Disease Control and Prevention in China. The aim of the study was to compare the efficacy of cloth masks to medical masks in hospital healthcare workers. The study, which was extensive, concluded that the results caution against the use of cloth masks.

> "'This is an important finding to inform occupational health and safety,' concluded the authors. 'Moisture retention, re-use of cloth masks and poor filtration may result in increased risk of infection.'"

If anyone tells you to wear a face mask, you know they are either stupid or up to no good. If they tell you to wear a cloth mask, you know they are really stupid or really up to no good.

Reason 133: Cloth Face Masks Are So Awful That They Should Never Be Recommended To Prevent The Spread Of A Virus

Scientists can be very staid in their writing style. Within the bounds of staid C. Raina MacIntyre, in "A cluster randomized trial of cloth masks compared with medical masks in healthcare workers,"[1] dismantles the narrative that cloth masks work:

> "In many parts of the world, cloth masks and medical masks may be the only options available for Healthcare Workers (HCWs.) Cloth masks have been used in West Africa during the Ebola outbreak in 2014, due to shortages of Personal Protective Equipment (PPE.) The use of cloth masks is recommended by some health organizations, with caveats.[2-4] In light of our study, and the obligation to ensure occupational health and safety of HCWs, cloth masks should not be recommended for HCWs, particularly during Aerosol-Generating Procedures (AGPs) and in high-risk settings such as emergency, infectious/respiratory disease and intensive care wards. Infection control guidelines need to acknowledge the widespread real-world practice of cloth masks and should comprehensively address their use."

Wearing a cloth mask is pure idiocy. Do not do it. A giant lie is being told to you. If you believe it, it is not the liar's fault that you are so gullible.

Reason 134: Double Masking May Cause Even Higher Risk Of Infection To The Wearer

We know face masks do not work.

We know they are bad for you to wear and can be bad when others wear them around you.

We know as well that cloth masks are even worse and come with powerfully harmful effects.

Would you believe it if I told you that a double mask is also awful for you?

As the Association of American Physicians and Surgeons points out:[1]

> "Observations during SARS suggested double-masking and other practices increased the risk of infection because of moisture, liquid diffusion."[2]

Single masks are bad for you and so are double masks. There is no reason you should be double masked and there is definitely no reason your children should be double masked.

MICRO ENVIRONMENTS, DEAD SPACE, OXYGEN, CARBON DIOXIDE, AND TEMPERATURE STRESS

Reason 135: Years Of Masking Precautions Meant To Benefit The Wearer Were Thrown Out The Window Suddenly In 2020

Germany's Social Accident Insurance (DGUV) has long had safety standards for masks on workers. Kai Kisielinski, in an April 20, 2021 article entitled "Is a Mask That Covers the Mouth and Nose Free from Undesirable Side Effects in Everyday Use and Free of Potential Hazards?" writes:[1]

> "The standards and norms prescribed in many countries regarding different types of masks to protect their workers are also significant from an occupational health point of view.[2] In Germany, for example, there are very strict safety specifications for masks from other international countries. These specify the requirements for the protection of the wearer.[3] All these standards and the accompanying certification procedures were increasingly relaxed with the introduction of mandatory masks for the general public. This meant that non-certified masks such as community masks were also used on a large scale in the work and school sectors for longer periods during the pandemic measures.[4] Most recently, in October 2020, the German Social Accident Insurance (DGUV) recommended the same usage time limits for community masks as for filtering half masks, namely, a maximum of three shifts of 120 minutes per day with recovery breaks of 30 minutes in between.

> "In Germany, FFP2 (N95) masks must be worn for 75 minutes, followed by a 30-minute break. An additional suitability examination by specialized physicians is also obligatory and stipulated for occupationally used respirators."[5]

Though it took them months to apply those standards to the general population, they finally did. In this regard the US is far behind. In the United States there is near silence from the institutions meant to protect people from dangerous masking orders. Though Germany is applying these more relaxed masking orders to the whole population and allowing people rest in between prolonged periods of masking, that approach is still not good enough. Face masks are unsafe and ineffective. They should not be forced on anyone, even if the person is given a long break.

Reason 136: OSHA Considers The Micro-Environment Of Face Masks As "Not Safe For Workers"

Breathing oxygen allows us to live. Even minor changes to the amount of oxygen we breathe can have powerful impacts on the body. Inside a face mask, there are pockets of reduced oxygen, despite the presence of a healthy amount of oxygen outside of that mask. Breathing through a face mask may, therefore, be harmful because of reduced oxygen. It may be harmful over the short-term as well as the long-term. In the article "Masks, false safety and real dangers, Part 1: Friable mask particulate and lung vulnerability," Boris Borovoy et al. write:[1]

> "Optimal oxygen intake in humans has been calculated in the absence of any obstruction to the airways. The US Occupational Safety and Health Administration (OSHA) has determined that the optimal range of oxygen in the air for humans is between 19.5 and 23.5%. In previous times, before the Covid-19 era OSHA required that any human-occupied airspace where oxygen measured less than 19.5% to be labelled as 'not safe for workers.'[2]

> "The percentage of oxygen inside a masked airspace generally measures 17.4% within several seconds of wearing. It has been observed that maximal voluntary ventilation and maximal inspiratory pressure increase during lower availability of oxygen at ascent in altitude,[3] as well as for those who live at high altitude.[4] Because oxygen is so essential to life, and in adequate amounts, humans and animals have developed the ability to sense changes in oxygen concentration, and to adapt to such challenges quickly. The medulla oblongata and carotid bodies are sensitive to such changes. Both lower ambient oxygen and increased ambient carbon dioxide stimulates ventilation, as the body quickly and steadfastly attempts to acquire more oxygen.[5] As a compensatory mechanism, inspiratory flow is measurably higher in mask-wearers than in controls."[6]

A great unanswered question of 2020 and beyond has been "Why has OSHA been so silent on masks?"

They have stringently regulated masks in the past. They knew exactly how harmful the masks were. They were willing to destroy small businesses in the past over nearly nothing. Now there is something important for OSHA to chime in about, an area of expertize for that government body, in fact. Yet this organization that exists allegedly to protect workers has been nearly silent on the topic of face masks on all workers and face masks on the general population.

As Congressman Thomas Massie has pointed out:

"The cloth mask is the only piece of government mandated medical equipment or safety gear for which there is no specification or certification."[7]

If any entity was prepared to present a case on what a supremely bad idea this was, it would be OSHA. Did they? Nope. Add that to a list of institutions that failed the American people and all people in 2020 and beyond. The best we have are some whistleblowers risking their lives and livelihoods to step forward and say how criminal this has all been. This is not just institutional failure. This is systemic failure.

Reason 137: Increased "Dead Space" Can Be Lethal

There is research and policy going back decades, that says any respiratory equipment worn on the face has to not produce a high physiological burden on the wearer.

In the *HSE Contract research report No. 27/1991* article, "Dead Space and inhaled carbon dioxide levels in respiratory protective equipment," L. A. Morris writes:[1]

> "One of the more important functions of respiratory protective equipment (RPE) standards has been to ensure that devices do not impose an excessive physiological burden upon the wearer. High levels of strain may lead to operator fatigue or, where other environmental stressors exist, to acute health damage."

This question has hardly been asked since the Ides of March 2020, at least not by those institutions tasked with asking them. It has hardly been asked by the elites tasked with asking them. It has hardly been asked by the scientific journalism community tasked with asking them. One purpose of this book is to more thoroughly ask that question. If it were asked properly, it would fail that test.

Does the mandatory masking of the general population impose an excessive physiological burden upon the wearer?

The answer is yes.

The response therefore, by all institutions and professionals tasked with this work must be to stand against such mandates.

They largely refuse to do the work they have been trusted by society to do for decades: ensuring that a respirator does not place an undue burden on the wearer.

Instead, they are largely silent.

In contrast, *Face Masks Hurt Kids* is filled with the accounts of heroes who refused to remain silent.

Morris continues, pointing to foundational and still very much relevant studies on the topic of "dead space" and the "rebreathing of carbon dioxide" from 1974 and 1984:

> "A review of the literature by Louhevaara[2] found that the re-breathing of carbon dioxide due to added dead space was a potential source of strain in RPE. In physiological terms, dead space can be defined as the volume of the airway in

which there is no significant exchange of oxygen and carbon dioxide."[3]

The term "dead space," is sometimes used in connection to face masks and other respiratory protective equipment.

Dead space is space in the respiratory system that is unable to engage in an efficient exchange of oxygen and carbon dioxide. It is part of your respiratory system, but it is not a part that efficiently exchanges oxygen and carbon dioxide. The wearing of a face mask increases the dead space by trapping air outside of the body, so near the mouth and nose that it can effectively be considered part of the body's respiratory system, part of the "dead space," in which air is present but does not engage in efficient oxygen and carbon dioxide exchange. Morris Continues:

> "Wearing a respirator face mask or mouthpiece increases the physiological dead space and hence the volume of the previous exhalation (with high carbon dioxide content) which is re-inhaled with each breath. The increased inhaled carbon dioxide levels which result from this effect lead to both increased lung ventilation and the retention of carbon dioxide in the lungs.[4,5] Initially the RPE wearer may only be aware of increased breathing effort but as inhaled carbon dioxide levels increase, the ability to compensate through hyperventilation diminishes, leading to the onset of adverse physiological reactions and symptoms. Limits must therefore be set for inhaled carbon dioxide in respirators if adverse health effects are to be avoided.[4]

> "A number of factors influence the dead space imposed by a respirator face mask. The design of the mask in terms of its internal volume, the location of openings and the paths of air into and out of the device, all have an influence on the dead space effect.[6] It is important to recognize that not all the dead space volume within the face mask is re-breathed. The volume closest to the mouth and nose will be, but there may also be static pockets of air around the edge of the facepiece. On this basis one can distinguish an effective dead space from the geometric dead space, the latter being the actual volume of the facepiece cavity. Physiological effects are dependent upon the effective dead space and it is this parameter which is evaluated either directly or indi-

rectly (through inhaled carbon dioxide levels) in standard test methods."

As can be seen, there is such intricacy of design that has long gone into the study of the safety of respiratory devices.

This was entirely done away with in 2020 and beyond. This leads one to ask "If it was so important then, why is it so *unimportant* now?"

The initial answer was "Because Covid is so dangerous." That was proven to be an inaccurate claim by February 2020 with the quarantined cruise ship known as the Grand Princess.

Very few died. The old and infirm were most likely to die. Those with serious comorbidities were an easy target for this virus.

My family and I were passengers aboard the Grand Princess in December 2019. My daughter, celebrating her first birthday, was a beloved passenger to many. We befriended dozens of crew members who were eventually quarantined off the coast of California as health officers and researchers figured out what was going on aboard that ship.

I could not help but notice as salacious and deceitful reports came off that ship. The media told lie after lie about an illness proven in February 2020 to have health outcomes comparable to the seasonal flu — a little worse in the sick and elderly, far better in the young and healthy.

Despite that near perfect closed environment for an experiment, that February 2020 data about how minor of a concern Covid was, both biologically and medically, it did not stop the March 17, 2020, lockdown of the San Francisco Bay Area adjacent to the ship and the April 3, 2020, face mask orders.

Everyone who signed those orders had access to how not serious Covid was because of the data from the Grand Princess and proceeded anyway with these brutal public health measures.

Our institutions, our professionals, our elites are either inept or up to no good. Either way, they need to be removed and never allowed a position of trust in our society again, as long as they live.

Reason 138: The Many Details Of Breathing Are Not One-Size-Fits-All, But Highly Individualized And Face Mask Policy Can Therefore Not Be One-Size-Fits-All

Mask policy needs to be entirely individualized, like all other medical care. Individual care is the foundation of medicine and medical ethics.

As mentioned in the previous chapter, in a 1991 landmark piece on the topic of dead space and respiratory protective equipment, L. A. Morris summarizes research on the topic. Morris writes:[1]

"It was found, not surprisingly, that breathing zone carbon dioxide concentrations increased in proportion to the wearer's metabolic rate. While carbon dioxide concentrations could be reduced to the 1% level by increasing the suit flow rate, this was less effective at high metabolic rates (>325 Wm^{-2})."

Metabolic rates and work rates both play a role in the appropriateness of a mask on a given individual. Morris continues:

"Comte,[2] measured breathing zone carbon dioxide concentrations in wearers of self contained breathing apparatus and a variety of air fed equipment. The protocol involved 30 minutes cycling at 50 W, followed by a 10-minute bout at 100 W. Carbon dioxide levels again increased with the wearer's work rate, ranging from 0.25% at rest to a peak value of 1.6% at 50 W. At 100 W there was some evidence of an increase in arterial carbon dioxide levels."

Morris cites a 1972 study and concludes that there is an individual amount of dead space created, even if everyone in a study wears the same model of mask:

"Leers[3] compared the physiological effects of a full face mask with an experimental dead space (split plastic tube). The protocol involved a 75 W bicycle ergometer workload (duration not specified) preceded by a rest period. Respiratory and blood gas parameters were recorded under steady state conditions. Breathing zone carbon dioxide concentrations were not measured directly but were estimated from an empirical formula based on the effective dead space: tidal volume ratio.

"The results showed that there was considerable inter-subject variation in effective dead space and hence in the ventilator responses to the mask or the tube. A mask with a given geometric volume could therefore have widely differing effects on a panel of wearers depending on individual breathing patterns."

Further uncertainty is created when workloads are added to studies.

As Morris shows, alongside concerns about dead space and breathing resistance, there are individual additional questions even on set tasks of metabolic rates for task — which can show considerable variation — based on factors such as working method, pace, and skill of the individual doing the work.

This research points to the need for a prohibition on one-size-fits-all approaches and considerable research to understand the impacts on the individual. No such effort has taken place to protect masked individuals in the general population, least of all children, who are far less likely to be able to explain difficulties they are having with masks.

This is a longstanding, established aspect of science, intended to protect those wearing a mask from harm, a subset of science that has been entirely done away with over the course of 2020 and beyond, while the common lie from public health officials "safe and effective" is plastered all over in its place.

Reason 139: Too Much Carbon Dioxide

Carbon dioxide is a natural, healthy part of life. We exhale carbon dioxide normally and also inhale some carbon dioxide normally. There is nothing wrong with that. It is when there is too much carbon dioxide inhaled that it becomes a problem. In the *HSE Contract research report No. 27/1991* article, "Dead Space and inhaled carbon dioxide levels in respiratory protective equipment," L. A. Morris writes:[1]

> "Carbon dioxide is a normal body constituent and has important physiological roles in the control of respiration and the regulation of cerebral blood flow.[2] It is readily taken up by the blood and can freely diffuse into the body tissues, leading to a rapid onset of toxic effects."[3]

Carbon dioxide so easily diffuses into the body's tissues, making too much inhaled carbon dioxide particularly toxic, with impacts that harm the entire body. Morris points out:

> "When ambient levels exceed a threshold of about 0.3 % CO_2, the partial pressure gradient from the blood to the lungs becomes less favorable to the elimination of metabolically generated carbon dioxide.[4] The body initially compensates for this by increasing pulmonary ventilation. However, as inhaled CO_2 levels increase further (beyond 1-2%) the effectiveness of this response falls off, with the result that arterial CO_2 levels increase beyond their normal range, 35-45 mm Hg.[2,5] If unchecked, the consequent acidosis can cause severe disruption to acid-base regulation with widespread effects on the respiratory, circulatory and central nervous systems."[4]

At high enough levels, carbon dioxide even creates a narcotic effect. Morris continues:

> "At concentrations in excess of 7.5%, carbon dioxide has a narcotic action leading to signs of intoxication and eventual loss of consciousness. While such levels are unlikely to be encountered in industrial RPE, they could be attained in the rare even of air supply failure in a positive pressure device."[6]

This narcotic effect can be felt in under two minutes in high enough concentrations. Morris writes about this further:

"The toxic effects of carbon dioxide are known to be related to the duration of exposure as well as the ambient concentration.[7] For example, an ambient level of 10% CO_2 can lead to the onset of neurological symptoms in less than two minutes.[8,9] On the other hand, concentrations in the range 1 to 1.5% have been tolerated for extended periods (up to 42 days) without adverse physiological effects or symptoms.[10,11] Indeed, during prolonged exposures at these levels there may be some adaptation or acclimatization which can modify the physiological and biochemical changes."[12,13]

You may ask, though, how much carbon dioxide is trapped behind a face mask. Without that information, after all, this data from Morris is not very helpful.

Michelle Rhea et al. in a somewhat dishonestly named April 2021 study "Carbon dioxide increases with face masks but remains below short-term NIOSH limits," cover that topic further.

A more fitting title for their paper would be "Carbon dioxide increases with face masks far above NIOSH limits." According to their research, KN95 masks are acceptable to wear for no more than 15 minutes, because they fall slightly below the National Institute for Occupational Safety and Health (NIOSH) 15 minute threshold for carbon dioxide. With the mandates everywhere to be found, no one who wears a face mask realistically wears a face mask for only 15 minutes. Your child at school is estimated to wear a face mask for more like 270 minutes.[14] Taking that into consideration, the title of Rhea's work is dishonest, in deed. 1% is the 8 hour NIOSH exposure limit for carbon dioxide. Wearing no mask, according to Rhea keeps one below that limit.

Rhea looks at the Chinese standard, KN95 mask in the study. 70% of KN95 mask sold in the United States do not meet the minimum standards for that product, according to a September 2020 study.[15] Had N95 masks been used in this study, that may have produced different results, likely with higher levels of carbon dioxide, since a higher standard mask would likely have less air transfer.

Rhea determined that KN95 masks create an environment between 2.5% and 3.0% carbon dioxide under the mask. Again 3% is the NIOSH 15 minute exposure limit for carbon dioxide. Though we must keep in mind the vast possibility of individual dead space, Rhea's research means that a KN95 mask can likely be worn by most people for less than 15 minutes without carbon dioxide levels becoming dangerous.

I have not seen those headlines or warnings flashed anywhere during Covid. The CDC is the parent organization of NIOSH. Would it be asking too much for the CDC to publicly state these limits and the dangerous conditions caused by wearing them for more than 15 minutes, seeing that the CDC is purporting to forcibly mask us and our children for our safety?

A dangerous environment is not just created by KN95 masks, but surgical masks also trap carbon dioxide in the dead space of the wearer.

According to Harald Walach et al. writing in a research letter for the *Journal of the American Medical Association Pediatrics* on June 30, 2021:

> "The normal content of carbon dioxide in the open is about 0.04% by volume (ie, 400 ppm). A level of 0.2% by volume or 2000 ppm is the limit for closed rooms according to the German Federal Environmental Office, and everything beyond this level is unacceptable."[16]

Walach's study has limited use in practical setting because it was conducted in a laboratory and after only a few minutes of mask use. This information is useful for demonstrating a trend, but does not describe real life scenarios well. Real life scenarios may prove far more harmful to wearers of face masks. Walach's conclusions were that face masks significantly exceed safe federal limits for carbon dioxide:

> "We measured means (SDs) between 13,120 (384) and 13,910 (374) ppm of carbon dioxide in inhaled air under surgical and filtering facepiece 2 (FFP2) masks, which is higher than what is already deemed unacceptable by the German Federal Environmental Office by a factor of 6. This was a value reached after 3 minutes of measurement. Children under normal conditions in schools wear such masks for a mean of 270 (interquartile range, 120-390) minutes.[17] The Figure shows that the value of the child with the lowest carbon dioxide level was 3-fold greater than the limit of 0.2 % by volume.[18] The youngest children had the highest values, with one 7-year-old child's carbon dioxide level measured at 25,000 ppm."

Even higher readings than these are likely to be noticed after longer periods of mask wearing and in environments of normal activity outside of a laboratory.

Nothing about these findings is surprising. This is research in a mainstream publication pointing to what occupational health professionals have long known: a dangerous amount of carbon dioxide accumulates behind a face mask.

The research letter from Walach was retracted by the editor of the journal, Dimitri Christakis, 17 days after it was first published in a July 16, 2021 letter Christakis writes:

> "Given fundamental concerns about the study methodology, uncertainty regarding the validity of the findings and conclusions, and the potential public health implications, the editors have retracted this Research Letter."[19]

Having not read the feedback received by Christakis, I am unable to comment on the validity of the criticism toward the methodology. The measurements reported in the results are approximately what could have been expected. I have no idea if Walach's work was faulty, which is unlikely since the range was inside the limit one would expect and which other research confirms. Even if Walach's research was faulty, could it possibly matter to you or me if the results were 2x, 5x, or 10x the German federal limit? The trend remains the same — too much carbon dioxide exists behind the face mask, so much as to be illegal for a grown man at work.

Walach's point is well taken. Face mask limits were put in place for safety. Carbon dioxide limits were put in place for safety. Those standards are being violated en masse across the globe, sacrificing the wellbeing of those wearing them, and for the sake of a face mask that does not work.

The likely reason for retraction is to be found in the Christakis letter. Walach and team attacked a topic they were not supposed to: mandatory masking of the population.

Walach had a second piece of research in a major publication retracted in the same month. It was a peer reviewed article illustrating that there may be more danger to taking the Covid vaccine than there is benefit of prevention.[20]

The successful publishing of that piece and the retraction likely also played a role in the retraction of the Walach face mask piece. The backlash was fierce.

Six members of the editorial board of the journal *Vaccines* threatened to resign if the study was published.[21] Walach was also fired from his university post as a punishment for publishing an article critical of Covid-19 vaccines. The University of Poznań, his former employer issuing a statement that it did not agree with Walach on his criticism of vaccines. It is unclear why anyone needs to agree with or disagree with Walach when it was data that he was presenting.

Given the poor post-marketing resources for Covid-19 vaccine data, it appears that Walach and his co-authors identified the best resources they could to determine that there is, in deed, a trend toward the Covid vaccines being unsafe.

In a letter from his former employer, Poznan University of Medical Sciences, signed by the press officer of the school, Rafał Staszewski, and the head of the College of Health Sciences, Jarosław Walkowiak, university leadership pays lip service to academic freedom before stating their opinion: "In our opinion, the study misleadingly used data to yield conclusions that are wrong and may lead to public harm."[22]

If Walach's research is such a danger to public health, proving him wrong with robust debate backed by solid data would be significantly more reassuring than silencing his work and pushing him out of his job.

Walach's former employers close their letter on the firing of Walach with this "Vaccinations are the most important weapon in the fight against the Sars-Cov-2 pandemic. This is the message that the Poznan University of Medical Sciences wishes to spread." They are terrified to appear to oppose the official narrative. Can such cowardly authors possibly be brave enough to actually support the academic freedom that they claim to support? That would be unusual.

Freedom is won by the brave and lost by the cowardly. In all ages, this one being no different, cowards pave the way for tyranny and exchange freedom for the ability to continue in their own comfortable cowardice.

Outlandish reactions to Walach's work, and the work of other honest and heroic scientists, in an attempt to use readily available data and the scientific method to open discussion on the topic is one reason why there has been so little scientific debate on the topic. Dissent has been dealt with harshly. Brave men, like Harald Walach, are in short supply. Scienticism — an obedience to authority — has replaced the scientific method — a process of research and question asking.

Reason 140: Increases In Exhalation Resistance, Inhalation Resistance, And Temperature May Be Harmful To One Wearing A Face Mask

Face masks cause additional strain while breathing. This may seem trivial, but is not. Adding additional strain to breathing has been well studied and leads to increased arterial carbon dioxide levels over and above the heightened carbon dioxide levels caused by increasing the dead space of the respiratory system, a phenomenon described in previous chapters.

As L. A. Morris points out in the *HSE Contract research report No. 27/1991* article, "Dead Space and inhaled carbon dioxide levels in respiratory protective equipment:"[1]

> "The interactions between the effects of breathing resistance and respirator dead space are relatively well documented. Increases in both inhalation and exhalation resistance above normal airway levels can result in hypoventilation and carbon dioxide retention.[2] This may be associated with a diminished ventilator response to increased arterial CO_2 levels[3,4] and hence may result in less effective compensation. The effects on strain are demonstrated by the following studies."

Morris cites a study in which people became weaker when breathing resistance was increased in the presence of 3% carbon dioxide, which is close to the level experienced in a face mask:

> "Craig et al.[5] studied the combined effects of elevated breathing resistance (inhalation resistance 1.5-15.5 cm $H_2O/\&/sec$, exhalation resistance 2.0-3.9 cm $H_2O/\&/sec$) and carbon dioxide levels (1.1-4.5%) on subjects undertaking heavy physical work. It was found that for a given level of breathing resistance, work endurance time was reduced with the inhaled CO_2 level exceeded 3%."

Heavy physical work is long known to not be tolerable above 3% carbon dioxide, yet we mask kids at play and pretend everything is okay. Morris continues:

> "Love et al.[6] examined the effects of 2 to 5% inhaled CO_2 on the ventilator responses of mineworkers breathing

through an inspiratory resistance of 10cm H_2O (at 100l min-^{1}). Several subjects were unable to complete the treadmill workload (VO_2 1.6l minute $^{-1}$) when the inhaled CO_2 level was 4% or more, this being associated with symptoms of headache and breathlessness. The authors concluded that inhaled CO_2 levels in excess of 3% were unlikely to be tolerated by industrial workers. It was considered that above this level the combined effects of physical workload, breathing resistance and inhaled CO_2 would cause severe discomfort due to high levels of pulmonary ventilation and/or carbon dioxide retention."

The same study also shows cause for concern on how increased external temperatures may affect a person in a face mask, as well as how increased body temperature may negatively affect a person in a face mask.

If someone in your life works in the field of occupational safety, I encourage you to go through this book with that person chapter by chapter and ask him to address every single concern raised in this book.

If someone in your life insists that you, or any of your loved ones, be masked, I encourage you to do the same — chapter by chapter.

This book was made for that. This book was made for you to be able to do exactly that. This book is not intended to have all the answers. It is intended to ask the questions that have gone unanswered and to provoke further inquiry beyond these pages.

Face masks are unsafe and ineffective. The body of scientific evidence out there shows that to be the case. They should not be worn. They should be vigorously questioned. All people who assert a face mask policy should be vigorously questioned — whether they attempt to impose it on you or not.

The very existence of any face mask policy whether it be voluntary or not, indicates a lack of knowledge or a lack of willingness to seek the knowledge.

Reason 141: Face Masks Induce Thermal Stress And Affect Heartrate, Even Among Healthy Adults And Likely Far More Among Children And The Infirm

The body has many intricate systems to provide stasis, so that everything can work appropriately. Stasis is a moderate condition which the body is able to properly function. When not in a sense of stasis, the human body, like any other biological system, can easily teeter out of control as a cascade of changes take place. Small initial changes can have large consequences.

The body has a sensitive mechanism to prevent overheating. We do not entirely understand that mechanism. We know that the nose and mouth play a role in it. We know that the humidity of the air in the nose and mouth play a role in it. We know that covering the nose and mouth with a face mask alters the ability for this system to properly function.

Sven Fikenzer writes in the July 2020 "Effects of surgical and FFP2/N95 face masks on cardiopulmonary exercise capacity," published in the journal *Clinical Research in Cardiology*:[1]

> "We discuss how N95 and surgical face masks induce significantly different temperature and humidity in the microclimates of the face masks, which have profound influences on heart rate and thermal stress and subjective perception of discomfort."[2]

More recent studies of healthy adults indicate the same. Fikenzer continues:

> "This first randomized cross-over study assessing the effects of surgical masks and FFP2/N95 masks on cardiopulmonary exercise capacity yields clear results. Both masks have a marked negative impact on exercise parameters such as maximum power output (Pmax) and the maximum oxygen uptake (VO2max/kg). FFP2/N95 masks show consistently more pronounced negative effects compared to surgical masks. Both masks significantly reduce pulmonary parameters at rest (FVC, FEV1, PEF) and at maximum load (VE, BF, TV). …"[3]

> "The data of this study are obtained in healthy young volunteers, the impairment is likely to be significantly greater,

e.g., in patients with obstructive pulmonary diseases (ref). From our data, we conclude that wearing a medical face mask has a significant impact on pulmonary parameters both at rest and during maximal exercise in healthy adults.[3]

"These data suggest a myocardial [relating to the muscular tissue of the heart] compensation for the pulmonary limitation in the healthy volunteers. In patients with impaired myocardial function, this compensation may not be possible."[4]

When wearing a face mask, the heart must work harder to compensate, this compensation may not be possible for those with heart problems. This is, of course, true whether or not the heart problem has been diagnosed. This further illustrates what a bad idea such one-size-fits-all public health approaches are.

Reason 142: Hypercapnia

Hypercapnia is a high level of carbon dioxide in the blood. This causes the blood to become more acidic. When hypercapnia occurs too quickly, it can even overwhelm the kidneys.

Wearing a face mask can lead to hypercapnia.

Vernon Coleman states in "Proof that Face Masks do More Harm than Good:"[1]

> "Some of the carbon dioxide exhaled with each breath is retained behind the mask and then breathed in again."

Excess carbon dioxide leads to: headaches, dizziness, drowsiness, fatigue, nausea, vomiting, tightness of the chest, among other symptoms.

The effects of hypercapnia can be far more severe than the above, with acute (sudden) hypercapnia being particularly dangerous.

Those who suffer from COPD, because of the inability to breathe sufficiently to clear carbon dioxide from the blood, may develop hypercapnia. The wearing of a face mask is akin to an artificial inducement of COPD, an artificial decrease in the functioning of the lungs and breathing mechanism, without any positive benefit, least of all the prevention of the spread of a respiratory virus.

To do this to oneself is senseless, harmful, and abusive. You deserve better. No child deserves to be treated in a senseless, harmful, or abuse way either.

Reason 143: Face Masks Increase "Dead Space"

Kai Kisielinski, in an April 20, 2021 article entitled "Is a Mask That Covers the Mouth and Nose Free from Undesirable Side Effects in Everyday Use and Free of Potential Hazards?" writes:[1]

> "As early as 2005, an experimental dissertation (randomized crossover study) demonstrated that wearing surgical masks in healthy medical personnel (15 subjects, 18–40 years old) leads to measurable physical effects with elevated transcutaneous carbon dioxide values after 30 minutes.[2] The role of dead space volume and CO_2 retention as a cause of the significant change ($p < 0.05$) in blood gases on the way to hypercapnia, which was still within the limits, was discussed in this article. Masks expand the natural dead space (nose, throat, trachea, bronchi) outwards and beyond the mouth and nose.

> "An experimental increase in the dead space volume during breathing increases carbon dioxide (CO_2) retention at rest and under exertion and correspondingly the carbon dioxide partial pressure pCO_2 in the blood ($p < 0.05$).[3]

> "As well as addressing the increased rebreathing of carbon dioxide (CO_2) due to the dead space, scientists also debate the influence of the increased breathing resistance when using masks."[4-6]

Breathing is such an intricate system that we barely understand. Within this field, the significance of the impact on dead space from surgical masks has only begun to come to light. Wearing a face mask increases the amount of space in and around your body that does not engage in gas exchange and which is not protected by your body's defenses. The increase of dead space has other effects on the body. This may be causal or correlated. It is unclear. It appears that harm to the body occurs when dead space is increased. This is yet another reason not to wear a face mask nor to put a face mask on your child.

Reason 144: Face Masks Increase Carbon Dioxide Dangerously And Decrease Oxygen Dangerously

Face masks lead to 12.4% reduction of oxygen in inhaled air and a 3,000% increase in carbon dioxide.

Kai Kisielinski, in an April 20, 2021 article entitled "Is a Mask That Covers the Mouth and Nose Free from Undesirable Side Effects in Everyday Use and Free of Potential Hazards?" writes:[1]

> "In a recent intervention study conducted on eight subjects, measurements of the gas content for oxygen (measured in O2 Vol%) and carbon dioxide (measured in CO_2 ppm) in the air under a mask showed a lower oxygen availability even at rest than without a mask. A Multi-Rae gas analyzer was used for the measurements (RaeSystems®) (Sunnyvale, California CA, United States). At the time of the study, the device was the most advanced portable multivariant real-time gas analyzer. It is also used in rescue medicine and operational emergencies. The absolute concentration of oxygen (O2 Vol%) in the air under the masks was significantly lower (minus 12.4 Vol% O2 in absolute terms, statistically significant with $p < 0.001$) at 18.3% compared to 20.9% room air concentration. Simultaneously, a health-critical value of carbon dioxide concentration (CO_2 Vol%) increased by a factor of 30 compared to normal room air was measured (ppm with mask versus 464 ppm without mask, statistically significant with $p < 0.001$)"[2]

This increased inhaled carbon dioxide leads to increased carbon dioxide in the blood. Kisielinski writes:

> "These phenomena are responsible for a statistically significant increase in carbon dioxide (CO_2) blood content in mask wearers,[3,4] on the one hand, measured transcutaneously via an increased $PtcCO_2$ value,[3,5-8] on the other hand, via endexpiratory partial pressure of carbon dioxide ($PET-CO_2$)[9,10] or, respectively, the arterial partial pressure of carbon dioxide ($PaCO_2$)."[11]

The decreased inhaled oxygen leads to decreased oxygen in the blood, increased respiratory rate, and increased pulse rate. Kisielinski continues:

"In addition to the increase in the wearer's blood carbon dioxide (CO_2) levels ($p < 0.05$),[3,5-15] another consequence of masks that has often been experimentally proven is a statistically significant drop in blood oxygen saturation (SpO_2) ($p < 0.05$).[2,3,7,9,16-21] A drop in blood oxygen partial pressure (PaO_2) with the effect of an accompanying increase in heart rate ($p < 0.05$)[5,9,16,17,21] as well as an increase in respiratory rate ($p < 0.05$)[5,7,9,22,23] have been proven.

"A statistically significant measurable increase in pulse rate ($p < 0.05$) and decrease in oxygen saturation SpO_2 after the first ($p < 0.01$) and second hour ($p < 0.0001$) under a disposable mask (surgical mask) were reported by researchers in a mask intervention study they conducted on 53 employed neurosurgeons."[17]

The harmful increase in carbon dioxide, decrease in oxygen, and increased pulse are another reason neither you nor your child should be masked.

Reason 145: Face Masks Dangerously Increase The Rebreathing Of Carbon Dioxide

As previously established, face masks trap carbon dioxide. That trapped carbon dioxide is breathed back in by the face mask wearer, creating higher rates of inhaled carbon dioxide than fresh air. This is called "rebreathing" of carbon dioxide. The level of rebreathing of carbon dioxide that takes place in a face mask is harmful to an adult and especially harmful to a developing child.

Kai Kisielinski published an April 20, 2021 article entitled "Is a Mask That Covers the Mouth and Nose Free from Undesirable Side Effects in Everyday Use and Free of Potential Hazards?"[1] Heart rate, blood carbon dioxide, and breathing difficulties during exercising are reported by Kisielinski:

> "These phenomena were reproduced in another experiment on 20 healthy subjects wearing surgical masks. The masked subjects showed statistically significant increases in heart rate ($p < 0.001$) and respiratory rate ($p < 0.02$) accompanied by a significant measurable increase in transcutaneous carbon dioxide $PtcCO_2$ ($p < 0.0006$). They also complained of breathing difficulties during the exercise."[2]

Increased rebreathing of carbon dioxide is caused by the face mask increasing dead space, which again is the part of the respiratory system that does not engage in gas exchange. Kisielinski continues:

> "The increased rebreathing of carbon dioxide (CO_2) from the enlarged dead space volume in mask wearers can reflectively trigger increased respiratory activity with increased muscular work as well as the resulting additional oxygen demand and oxygen consumption.[3] This is a reaction to pathological changes in the sense of an adaptation effect. A mask-induced drop in blood oxygen saturation value (SpO_2)[4] or the blood oxygen partial pressure (PaO_2)[5] can in turn additionally intensify subjective chest complaints."[5,6]

This may also harm the mind. Kisielinski points out:

> "The documented mask-induced changes in blood gases towards hypercapnia (increased carbon dioxide/CO_2 blood levels) and hypoxia (decreased oxygen/O_2 blood levels) may result in additional nonphysical effects such as confu-

sion, decreased thinking ability and disorientation[7-11] including overall impaired cognitive abilities and decrease in psychomotoric abilities.[10-15] This highlights the importance of changes in blood gas parameters (O_2 and CO_2) as a cause of clinically relevant psychological and neurological effects. The above parameters and effects (oxygen saturation, carbon dioxide content, cognitive abilities) were measured in a study on saturation sensors (Semi-Tec AG, Therwil, Switzerland), using a Borg Rating Scale, Frank Scale, Roberge Respirator Comfort Scale and Roberge Subjective Symptoms-during-Work Scale, as well as with a Likert scale.[12] In the other main study, conventional ECG, capnography and symptom questionnaires were used in measuring carbon dioxide levels, pulse and cognitive abilities.[7] Other physiological data collection was done with pulse oximeters (Allegiance, MCGaw, USA), subjective complaints were assessed with a 5-point Likert scale and motoric speed was recorded with linear-position transducers (Tendo-Fitrodyne, Sport Machins, Trencin, Slovakia).[13] Some researchers used standardized, anonymized questionnaires to collect data on subjective complaints associated with masks."[7]

For those who claim masks are not harmful to the young, Kisielinski proves yet another example of the harm of face mask wearing to children:

"In an experimental setting with different mask types (community, surgical, N95) a significant increase in heart rate ($p < 0.04$), a decrease in oxygen saturation SpO_2 ($p < 0.05$) with an increase in skin temperature under the mask (face) and difficulty of breathing ($p < 0.002$) were recorded in 12 healthy young subjects (students). In addition, the investigators observed dizziness ($p < 0.03$), listlessness ($p < 0.05$), impaired thinking ($p < 0.03$) and concentration problems ($p < 0.02$), which were also statistically significant when wearing masks."[16]

Carbon dioxide is your body's waste. Why would you force waste back into your body? Why would you force waste back into your child's body? When you put your child into a face mask you do exactly that.

Masks are harmful to all who wear them. They are especially harmful to children. No child should ever be put into a face mask.

339

Reason 146: Increased Dead Space Is Significant, And So Is Increased Breathing Resistance

Dead space volume is increased by mask wearing. It even doubles for some face mask wearers.

Kai Kisielinski, in an April 20, 2021 article entitled "Is a Mask That Covers the Mouth and Nose Free from Undesirable Side Effects in Everyday Use and Free of Potential Hazards?" writes:[1]

> "The average dead space volume during breathing in adults is approximately 150–180 mL and is significantly increased when wearing a mask covering the mouth and nose.[2] With an N95 mask, for example, the dead space volume of approximately 98–168 mL was determined in an experimental study.[3] This corresponds to a mask-related dead space increase of approximately 65 to 112% for adults and, thus, almost a doubling."

This amount of increase in dead space by wearing an allegedly "safe" N95 mask, reduced the gas exchange volume available to the lungs by 37%. Kisielinski continues:

> "At a respiratory rate of 12 per minute, the pendulum volume respiration with such a mask would, thus, be at least 2.9–3.8 L per minute. Therefore, the dead space amassed by the mask causes a relative reduction in the gas exchange volume available to the lungs per breath by 37%.[4] This largely explains the impairment of respiratory physiology reported in our work and the resulting side effects of all types of masks in everyday use in healthy and sick people (increase in respiratory rate, increase in heart rate, decrease in oxygen saturation, increase in carbon dioxide partial pressure, fatigue, headaches, dizziness, impaired thinking, etc.)."[2,6]

The dead space volume is significant, but so is the added breathing resistance, as stated elsewhere in these pages. Kisielinski writes:

> "In addition to the effect of increased dead space volume breathing, however, maskrelated breathing resistance is also of exceptional importance.[6,7]

"Experiments show an increase in airway resistance by a remarkable 126% on inhalation and 122% on exhalation with an N95 mask.[4] Experimental studies have also shown that moisturization of the mask (N95) increases the breathing resistance by a further 3%[5] and can, thus, increase the airway resistance up to 2.3 times the normal value.

"This clearly shows the importance of the airway resistance of a mask. Here, the mask acts as a disturbance factor in breathing and makes the observed compensatory reactions with an increase in breathing frequency and simultaneous feeling of breathlessness plausible (increased work of the respiratory muscles). This extra strain due to the amplified work of breathing against bigger resistance caused by the masks also leads to intensified exhaustion with a rise in heart rate and increased CO_2 production. Fittingly, in our review of the studies on side effects of masks, we also found a percentage clustering of significant respiratory impairment and a significant drop in oxygen saturation (in about 75% of all study results)."

The mask acts as "a disturbance factor in breathing," affecting heart, lungs, and beyond. There is no good reason to wear a mask and plenty of good reasons not to wear a mask.

Reason 147: Increased Dead Space Increases Breathing Resistance, Leading To Decreased Gas Exchange Of The Respiratory System — And A Cascade Of Other Physiological Side Effects

Face masks make it harder to breathe, cause less gas to be exchanged during the breathing process, and decrease breathing depth and volume.

Kai Kisielinski, in an April 20, 2021 article entitled "Is a Mask That Covers the Mouth and Nose Free from Undesirable Side Effects in Everyday Use and Free of Potential Hazards?" writes:[1]

> "When breathing, there is an overall significantly reduced possible gas exchange volume of the lungs of minus 37% caused by the mask[2] according to a decrease in breathing depth and volume due to the greater breathing resistance of plus 128%[3] (exertion when inhaling greater than when exhaling) and due to the increased dead space volume of plus 80%,[4] which does not participate directly in the gas exchange and is being only partially mixed with the environment."

Face masks should not be worn.

Reason 148: Suprathreshold Stimuli Can Cause Pathological Consequences, But So Can Subthreshold Stimuli

Those behaviors that cause medical symptoms can harm you. We all know that. We each know when something is unmistakably wrong with us.

However, those behaviors that do not cause noticeable medical symptoms, those behaviors can harm you too.

That can be easier to forget.

Just because something does not immediately feel like it hurts, does not mean it is not doing harm to you. In fact, with face masks, we know the very opposite to be true.

We know that long before most people realize physical symptoms of masking, the face mask has already done them considerable harm.

Only time will tell how reversible or repairable that harm is, but the existence of harm — or subthreshold stimuli pathological consequences — is unquestionable.

Kai Kisielinski, in an April 20, 2021 article entitled "Is a Mask That Covers the Mouth and Nose Free from Undesirable Side Effects in Everyday Use and Free of Potential Hazards?" writes:[1]

> "It is known from pathology that not only supra-threshold stimuli exceeding normal limits have disease-relevant consequences. Subthreshold stimuli are also capable of causing pathological changes if the exposure time is long enough. Examples occur from the slightest air pollution by hydrogen sulfide resulting in respiratory problems (throat irritation, coughing, reduced absorption of oxygen) and neurological diseases (headaches, dizziness).[2]

> "Furthermore, subthreshold but prolonged exposure to nitrogen oxides and particulate matter is associated with an increased risk of asthma, hospitalization and higher overall mortality.[3,4] Low concentrations of pesticides are also associated with disease-relevant consequences for humans such as mutations, development of cancer and neurological disorders.[5] Likewise, the chronic subthreshold intake of arsenic is associated with an increased risk of cancer,[6] subthreshold intake of cadmium with the promotion of heart failure,[7] subthreshold intake of lead is associated with hy-

pertension, renal metabolic disorders and cognitive impairment[8] or subthreshold intake of mercury with immune deficiency and neurological disorders.[9] Subliminal UV radiation exposure over long periods is also known to cause mutation-promoting carcinogenic effects (especially white skin cancer)."[10]

These well-established examples of harm done to people who report feeling fine, also applies to face masks. Kisielinski continues:

"The mask-induced adverse changes are relatively minor at first glance, but repeated exposure over longer periods in accordance with the above-mentioned pathogenetic principle is relevant. Long-term disease-relevant consequences of masks are to be expected. Insofar, the statistically significant results found in the studies with mathematically tangible differences between mask wearers and people without masks are clinically relevant. They give an indication that with correspondingly repeated and prolonged exposure to physical, chemical, biological, physiological and psychological conditions, some of which are subliminal, but which are significantly shifted towards pathological areas, health-reducing changes and clinical pictures can develop such as high blood pressure and arteriosclerosis, including coronary heart disease (metabolic syndrome) as well as neurological diseases. For small increases in carbon dioxide in the inhaled air, this disease-promoting effect has been proven with the creation of headaches, irritation of the respiratory tract up to asthma as well as an increase in blood pressure and heart rate with vascular damage and, finally, neuropathological and cardiovascular consequences.[11] Even slightly but persistently increased heart rates encourage oxidative stress with endothelial dysfunction, via increased inflammatory messengers, and finally, the stimulation of arteriosclerosis of the blood vessels has been proven.[12] A similar effect with the stimulation of high blood pressure, cardiac dysfunction and damage to blood vessels supplying the brain is suggested for slightly increased breathing rates over long periods.[13,14] Masks are responsible for the aforementioned physiological changes with rises in inhaled carbon dioxide,[15-25] small sustained increases in heart rate[20,26-29] and mild but sustained increases in respiratory rates."[18,20,26,30,31]

Even when symptoms are not felt, the existence of sub-threshold stimuli causing physiological harm is enough to suggest the same could be true for a face mask. Even those who believe face masks do them no harm, because they feel fine, may, in fact, be harming themselves.

SELF-INDUCED ILLNESS AND EXACERBATION OF ILLNESS

Reason 149: Everyone In A Face Mask Induces A Condition Similar On The Body To Sleep Apnea

You can argue positive and negative effects of masking on the brain. What you cannot argue is that it affects the brain, that it affects the brain negatively, and that its effects on the brain are significant.

To say otherwise is to speak contrary to the truth.

In the *Medical Hypotheses* article, "Exercise with face mask; Are we handling a devil's sword?" Baskaran Chandrasekaran and Shifra Fernandes write:[1]

> "Brain metabolism and mental health. Acute hypercapnia, a double-edged sword, on the one hand, elevates intracranial pressure, lowers cerebral perfusion, and triggers cerebral ischemia and, on the other hand, it is found to be neuroprotective decreasing the excitatory amino acids and minimizing the cerebral metabolism."[2]

Hypercapnia, is abnormally high levels of carbon dioxide, acute hypercapnia is high levels of carbon dioxide that comes on suddenly. Chandrasekaran and Fernandes continue:

> "Studies from obstructive sleep apnea[3] provide irrefutable evidence of hypercapnic hypoxemia affecting the postural stability, proprioception, altered gait velocities and falls. The above findings can be extrapolated to elderly persons as well as individuals with established respiratory diseases exercising with N95 respirator masks."

Low oxygen in the presence of high carbon dioxide causes an impact on the body and mind similar to sleep apnea. The symptoms of mask wearing are likely so similar to the symptoms of sleep apnea, precisely because sleep apnea creates the same low oxygen and high carbon dioxide environment in the body.

Wearing a face mask is like an artificial inducement of sleep apnea on the wearer. Why would you do that to yourself? Why would you do that to anyone else? Why would you do that to a child?

Reason 150: Exercising In A Face Mask Induces An Artificial Version Of COPD

As if self-induced sleep apnea is already not bad enough, Chandra-sekaran and Fernandes take it further. A face mask also creates an impact on the body similar to artificially induced COPD.

In the *Medical Hypotheses* article, "Exercise with face mask; Are we handling a devil's sword?" Baskaran Chandrasekaran and Shifra Fernandes write:[1]

> "The face mask forms a closed circuit for the inspired and expired air, though not completely airtight. Rebreathing of the expired air increases arterial CO_2 concentrations and increases the intensity of acidity in the acidic environment."[2]

Chandrasekaran and Fernandes specifically point to COPD-like symptoms being a problem when exercising in a face mask:

> "Thus individuals exercising with a mask would have physiological effects similar to a Chronic Obstructive Pulmonary Disease (COPD) person exercising such as discomfort, fatigue, dizziness, headache, shortness of breath, muscular weakness and drowsiness."[3]

However, these same COPD-like symptoms take place with activity as light as walking. Chandrasekaran and Fernandes continue:

> "Besides, light activity, like walking with a MET value of 2, could increase the amount of inhaled CO_2 and decrease the amount of O_2 via an N95 mask, increasing the work of breathing. Therefore, we could assume this effect to magnify when performing any aerobic or resistance exercise at a higher workload. The resistance offered to the inspiratory and expiratory flow, for prolonged periods (about 10 minutes), could result in respiratory alkalosis, increased lactate levels and early fatigue.[4] The aforementioned symptoms affect the exercising individuals psychologically as well as bring about physiological alterations such as muscle damage, muscle fiber switch and fast-twitch fibers size."

Again, to exercise in a face mask has psychological and physiological impact on the wearer.

COPD is an awful disease. Almost 15.7 million Americans suffer from it.[5] Why would anyone seek to induce COPD-like symptoms in themselves? Why would they want to do it to another? Why would they want to do it to their own child?

No one should exercise in a face mask, not even if that exercise is light walking.

Reason 151: Face Masks Are Definitely Not Suitable For Those With Epilepsy

Face masks increase the respiratory rate of the wearer above the natural respiratory rate of the same wearer engaging in the same activity unmasked. Respiratory rate is how many breathes a person takes per minute. This detail is especially significant for those with epilepsy.

Kai Kisielinski, in an April 20, 2021 article entitled "Is a Mask That Covers the Mouth and Nose Free from Undesirable Side Effects in Everyday Use and Free of Potential Hazards?" writes:[1]

> "In their level III evidence review, neurologists from Israel, the UK and the USA state that a mask is unsuitable for epileptics because it can trigger hyperventilation.[2]

> "The use of a mask significantly increases the respiratory rate by about plus 15 to 20%. However, an increase in breathing frequency leading to hyperventilation is known to be used for provocation in the diagnosis of epilepsy and causes seizure equivalent EEG changes in 80% of patients with generalized epilepsy and in up to 28% of focal epileptics."[3]

Wearing a face mask can trigger hyperventilation, which can trigger a seizure. The CDC tracks these numbers:

> "In 2015, 1.2% of the US population had active epilepsy. This is about 3.4 million people with epilepsy nationwide: 3 million adults and 470,000 children."[4]

That is a measure of active epilepsy.[5] More than that actually have epilepsy.

This is a public health concern you think would be screamed from the rooftops: this group of 1 out of 100 Americans cannot safely wear a face mask because it may trigger a seizure. They must never be forced into one. They must be very careful when wearing one. It may even be best if no epileptic ever wears a face mask for any reason. These would be reasonable statements from the CDC that could have been made alongside every face mask order announcement.

Were they?

No.

This is a further indication that the face mask is not about health at all.

In a hospital, in fact, epileptics who say "I am unable to wear a face mask safely, because I have epilepsy," are more likely to hear "That is okay; you must wear it anyway; we will just treat your seizure with medicine if you have one," than to hear "You do not have to wear one then, because this is a hospital and we care for the individual wellbeing of our patients." All wellbeing is, of course, individual. There is no collective wellbeing. It is redundant to say "individual wellbeing."

In our era however, great effort is put into confusing that idea. Therefore, in our era, that individual nature of one's wellbeing, may be necessary to emphasis.

If one can believe that there is collective wellbeing, then many people can be made to suffer individually for a non-existent collective wellbeing.

Good people suffer for lack of wisdom. Impoverished philosophy opens the door to massive tyranny. You are an individual. Your wellbeing is individual. If someone can get you to embrace an impoverished philosophy, in which you grow confused about your importance as an individual, then many horrible things can be done to you.

The harm a face masks can do to a person with epilepsy by triggering seizures is another of many reasons that a face mask should not be worn.

Reason 152: Face Mask Wearing Affects The Central Nervous System And May Increase Sleep Apnea

As already abundantly demonstrated, masks lead to lower blood oxygen and higher blood carbon dioxide levels.

In an April 20, 2021 article entitled "Is a Mask That Covers the Mouth and Nose Free from Undesirable Side Effects in Everyday Use and Free of Potential Hazards?"[1] Kai Kisielinski writes:

> "In our work, we have identified scientifically validated and numerous statistically significant adverse effects of masks in various fields of medicine, especially with regard to a disruptive influence on the highly complex process of breathing and negative effects on the respiratory physiology and gas metabolism of the body. The respiratory physiology and gas exchange play a key role in maintaining a health-sustaining balance in the human body.[1,2] According to the studies we found, a dead space volume that is almost doubled by wearing a mask and a more than doubled breathing resistance[3-5] lead to a rebreathing of carbon dioxide with every breathing cycle[6-10] with — in healthy people mostly — a subthreshold but, in sick people, a partly pathological increase in the carbon dioxide partial pressure ($PaCO_2$) in the blood.[11-13] According to the primary studies found, these changes contribute reflexively to an increase in respiratory frequency and depth[12,14-16] with a corresponding increase in the work of the respiratory muscles via physiological feedback mechanisms."[16,17]

These lead to additional changes in breathing and heart function. Kisielinski continues:

> "Thus, it is not, as initially assumed, purely positive training through mask use. This often increases the subliminal drop in oxygen saturation SpO_2 in the blood,[15,18-21] which is already reduced by increased dead space volume and increased breathing resistance.[8,17] The overall possible resulting measurable drop in oxygen saturation O_2 of the blood on the one hand[8,15,18-21] and the increase in carbon dioxide (CO_2) on the other,[14,15,18,22-,28] contribute to an increased

noradrenergic stress response, with heart rate increase[19,20,31] and respiratory rate increase,[12,14,15,23] in some cases also to a significant blood pressure increase."[11,31]

These changes impact deep in the brain stem. Kisielinski continues:

"In panic-prone individuals, stress-inducing noradrenergic sympathetic activation can be partly directly mediated via the carbon dioxide (CO_2) mechanism at the locus coeruleus in the brainstem,[2,9,32,33] but also in the usual way via chemosensitive neurons of the nucleus solitarius in the medulla.[1,34] The nucleus solitarius[1] is located in the deepest part of the brainstem, a gateway to neuronal respiratory and circulatory control.[34] A decreased oxygen (O_2) blood level there causes the activation of the sympathetic axis via chemoreceptors in the carotids."[35,36]

This disturbed breathing in a face mask, causes additional harm and is linked to hypertension, sleep apnea, and metabolic syndrome. Kisielinski continues:

"Even subthreshold changes in blood gases such as those provoked when wearing a mask cause reactions in these control centers in the central nervous system. Masks, therefore, trigger direct reactions in important control centers of the affected brain via the slightest changes in oxygen and carbon dioxide in the blood of the wearer.[1,34,35]

"A link between disturbed breathing and cardiorespiratory diseases such as hypertension, sleep apnea and metabolic syndrome has been scientifically proven.[37,38] Interestingly, decreased oxygen/O_2 blood levels and also increased carbon dioxide/CO_2 blood levels are considered the main triggers for the sympathetic stress response.[1,39] The aforementioned chemo-sensitive neurons of the nucleus solitarius in the medulla are considered to be the main responsible control centers.[1,34,35] Clinical effects of prolonged maskwearing would, thus, be a conceivable intensification of chronic stress reactions and negative influences on the metabolism leading towards a metabolic syndrome. The mask studies we found show that such disease-relevant respiratory gas changes (O_2 and CO_2)[1,39] are already achieved by wearing a mask." [8,11,12,14,15,17-30,40]

Mask wearing during the day may even increase sleep apnea at night and other physiological problems. Kisielinski continues:

> "According to the scientific results and findings, masks have measurably harmful effects not only on healthy people, but also on sick people and their relevance is likely to increase with the duration of use.[41] Further research is needed here to shed light on the long-term consequences of widespread mask use with subthreshold hypoxia and hypercapnia in the general population, also regarding possible exacerbating effects on cardiorespiratory lifestyle diseases such as hypertension, sleep apnea and metabolic syndrome. The already often elevated blood carbon dioxide (CO_2) levels in overweight people, sleep apnea patients and patients with overlap-COPD could possibly increase even further with everyday masks. Not only a high body mass index (BMI) but also sleep apnea are associated with hypercapnia during the day in these patients (even without masks).[24,42] For such patients, hypercapnia means an increase in the risk of serious diseases with increased morbidity, which could then be further increased by excessive mask use."[8,39]

The body is an intricately balanced mechanism. Breathing is poorly understood by science. At this point in the great masking of society, we do not understand breathing much better, but we know this much: putting a face mask on a person is harmful to that person in many ways.

Those with existing risk of sleep apnea, metabolic syndrome, obesity, and high blood pressure are particularly vulnerable from the harm done by wearing a face mask.

Reason 153: Face Masks Harm Cancer Patients

The high carbon dioxide, low oxygen environment created inside the body by face mask wearing helps promote the growth of cancer cells.

Russel Blaylock warns of the danger to patients with cancer:[1]

"People with cancer, especially if the cancer has spread, will be at a further risk from prolonged hypoxia as the cancer grows best in a microenvironment that is low in oxygen. Low oxygen also promotes inflammation which can promote the growth, invasion and spread of cancers. Repeated episodes of hypoxia have been proposed as a significant factor in atherosclerosis and hence increases (the risk of) all cardiovascular and cerebrovascular diseases."

Long-terms studies done with face masks may identify correlation with cancer. The basic principles for why that may be the case are identified above by Blaylock.

In addition to cancer, the low oxygen environment of the face mask is also harmful to the heart and brain, as demonstrated in other places in this book.

This is further clarification as to why no one should be wearing a face mask. Those at risk for cancer, those with cancer, those with risk of heart disease or other vascular illness, should not be masked.

Heart disease is the top killer of Americans. Cancer is the second biggest killer of Americans. 659,041 died of the former and 599,601 died of the latter in 2019.[2]

An honest discussion of how the face mask impacts these two diseases is a major public health concern.

THE IMMUNE SYSTEM

Reason 154: Face Masks Weaken Immunity, And Therefore May Make Children MORE Susceptible To Covid-19

Far from benefiting the immune system, as must be claimed for a face mask to be safe and effective, wearing a face mask does the exact opposite. It has the impact of harming the immune system.

Russel Blaylock writes about a drop in oxygen levels being associated with an impairment in immunity:[1]

> "Studies have shown that hypoxia can inhibit the type of main immune cells used to fight viral infections called the CD4+T-lymphocyte. This occurs because the hypoxia increases the level of a compound called hypoxia inducible factor-11 (HIF-11) which inhibits T-lymphocytes and stimulates a powerful immune inhibitor cell. This sets the stage for contracting any infection, including Covid-19, and making the consequences of that infection much graver. In essence, your mask may very well put you at an increased of infections and if so, having a much worse outcome."

Throughout this book, we see what we already know: breathing is vital to health. Obstructing breathing harms health. Of course, the immune system is harmed by the obstruction of breathing, the entire body is harmed.

The mask understandably causes the immune system to be harmed and makes the outcome of any illness suffered worse for the patient. But remember, it also, however, harbors pathogenic bacteria near the mouth and nose in unnatural quantities, much like a person were walking around inhaling and exhaling over a petri dish filled with pathogens. The face mask presents this double threat to your body: it weakens the body and grows pathogens near the nose and mouth.

Even if the face mask did work to prevent the spread of a respiratory virus, the strategy behind it remains faulty. The strategy is to protect a healthy person from a virus that is not going to do him harm. It is a strategy of denying challenge to an immune system. The immune system — if such a system can even be distinguished from the rest of the body, for it is integral to all parts of the body and even includes the non-human microbiota throughout the body — is comprised of a series of challenges from conception to the present. Exposure to all manner of microorganisms takes place with little harm to the individual, making that person's immune system increasingly robust. To deny a person that challenge is to deny a person a robust immune system.

Though masks do not work, they are effective at depressing the immune system, as one would expect from any strategy that denies a person a microbiotic challenge to their immune system. Instead, the way face masks so effectively appear to depress the immune system is by disturbing healthy breathing and producing an unbalanced and harmful condition in the body.

Reason 155: Face Masks Reduce Healthy Functioning Of The Immune System

We understand from randomized controlled trials that wearing masks does not lead to fewer illnesses from a respiratory virus.

Masks may limit antibody formation, however, in those who wear them. As the Association of American Physicians and Surgeons points out,[1] a September 2020 CDC review of mask and antibody presence in healthcare workers (HCWs) shows a higher prevalence of antibodies in those healthcare workers who do not wear masks:

> "3,248 HCWs observed. 6% had antibodies to Sars-Cov-2; 29% were asymptomatic; 69% had not had a diagnosis of SARS-Co-V-2 infection. Prevalence of antibodies was lower (6%) in HCWs who wore masks that those who did not (9%)."[2]

Mask wearing may limit antibody formation, though the reason this takes place is unclear from the studies cited above.

As was demonstrated in the previous chapter, with other immune system responses, a hypoxic environment may also inhibit antibody production. There may be additional uncontrolled variables at play in this study.

We have here yet another difficult to ignore detail as to why a person concerned with his health and the health of others would want anyone masked, least of all his own child.

Reason 156: Face Mask Wearing Increases Leptin Release

Face masks even have an impact on the hormones in your body such as leptin. Kai Kisielinski, in an April 20, 2021 article entitled "Is a Mask That Covers the Mouth and Nose Free from Undesirable Side Effects in Everyday Use and Free of Potential Hazards?" writes:[1]

> "A connection between hypoxia, sympathetic reactions and leptin release is scientifically known."[2]

Leptin is one of many hormones that help to regulate metabolism. It gets attention in the media for being linked with weight loss. This focus on that single function is troubling, though, and avoids the realization that if an artificially induced hypoxia with an allegedly safe and effective face mask leads to a change in this key hormone, how many other hormones are brought into sudden imbalance by face mask wearing and with what impact on the body?

The sympathetic nervous system is responsible for maintaining many aspects of homeostasis in the body. From the digestive track, to the eyes, to the heart, it is constantly at work keeping your body properly functioning.

It is not a question whether or not the mask harms you and your child. It is a question of "How far reaching is the harm caused by a face mask?"

Reason 157: Face Mask Wearing May Negatively Influence Metabolism All The Way Down To The Cellular Level

On a molecular level, face masks harm your body, right down to every cell. Kai Kisielinski, in an April 20, 2021 article entitled "Is a Mask That Covers the Mouth and Nose Free from Undesirable Side Effects in Everyday Use and Free of Potential Hazards?" writes:[1]

"According to the latest scientific findings, blood-gas shifts towards hypoxia and hypercapnia not only have an influence on the described immediate, psychological and physiological reactions on a macroscopic and microscopic level, but additionally on gene expression and metabolism on a molecular cellular level in many different body cells."

The cellular impact may have further cancer promoting effects. Yes, face mask wearing may promote cancer growth in the wearer. Kisielinski continues:

"Through this, the drastic disruptive intervention of masks in the physiology of the body also becomes clear down to the cellular level, e.g., in the activation of hypoxia-induced factor (HIF) through both hypercapnia and hypoxia-like effects.[2] HIF is a transcription factor that regulates cellular oxygen supply and activates signaling pathways relevant to adaptive responses. e.g., HIF inhibits stem cells, promotes tumor cell growth and inflammatory processes."[2]

The face mask impacts your entire body, down to the cellular level, brain and metabolism included. Kisielinski continues:

"Based on the hypoxia- and hypercapnia-promoting effects of masks, which have been comprehensively described for the first time in our study, potential disruptive influences down to the intracellular level (HIF-a) can be assumed, especially through the prolonged and excessive use of masks. Thus, in addition to the vegetative chronic stress reaction in mask wearers, which is channeled via brain centers, there is also likely to be an adverse influence on metabolism at the cellular level. With the prospect of continued mask use in everyday life, this also opens up an interesting field of research for the future."

Every cell in your body may be harmed by the wearing of a face mask. It is the opposite of safe and ineffective.

Reason 158: Immunity Debt

Even if face masks did help to stop the spread of Sars-Cov-2, or any other respiratory virus — which they do not — and if they were safe to wear — which they are not — there would still be another question that needs answering: "Are these non-existent safe and effective face masks beneficial in the long-term for my child?"

The answer might still be a resounding "No!"

More and more we are seeing that human beings are part of the ecosystem they live in. It is an ecosystem that is so diverse and carefully constructed, that we cannot even begin to make sense of it. Anyone trusting a doctor or public health bureaucrat claiming that he can control something that he cannot even begin to understand is in for a world of pain.

We are increasingly coming to see that not a single part of this approach to Covid-19 focused on germs rather than hosts work. As far as we can tell, the interplay with germs is not only beneficial to us, but is a vital part of our existence. Not only is there a massive amount of bacteria in and on our bodies, there are believed to be many times more viruses in and on our bodies than human cells. This includes pathogenic organisms that could severely harm us. They are constantly in, on, and around us, and so seldom are any of us harmed by them. Are viruses, then, really our enemy?

As we spend this year experimenting on our children, our canaries in the mine, we are increasingly seeing how much harm is done to them by this nonsensical war on germs.

Ebola does not kill. Tuberculosis does not kill. Flu does not kill. Covid-19 does not kill. HIV does not kill. Weakened hosts succumb.

Be strong. Do not fear germs. Strengthen your body against them. Be strong. Do not fear illness. Strengthen your body against it. Have faith. Do the things that years of wisdom have counseled us to do to be strong and of faith. There is no need to fear the gravest plague if you do that. You are on the right side of history during Covid-19 if you have done exactly that.

Thank you for your efforts.

FACE MASK USE HARMS THE MOUTH

Reason 159: Face Masks Harm Teeth And Gums And Cause A Condition Known As "Mask Mouth"

The mouth is a difficult body part to make sense of. Why does a child in the remote Atlas Mountains of Morroco, who has never seen a dentist, have better teeth than his peer in Cupertino, California, who has seen a dentist with the most high tech tools at his disposal, twice each year for the last 12 years?

Researcher and dentist, Weston Price, linked the difference to diet: a Western diet rots the teeth and leads to a deformed face and teeth, while a traditional diet leads to dental and cranial health.

Teeth may be early indicators of the health of other parts of the body.

Even after decades of this intuitive work by Price and others of a similar perspective, the dental profession is no closer to adopting these ideas. Superficiality reigns supreme and the importance of the mouth as little more than an inconvenience is seldom considered.

As with many other health considerations, the mouth is an early indication of the harm being done to the body by mandatory masking. Masks are devastating to oral health.

Vernon Coleman writes in the January 11, 2021 article: "Masks And Mask Wearing: 100 Facts You Must Know:"

> "Two dentists in New York have reported seeing a number of patients with inflamed gums and other problems. The news story was reported in the *New York Post*. 'We are seeing inflammation in people's gums that have been healthy forever, and cavities in people who have never had them before,' said dentist Rob Ramondi. 'About 50% of our patients are being impacted by this, (so) we decided to name it 'mask mouth'.' Another dentist, Marc Sclafani, told the *New York Post* that 'gum disease, or periodontal disease, will eventually lead to strokes and an increased risk of heart attacks.' The dentists said that the problem is caused by the fact that face coverings increase mouth dryness and contribute to a build-up of bad bacteria. 'People tend to breathe through their mouth instead of through their nose while wearing a mask,' said Sclafani. 'The mouth breathing is causing the dry mouth, which leads to a de-

crease in saliva — and saliva is what fights the bacteria and cleanses your teeth.'"[1]

The Association of American Physicians and Surgeons concurs:

"Wearing masks increases dryness, which leads to decrease in saliva. It is the saliva that fights bacteria. Result is decaying teeth, receding gum lines and seriously sour breath. Gum disease — or periodontal disease — will eventually lead to strokes and an increased risk of heart attacks."[2]

Wearing a face mask even harms the teeth and gums, two parts of the body that are indicators of overall health of the body.[3-5]

Reason 160: Face Mask Wearing Causes "Mask Mouth" And Other Harm

Wearing of a face mask harms the lips and areas around the mouth.

Kai Kisielinski, in an April 20, 2021 article entitled "Is a Mask That Covers the Mouth and Nose Free from Undesirable Side Effects in Everyday Use and Free of Potential Hazards?" writes:[1]

"There are reports from dental communities about negative effects of masks and are accordingly titled 'mask mouth.'[2] Provocation of gingivitis (inflammation of the gums), halitosis (bad breath), candidiasis (fungal infestation of the mucous membranes with Candida albicans) and cheilitis (inflammation of the lips), especially of the corners of the mouth, and even plaque and caries are attributed to the excessive and improper use of masks. The main trigger of the oral diseases mentioned is an increased dry mouth due to a reduced saliva flow and increased breathing through the open mouth under the mask. Mouth breathing causes surface dehydration and reduced salivary flow rate (SFR).[2] Dry mouth is scientifically proven due to mask wear.[3] The bad habit of breathing through the open mouth while wearing a mask seems plausible because such breathing pattern compensates for the increased breathing resistance, especially when inhaling through the masks.[4,5] In turn, the outer skin moisture[6-8] with altered skin flora, …is held responsible as an explanation for the inflammation of the lips and corners of the mouth (cheilitis).[2] This clearly shows the disease-promoting reversal of the natural conditions caused by masks. The physiological internal moisture with external dryness in the oral cavity converts into internal dryness with external moisture."

The wearing of a face mask harms the mouth, lips, and areas around the mouth.

Reason 161: Face Mask Wearing Exacerbates Existing Voice Disorders And May Trigger New Voice Disorders

The wearing of the mask also harms the voice and exacerbates existing voice disorders.

In an April 20, 2021 article entitled "Is a Mask That Covers the Mouth and Nose Free from Undesirable Side Effects in Everyday Use and Free of Potential Hazards?" Kai Kisielinski writes:[1]

> "In a study of 221 healthcare workers, Ears, Nose and Throat (ENT) physicians objectified a voice disorder in 33% of mask users. The VHI-10 score of 1 to 10, which measures voice disorders, was on average 5.72 higher in these mask users (statistically significant with $p < 0.001$)."

This is not just because the mask muffles sound, making it harder for the mask wearer to be heard and understood, but it disturbs speech by impacting the pressure gradients required of normal speech. Kai Kisielinski continues:

> "The mask not only acted as an acoustic filter, provoking excessively loud speech, it also seems to trigger impaired vocal cord coordination because the mask compromises the pressure gradients required for undisturbed speech."[2]

Not only does a face mask impact those with existing voice disorders, it may impact those as well who have otherwise normal speech, thereby triggering new voice disorders. Kisielinski continues:

> "The researchers concluded from their findings that masks could pose a potential risk of triggering new voice disorders as well as exacerbating existing ones."

Voice disorders exacerbated by masking and triggered by masking are another reason not to wear a mask and not to put one on your child.

Reason 162: Face Mask Wearing Has Caused A New Condition, A Form Of Face Mask-Induced Rhinitis

Mask wearing has caused a new disease, a form of mask-induced rhinitis. Kai Kisielinski, in an April 20, 2021 article entitled "Is a Mask That Covers the Mouth and Nose Free from Undesirable Side Effects in Everyday Use and Free of Potential Hazards?" writes:[1]

> "Ear, Nose, and Throat (ENT) physicians recently discovered a new form of irritant rhinitis due to N95 mask use in 46 patients. They performed endoscopies and nasal irrigations on mask wearers, which were subsequently assessed pathologically. Clinical problems were recorded with standardized questionnaires. They found statistically significant evidence of mask-induced rhinitis and itching and swelling of the mucous membranes as well as increased sneezing ($p < 0.01$). Endoscopically, it showed an increased secretion and evidence of inhaled mask polypropylene fibers as the trigger of mucosal irritation."[2]

A new disease has been identified, caused by the wearing of a mask. A mask induced rhinitis — a swelling of the nose. The nose is an entry to the respiratory system. What occurs there may eventually occur in other parts of the respiratory system.

Also mentioned above, are polypropylene particles in the nose, irritating the nasal passage. These polypropylene particles come from wearing face masks. These fibers do not stop at the nose. As we have seen elsewhere in this book, those same polypropylene particles make their way into the rest of the respiratory system, likely leading to pulmonary fibrosis.

Additionally, among those that wear masks, the nose runs more, the nose is irritated more, the nose itches more, and the wearer sneezes more.

We have, here, additional evidence of the harm done by face mask wearing, additional reasons why you should not wear them, and additional reasons why your children should not either.

FACE MASK USE HARMS
THE EARS AND THE SKIN

Reason 163: Face Masks Deform Children's Ears

The outer ear, or auricle, is made of cartilage and skin. Cartilage and skin are flexible materials. Like all parts of our body, they are able to be shaped by long-term pressure.

The three parts of the outer ear are the lobule (ear lobe), tragus (the piece of flesh that sticks out next to your ear canal), and the helix (the remainder of the ear). All three parts are subject to change under long-term pressure.

The loops of face masks most notably impact the shape of the helix — the major portion of the external ear. This may distort a person's appearance over the long-term and may also have lasting functional impact on the process of hearing, even long after the individual has stopped wearing a mask.

In the August 20, 2020 article "Review of scientific reports of harms caused by face masks," Dina Karvounides writes:[1,2]

> "Among those on the market, surgical masks with elastic loops are the ones most chosen by parents for their children. These elastics cause constant compression on the skin and, consequently, on the cartilage of the auricle, leading to erythematous and painful lesions of the retroauricular skin when the masks are used for many hours a day. Pre-adolescent children have undeveloped auricular cartilage with less resistance to deformation; prolonged pressure from the elastic loops of the mask at the hollow or, even worse, at the anthelix level can influence the correct growth and angulation of the outer ear. In fact, unlike when using conservative methods for the treatment of protruding ears, this prolonged pressure can increase the cephaloauricular angle of the outer auricle. It is important for the authorities supplying the masks to be aware of this potential risk and for alternative solutions to be found ..."

Do not wear a face mask, because it will deform your developed ears, but even worse, it will deform your child's undeveloped ears. It has far more impact on the correct growth of a child's ears. Poorly formed ears may look strange, a concern worth considering, but may also cause hearing impairment that otherwise would not exist. We do not know how badly this impact occurs. We only know that it occurs.

Again, here we are, experimenting on our children. If we do not know the answers to questions of harm — both long-term and short-term — then we are conducting an experiment on children — on a societal level, but also on an individual level — every time you put a face mask on your child.

Additionally, it leads to painful lesions. Why would anyone put their child through pain with no benefit to the child or anyone else? Such sadism visited upon a child is demented.

Reason 164: Face Masks
Are Bad For Your Face

Face masks seem to harm every organ of the body, including your biggest organ — the skin.

The health of the skin is an indicator of the health of the body. If face masks were unable to harm heart, kidneys, and brain, an argument could be made for any damage to the skin being only acute and localized. However, it is evident that the harm done by face masks is systemic rather than isolated.

Contemporary medicine is so eager to look at everything in isolated fashion, much as contemporary academia seeks to do. Inter-relatedness is much more significant than either field recognizes. Is a case of acne from a face mask isolated to just being a case of acne from a face mask? I doubt it. Whether or not I am right, this is a question that should have been answered long before a mask mandate was imposed.

Vernon Coleman writes in the January 11, 2021 article: "Masks And Mask Wearing: 100 Facts You Must Know":[1]

> "'The face mask traps warm moisture that is produced when we exhale,' says dermatologist Dr. Maggie Kober. 'For those with acne, this can lead to acne flares. For many others, this warm, moist environment surrounding skin creates the perfect condition for naturally occurring yeast and bacteria to flourish and grow more abundant. This overgrowth of yeast and bacteria can produce angular cheilitis, the cracking and sores at the corners of the mouth.' Face masks can also present a risk of contact dermatitis and can increase the risk of staph infections."

Many a teenager with acne knows the effort that goes into combatting acne, and the troubles a teenager faces. What parent would place that burden upon their child unnecessarily? And for what? For no benefit to the child.

As we see from the face mask symptoms of mouth sores, skin infection, and acne — the skin under and around the face mask is harmed by the face mask, just as the rest of the body is harmed by the face mask.

Reason 165: Face Mask Wearing Harms The Skin

The harm done to the skin and face by a face mask, goes far beyond acne.

Kai Kisielinski, in an April 20, 2021 article entitled "Is a Mask That Covers the Mouth and Nose Free from Undesirable Side Effects in Everyday Use and Free of Potential Hazards?" writes:[1]

"Unlike garments worn over closed skin, masks cover body areas close to the mouth and nose, i.e., body parts that are involved with respiration.

"Inevitably, this leads not only to a measurable temperature rise,[2-5] but also to a severe increase in humidity due to condensation of the exhaled air, which in turn changes the natural skin milieu considerably of perioral and perinasal areas.[5-7] It also increases the redness, pH-value, fluid loss through the skin epithelium, increased hydration and sebum production measurably.[8] Pre-existing skin diseases are not only perpetuated by these changes, but also exacerbated. In general, the skin becomes more susceptible to infections and acne."

The skin provides a protective function to the body, a function disturbed within 4 hours of mask wearing. Kisielinski continues:

"The authors of an experimental study were able to prove a disturbed barrier function of the skin after only 4 hours of wearing a mask in 20 healthy volunteers, both for surgical masks and for N95 masks.[8] In addition, germs (bacteria, fungi and viruses) accumulate on the outside and inside of the masks due to the warm and moist environment."[9-12]

Increased infection and mechanical damage to the skin occurs. Kisielinski writes:

"They can cause clinically relevant fungal, bacterial or viral infections. The unusual increase in the detection of rhinoviruses in the sentinel studies of the German Robert Koch Institute (RKI) from 2020[13] could be another indication of this phenomenon.

"In addition, a region of the skin that is not evolutionarily adapted to such stimuli is subjected to increased mechanical stress. All in all, the above-mentioned facts cause the unfavorable dermatological effects with mask related adverse skin reactions like acne, rashes on the face and itch symptoms."[14]

That damage to the skin can be quite significant. Kisielinski writes:

"A Chinese research group reported skin irritation and itching when using N95 masks among 542 test participants and also a correlation between the skin damage that occurred and the time of exposure (68.9% at ≤6 hours/day and 81.7% at >6 hours/day)."[15]

In this Chinese study, 68.9% of study participants had skin damage in under 6 hours of mask wearing, while 81.7% of the participants had skin damage when masks were worn for 6 hours or more. In New York, even greater impact was recorded. Kisielinski writes:

"A New York study evaluated in a random sample of 343 participants the effects of frequent wearing of surgical mask type and N95 masks among healthcare workers during the Covid-19 pandemic. Wearing the masks caused headache in 71.4% of participants, in addition to drowsiness in 23.6%, detectable skin damage in 51% and acne in 53% of mask users.[16]

"On the one hand, direct mechanical skin lesions occur on the nose and cheekbones due to shear force, especially when masks are frequently put on and taken off.[15,16] On the other hand, masks create an unnaturally moist and warm local skin environment.[5,7,17] In fact, scientists were able to demonstrate a significant increase in humidity and temperature in the covered facial area in another study in which the test individuals wore masks for one hour.[4] The relative humidity under the masks was measured with a sensor (Atmo-Tube, San Francisco, CA, USA). The sensation of humidity and temperature in the facial area is more crucial for well-being than other body regions.[3,5] This can increase discomfort under the masks. In addition, the increase in temperature favors bacterial optimization."

More than half of mask wearers report acne from the face mask, but it also causes harm below the skin. The normal functioning of lymph nodes and blood vessels are impeded by the wearing of a face mask. Kisielinski writes:

> "The pressure of the masks also causes an obstruction of the flow physiology of lymph and blood vessels in the face, with the consequence of increased disturbance of skin function[8] and ultimately also contributing to acne in up to 53% of all wearers and other skin irritations in up to 51% of all wearers.[5,7,16]

> "Other researchers examined 322 participants with N95 masks in an observational study and detected acne in up to 59.6% of them, itching in 51.4% and redness in 35.8% as side effects.[18]

> "In up to 19.6% (273) of the 1393 wearers of different masks (community masks, surgical, N95 masks), itching could be objectified in one study, in 9% even severely. An atopic predisposition (allergy tendency) correlated with the risk of itching. The length of use was significantly related to the risk of itching (p < 0.0001)."[19]

Fogged glasses can occur among those who wear glasses with a face mask, but so does slurred speech and breathing problems. Kisielinski continues:

> "In another dermatological study from 2020, 96.9% of 876 users of all mask types (community masks, surgical masks, N95 masks) confirmed adverse problems with a significant increase in itching (7.7%), accompanied by fogging-up of glasses (21.3%), flushing (21.3%), slurred speech (12.3%) and difficulty breathing (35.9%) (p < 0.01)."[20]

Potent, harmful chemicals are used in the manufacturing of masks, chemicals not intended for prolonged contact with humans. Kisielinski writes:

> "Apart from an increased incidence of acne[14,16,18] under masks, contact eczema and urticaria[22] are generally described in connection with hypersensitivities to ingredients of the industrially manufactured masks (surgical mask and N95) such as formaldehyde (ingredient of the textile) and thiram (ingredient of the ear bands).[8,21] The hazardous substance thiram, originally a pesticide and corrosive, is used in the rubber industry as a optimization accelerator. For-

maldehyde is a biocide and carcinogen and is used as a disinfectant in the industry."

Mask use can even permanently change the color of your skin, due to the repeated damaged caused by using them. Kisielinski writes:

"Even isolated permanent hyperpigmentation as a result of post-inflammatory or pigmented contact dermatitis has been described by dermatologists after prolonged mask use."[14,18]

This chapter provides another several dozen reasons face masks should not be worn — not by you, and certainly not by your children.

FACE MASK USE HARMS THE EYES

Reason 166: Face Mask Use Is Harmful To Eyes

Face masks redirect breathe onto the eyes. This is breathe that the eyes are not made to handle. This chronic breathe blowing is harmful and leads to damage to the eyes, which the below authors refer to as "mask-associated ocular irritation."

A paper in the journal, *Ophthalmology and Therapy*, "Face Mask-Associated Ocular Irritation and Dryness," written by Majid Moshirfar, William B. West Jr., and Douglas P. Marx warned of an increase in dry eye symptoms among mask wearers. Those using masks regularly for extended periods are more likely to show symptoms. The condition is caused by exhaled air blowing upwards from the mask into the eyes. The increased airflow causes irritation or inflammation. The authors conclude:[1]

> "This mask-associated ocular irritation raises concerns about eye health and increased risk of disease transmission in prolonged mask users."

Their advice is that lubricant eye drops should be used and goggles should be worn. Dry eyes lead to individuals rubbing their eyes which will lead to an increase in the risk of infection. Doctors and opticians are also reporting an increase in the number of patients complaining of persistent headaches — because of mask wearing.

In the true spirit of a cascade of medical intervention, Moshirfar, West, and Marx recommend goggles and eye drops. A better idea is to just stop wearing the unsafe and ineffective face mask.

If you never say "No!" to the medical community, you will end up with medicines and procedures which cause side effects. Some less than scrupulous doctors will provide you with more medicines and procedures to address those side effects that they caused, which will lead to more side effects and more intervention.

Doctors, public health officials, and politicians all have something in common — they need to clearly be told "No!" or else they will walk all over you.

A very clear way to say "No!" to them all is to never wear the unsafe and ineffective face mask and to never put one on your child.

Reason 167: Face Mask Use Impairs Vision

I never wear a face mask, so it never occurred to me how much worse ones vision becomes in a mask. A wearer of a face mask suffers from artificially induced downward peripheral vision loss. A student at a school board meeting I recently attended, during public comment, addressed this topic. She pointed to her newfound propensity to trip while walking down stairs in a face mask.

With our myopic medical community, myopic academic community, and myopic technocratic community leading the way in our vast society, it is easy to forget how the various parts of our body work so well in coordination with each other. Entire swaths of the American intelligentsia are obsessed with myopic views on life, from overspecialization in academia at the exclusion of all other fields, to symptom-focused medical treatment.

Say "No!" to such myopia. Say no to their intellectual tunnel vision. Refuse the mask. It is systemically harmful to you. Only someone with intellectual tunnel vision can justify the mask to themselves and others, even their children.

FACE MASK USE HARMS THE KIDNEYS

Reason 168: Face Masks
Are Hard On The Kidneys

Face masks lead to altered renal function. In the *Medical Hypotheses* article, "Exercise with face mask; Are we handling a devil's sword?" Baskaran Chandrasekaran and Shifra Fernandes write:[1]

> "Hypercapnic hypoxia reduces renal blood flow and glomerular filtration rate posing a risk of reduced renal functions. Thus, aciduria and resulting tubular damage may potentially aggravate the compromised renal functions in individuals with established chronic diseases.[2] Further, the autonomic dysfunction and reduced immune responses, increase the inflammatory substances such as C reactive protein, interleukins (IL-6, IL-12) resulting in generalized nephritis in chronic kidney failure patients.[3] Additionally, poor renal artery flow causes hypoxemia in nephrons perpetuating the pathophysiology of poor renal functions."

Low oxygen and high carbon dioxide is harmful to many people. Face masks artificially create that environment.

Those with weak kidneys should not wear a face mask, because it can exacerbate existing kidney problems. Though millions of Americans suffer from kidney disease, I have yet to see that warning anywhere. It has certainly not been plastered across society the way the harmful one-size-fits-all face mask directives have been.

Quite to the contrary, even patients on dialysis are forced to wear a face mask. What more evidence do we need to see that the people forcing the face mask on society do not care about individual health?

They do not care about you. They do not care about your family. They do not care about the health of your children.

You must not wear the face mask nor allow anyone to place your child in one.

Reason 169: N95 Respirators
Are Bad For Your Kidneys As Well

N95 Respirators are also bad for your kidneys, Baruch Vainshelboim writes in "Face masks in the Covid-19 era: A health hypothesis:"[1]

> "A study on 39 patients with renal disease found that wearing N95 face mask during hemodialysis significantly reduced arterial partial oxygen pressure (from PaO_2 101.7 to 92.7 mm Hg), increased respiratory rate (from 16.8 to 18.8 breaths/minute), and increased the occurrence of chest discomfort and respiratory distress.[2] Respiratory Protection Standards from Occupational Safety and Health Administration, US Department of Labor states that breathing air with O_2 concentration below 19.5% is considered oxygen-deficiency, causing physiological and health adverse effects. These include increased breathing frequency, accelerated heart rate and cognitive impairments related to thinking and coordination.[3] A chronic state of mild hypoxia and hypercapnia has been shown as primarily mechanism for developing cognitive dysfunction based on animal studies and studies in patients with chronic obstructive pulmonary disease."[4]

Dialysis patients should not be made to wear an N95 mask, nor any face mask at all. Both N95 masks and face masks are harmful to them in their compromised and fragile condition.

Some in public health say that is exactly who should be in a face mask: those most frail.

We see here, however, yet another example of how face masks hurt the most frail the most.

No one belongs in a face mask, least of all the most physiologically frail in society: the elderly, the infirm, and children.

FACE MASK USE HARMS THE LUNGS

Reason 170: You Need To Breathe, Everyone Needs To Breathe, Your Child Even Needs To Breathe

There was a time in which this chapter would have been considered absolute idiocy, because the ideas contained within are so obvious to anyone operating with a rational mind devoid of any agenda other than discovering the truth.

There will again, one day in the future, be a time in which this chapter will be considered absolute idiocy because the ideas contained within are so obvious to anyone operating with a rational mind devoid of any agenda other than discovering the truth.

This time we are in, this madness, this too shall pass.

Baruch Vainshelboim writes about the need to breathe in "Face masks in the Covid-19 era: A health hypothesis:"[1]

> "Breathing is one of the most important physiological functions to sustain life and health. Human body requires a continuous and adequate oxygen (O_2) supply to all organs and cells for normal function and survival. Breathing is also an essential process for removing metabolic byproducts [carbon dioxide (CO_2)] occurring during cell respiration.[2,3] It is well established that acute significant deficit in O_2 (hypoxemia) and increased levels of CO_2 (hypercapnia) even for few minutes can be severely harmful and lethal, while chronic hypoxemia and hypercapnia cause health deterioration, exacerbation of existing conditions, morbidity and ultimately mortality.[4-7] Emergency medicine demonstrates that 5–6 minutes of severe hypoxemia during cardiac arrest will cause brain death with extremely poor survival rates.[8-11] On the other hand, chronic mild or moderate hypoxemia and hypercapnia such as from wearing face masks resulting in shifting to higher contribution of anaerobic energy metabolism, decrease in pH levels and increase in cells and blood acidity, toxicity, oxidative stress, chronic inflammation, immunosuppression and health deterioration."[12-15]

Quite logically, restricting one's breathing leads to fundamental unhealthful and harmful changes in the body with far reaching consequences. Vainshelboim continues:

"Wearing face mask mechanically restricts breathing by increasing the resistance of air movement during both inhalation and exhalation process.[16,17] Although, intermittent (several times a week) and repetitive (10–15 breaths for 2–4 sets) increase in respiration resistance may be adaptive for strengthening respiratory muscles,[18,19] prolonged and continues effect of wearing face mask is maladaptive and could be detrimental for health.[20-22] In normal conditions at the sea level, air contains 20.93% O_2 and 0.03% CO_2, providing partial pressures of 100 mmHg and 40 mmHg for these gases in the arterial blood, respectively. These gas concentrations significantly altered when breathing occurs through face mask. A trapped air remaining between the mouth, nose and the face mask is rebreathed repeatedly in and out of the body, containing low O_2 and high CO_2 concentrations, causing hypoxemia and hypercapnia.[23-27] Severe hypoxemia may also provoke cardiopulmonary and neurological complications and is considered an important clinical sign in cardiopulmonary medicine.[28-33]

Wearing a face mask may, over time, lead to trouble with the cardiovascular system. Vainshelboim continues:

"Low oxygen content in the arterial blood can cause myocardial ischemia, serious arrhythmias, right or left ventricular dysfunction, dizziness, hypotension, syncope and pulmonary hypertension."[34]

Wearing a face mask may exacerbate existing conditions throughout the body, effectively making the sick sicker. Vainshelboim continues:

"Chronic low-grade hypoxemia and hypercapnia as result of using face mask can cause exacerbation of existing cardiopulmonary, metabolic, vascular and neurological conditions.[35-40] [The table below] summarizes the physiological, psychological effects of wearing face mask and their potential long-term consequences for health."

Below is a useful table from Vainshelboim that, as can be seen from the rest of this book, just begins to touch the surface on potential physiological and psychological effects of wearing a face mask and their potential health consequences.

Table 1

Physiological and Psychological Effects of Wearing Face mask and Their Potential Health Consequences.

Physiological Effects	Psychological Effects	Health Consequences
• Hypoxemia • Hypercapnia • Shortness of breath • Increase lactate concentration • Decline in pH levels • Acidosis • Toxicity • Inflammation • Self-contamination • Increase in stress hormones level (adrenaline, noradrenaline and cortisol) • Increased muscle tension • Immunosuppression	• Activation of "fight or flight" stress response • Chronic stress condition • Fear • Mood disturbances • Insomnia • Fatigue • Compromised cognitive performance	• Increased predisposition for viral and infection illnesses • Headaches • Anxiety • Depression • Hypertension • Cardiovascular disease • Cancer • Diabetes • Alzheimer disease • Exacerbation of existing conditions and diseases • Accelerated aging process • Health deterioration • Premature mortality

Wearing the face mask, as previously discussed, leads to additional pathogenic load on the body, as the face mask collects germs on its surface. In addition to the release of those toxic biological particles, it also leads to the release of toxic chemical particles. Vainshelboim continues:

> "In addition to hypoxia and hypercapnia, breathing through face mask residues bacterial and germs components on the inner and outside layer of the face mask. These toxic components are repeatedly rebreathed back into the body, causing self-contamination. Breathing through face masks also increases temperature and humidity in the space between the mouth and the mask, resulting a release of toxic particles from the mask's materials.[41-46] A systematic literature review estimated that aerosol contamination levels of face masks including 13 to 202,549 different viruses.[47] Rebreathing contaminated air with high bacterial and toxic particle concentrations along with low O_2 and high CO_2 levels continuously challenge the body homeostasis, causing self-toxicity and immunosuppression."[48-53]

Again, reports among surgeons and healthcare workers further highlight these findings. Vainshelboim continues:

> "The adverse physiological effects were confirmed in a study of 53 surgeons where surgical face mask were used during a major operation. After 60 minutes of face mask wearing the oxygen saturation dropped by more than 1% and heart rate increased by approximately five beats/minute.[54] Another study among 158 healthcare workers using protective personal equipment primarily N95 face masks reported that 81% (128 workers) developed new headaches during their work shifts as these become mandatory due to Covid-19 outbreak. For those who used the N95 face mask greater than 4 hours per day, the likelihood for developing a headache during the work shift was approximately four times higher [Odds ratio = 3.91, 95% CI (1.35–11.31) p = 0.012], while 82.2% of the N95 wearers developed the headache already within ≤10 to 50 minutes."[55]

You need to breathe, everyone needs to breathe, your child even needs to breathe. Such simple truth is being ignored in the face mask policies being issued across society and which many consent to in their own lives. Many claim to want to see those policies brought to an end. Such individual consent makes the end of such policies nearly impossible.

FACE MASK USE HARMS THE HEART

Reason 171: Face Masks Affect The Heart

Research has shown since at least 2005 face masks affect the hearts of healthy individuals. In the article "Review of scientific reports of harms caused by face masks," Denis Rancourt writes:[1]

> "We discuss how N95 and surgical face masks induce significantly different temperature and humidity in the microclimates of the face masks, which have profound influences on heart rate and thermal stress and subjective perception of discomfort."

In individuals with heart problems, the wearing of a face mask may be far worse, since the heart may not be able to compensate for the additional stress of the face mask. Rancourt continues:

> "These data suggest a myocardial [relating to the muscular tissue of the heart] compensation for the pulmonary limitation in the healthy volunteers. In patients with impaired myocardial function, this compensation may not be possible."

Heart disease is a top killer of Americans. Much effort goes into protecting people from heart conditions. Diet and exercise are important preventative approaches. Another way to protect your heart is to not wear a face mask, a device which has notable harmful impact upon the heart.

Reason 172: Face Masks Lead To Exhaustion And An Increased Stress On The Heart

Kai Kisielinski, in an April 20, 2021 article entitled "Is a Mask That Covers the Mouth and Nose Free from Undesirable Side Effects in Everyday Use and Free of Potential Hazards?" writes:[1]

> "In another experimental study (comparative study), surgical and N95 masks caused a significant increase in heart rate ($p < 0.01$) as well as a corresponding feeling of exhaustion ($p < 0.05$). These symptoms were accompanied by a sensation of heat ($p < 0.0001$) and itching ($p < 0.01$) due to moisture penetration of the masks ($p < 0.0001$) in 10 healthy volunteers of both sexes after only 90 minutes of physical activity.[2] Moisture penetration was determined via sensors by evaluating logs"

Face masks lead to exhaustion and increased stress on the heart. This is another reason not to wear them.

Literally, every single situation in which a person's body is under a high amount of stress, the introduction of a face mask should be an immediate red flag and should be challenged. Given the data above, no other option is logical.

If one is sick and fatigued, does it make sense to place that person in a medical device that causes additional sickness and fatigue? Absolutely not, this is a bad idea as a general principle and is unlikely to be a good idea in virtually all cases. Yet, as soon as one enters a hospital in a sick and fatigued condition, that is exactly what hospital staff force on the patient. For those who resist, staff may often go so far as to deny treatment to those who refuse to wear one.

This is not done in the interest of the patient, but out of a spirit of control. This behavior is sick and illogical and must be brought to a prompt end. Societally it must come to an end, but in your own life you must never say yes in such a situation again.

ENVIRONMENTAL CONCERNS

Reason 173: Environmental Harm

I have never been one to make plastic drinking straws or plastic bottles polluting waterways a high priority issue and I will not make face masks in waterways a high priority issue. There are more important issues around face masks for me.

Anyone who cared about straw and water bottle pollution, however, and does not care about the even greater harm face masks have to pollute and do harm to wildlife is being hypocritical on the topic, divulging that the issue of harm to wildlife and nature was likely not the key issue for them to begin with.

Environmentalism, just like any other field of activism that can tug at the heartstrings, is able to be used as a method of controlling others. Giving in to that spirit of control must be watched for carefully and avoided at all cost.

He who seeks to control, will only push further once his demands are met. He who acts out of sincerity, does not exhibit such an impulse.

Reason 174: Face Mask Wearing Comes With Environmental Effects

Masks break down easily, but their component fibers last a long time. Despite the relatively quick breakdown, the sheer quantities of masks create a huge environmental hazard. Kai Kisielinski, in an April 20, 2021 article entitled "Is a Mask That Covers the Mouth and Nose Free from Undesirable Side Effects in Everyday Use and Free of Potential Hazards?" writes:[1]

> "According to WHO estimates of a demand of 89 million masks per month, their global production will continue to increase under the Corona pandemic.[2] Due to the composition of, e.g., disposable surgical masks with polymers such as polypropylene, polyurethane, polyacrylonitrile, polystyrene, polycarbonate, polyethylene and polyester,[3] an increasing global challenge, also from an environmental point of view, can be expected, especially outside Europe, in the absence of recycling and disposal strategies."[2]

A common technocratic approach to a problem like this is to create another intervention in order to cure the problem caused by the original intervention. Creating a society-wide mask recycling program, providing it with a massive budget, and punishing those who do not comply would be an example of such an intervention built atop an already bad intervention. Medicine, as previously described, increasingly behaves this way. It is difficult to find a doctor who does not operate in this technocratic fashion. Medical researchers have described this tendency in the term "cascade of interventions," and have cautioned doctors against this approach.

A far more reasonable approach is to abandon the original intervention, especially when that intervention — mandatory masking of the general population — is both unsafe and ineffective.

This can be accomplished in this situation and others with questions like these.

1. **"What is causing this problem?"**

The answer to this question helps focus the inquiry.

2. **"Is it an approach advocated for by individuals in their own lives or is it being imposed upon them?"**

If imposed, the answer is almost always to lift the imposition, for it is an approach that will inevitably fail the individual.

3. "What are the risks and rewards of this approach?"

Do the benefits outweigh the costs? If not, what special interest is preventing this matter from being clearly examined?

With these three questions, you will almost always get to the root of any problem caused by an intervention, rather than piling intervention upon intervention in an attempt to cure the problems of previous interventions.

Face mask recycling programs are not the solution to this government created environmental catastrophe. Ending the unsafe and ineffective face mask mandates is the solution.

Not only do these fibers fill our oceans, which we treat as a dumping ground, the polymers in face masks are a pollutant in all of our water, including the water we drink. Kisielinski continues:

> "The aforementioned single use polymers have been identified as a significant source of plastic and plastic particles for the pollution of all water cycles up to the marine environment."[4]

Nor does it stop there with our drinking water. These polymers contained in face masks make their way into our food. Kisielinski continues:

> "A significant health hazard factor is contributed by mask waste in the form of microplastics after decomposition into the food chain."

We are eating plastic. This is not purely because of face masks, but we would be lying to ourselves if we pretended this massive amount of unsafe and ineffective single-use face masks produced, used, and dumped into the environment around us does not add to the amount of plastic in our water, in our food, and in our bodies.

Additionally, face masks are a biohazard in our immediate environment. They are a biohazard in a way other humans are not to us. They provide a breeding ground for harmful pathogens. Kisielinski continues:

> "Likewise, contaminated macroscopic disposable mask waste — especially before microscopic decay — represents a widespread medium for microbes (protozoa, bacteria, viruses, fungi) in terms of invasive pathogens.[5-9] Proper disposal of bio-contaminated everyday mask material is insufficiently regulated even in western countries."

Of course, we could again implement another protocol for proper waste disposal atop the already senseless, unsafe, and ineffective face mask mandates, but that would just be a predictably poor and knee-jerk reaction to a problem caused by mandatory masking. This intervention would doubtlessly lead to its own problems requiring the need for further intervention. Far better is to play no part in this and to not wear the unsafe and ineffective face mask.

This is yet another reason to not wear a face mask and to politely share your knowledge on this topic with others, so that they do not add to the environmental harm caused by wearing a face mask.

All of us who realize how unsafe and ineffective face masks are, must bravely share this knowledge face to face with people. Without you educating them on this topic, how would they ever find it?

This craziness did not start today, but in your life, this can end with you.

Reason 175: The Great Pacific Face Mask Patch

By the end of April 2020, China was producing 450 million masks daily.[1]

"Given an annual production figure of 52 billion disposable masks and a loss rate of 3% (the percentage of masks that escape water management systems),"[2] Teale Phelps Bondaroff,[3] Director of Research for OceansAsia, and his team, concluded, "Nearly 1.6 billion face masks wound up in our oceans in 2020. This amounts to approximately 5,500 tons of plastic pollution."

That means masks released into the oceans in 2020 alone represent the equivalent of 7% of the 80,000 ton Great Pacific Garbage Patch, a mass of plastic debris that floats in the Pacific Ocean.[2]

Based on widely available estimates, writer Marcus Lu points to an additional area of concern — the amount of time it takes a single-use face mask to biodegrade:

"Despite their single-use nature, disposable masks are expected to take more than four centuries to decompose while in the ocean. Here's how this compares to other items we use on a day-to-day basis."[2]

It takes 10 years for a cigarette butt to biodegrade, 20 years for a plastic grocery bag to biodegrade, 50 years for a styrofoam cup to biodegrade, and 200 years for an alumnim can to biodegrade, but 450 years for a face mask to biodegrade.[2]

Garbage in the Pacific was not a prime concern in my life prior to 2020 and it is not now. For those who had that as a prime concern then, but who are now silent on the topic, red flags should be raised about the sincerity of their motivation. The simplest way to alleviate this component of the Pacific Ocean pollution problem is to stop mandating face masks. Given the fact that there is no upside to face mask mandates, this would be a policy move with significant upside.

Those who seek to create more jobs for their environmental policy friends, will instead talk about face mask recapture programs and face mask recycling programs. Such talk is a sure sign that the speaker has no interest in doing the hard work of dealing with the root cause of the problem — the entirely senseless government mandated face mask orders and the corresponding media-driven fear campaigns on the topic.

Despite those sensible or senseless changes at the governmental level, you do not have to comply in your own life. Many people, such as myself, despite my existence in a most locked down place, live a normal life and do not comply. If pollution is a concern of yours, in your own life, you can stop feeding into such madness by no longer complying with face mask orders. Far from being a mere uncomfortable sacrifice that you make to benefit others, face masks are harmful to the life of the wearer, harmful to the lives of those whom it is worn around, and harmful to aquatic life. Better can and should be expected of each of us.

Reason 176: Kids Are Not A Biohazard — Dirty Face Masks On The Ground Are The True Biohazard

Children are not a biohazard. Used face masks are a biohazard and suddenly they seem to appear in every grocery store parking lot and every busy urban sidewalk. We are supposed to treat this as acceptable, when this is really another reason these awful one-size-fits-all, heavy-handed public health policies should be done away with, and those who implemented them permanently removed from all positions of public trust.

Further elaborating on the concerns of the previous chapter, in the article "Covid-19: Each discarded face mask is a potential biohazard," James H. Bamber and Tracey Christmas state:[1]

> "Javid and colleagues say that 'population benefits are plausible and harms unlikely' if the public are encouraged to wear face masks.[2] In one week (17-24 April) both of us, however, came across discarded surgical face masks on public roads on our way to work. On a single day, one of us (TC) came across six discarded masks on a cycleway. This is before any encouragement from the government for the public to wear masks. Each of these discarded masks represents a potential biohazard[3] that must be managed in a similar way to discarded hypodermic needles and syringes."

These authors properly point to the biohazard that face masks are. They are a breeding ground on which normal bacterial load in, on, and around a person is concentrated. Without face masks, this biohazard would not exist. Normal human interaction is not dangerous the way face masks are. Without face mask mandates, these biohazards would be far less in number. The policy creates biohazards all around us, which would otherwise not exist. If face masks are to be worn, they should be treated as the biohazard that they are. Even better, though, is to not wear the unsafe and ineffective things.

Bamber and Christmas also point to other concerns with this biohazard:

> "Such as contamination by touching the mask then touching other surfaces and fomites."

And while the incorrect wearing of a mask has been covered elsewhere in this book, Bamber and Christmas point to their own experiences in hospital settings with improper mask use among trained personnel.

"Additionally, the value of masks to protect other members of the public is diminished if they are incorrectly worn. As anesthetists we have seen other health professionals in our hospital wear masks in a variety of ways — below the nose, on the chin — because of the discomfort they cause."[4]

Appropriately, given this firsthand experience Bamber and Christmas cite, they seek to limit expectations for anyone who thinks the general public is going to wear a mask properly when highly trained professionals do not:

"Why should we expect the public to exhibit greater care in their mask wearing to ensure that the benefits outweigh the risks?"

The face mask biohazard is harmful to the wearer and to others in a way that a healthy human simply is not. Here is yet another reason why no one should wear, or be around, an unsafe and ineffective face mask, least of all your children.

FACE MASK USE LEADS TO MASK-INDUCED EXHAUSTION SYNDROME AND OTHER SYSTEMIC CONDITIONS

Reason 177: Symptoms Of Face Mask Wearing Are Now Being Blamed On Covid-19

Covid-19 is a bad cold for some. Covid-19 is asymptomatic or mild in 99% of people. That means it is not even a bad cold for them. The percent it harms are obese, overweight, seriously ill, or well past their life expectancy. Such people are badly harmed by the common cold too. The antigen and PCR tests used to determine Covid-19 infection are terribly inaccurate, so at best what can be said is that "The variety of cold and flu bugs that went around in late 2019 and early 2020 were rough on some." We cannot pinpoint which coronaviruses, which rhinoviruses, which influenza viruses did the damage in individual cases.

That is something that should really get people worked up.

My entire life, I have heard people say things like "I have been sicker for weeks than I have ever been," or "I caught something that floored me," or "My neighbor's grandmother died of pneumonia." Every single year a few hundred thousand Americans die from a respiratory virus and some hundreds of thousands more die with a respiratory virus hitting them hard. 2020 was the same. The difference was the insanity of the reaction, a reaction that shows Americans to be a far more frivolous people than I had ever thought possible. 2019 to 2020 was a regular cold and flu season. 2020 to 2021 was as well.

Very few healthy Americans wore a face mask before April 3, 2020. If you have an unusual symptom from this book and you wear a face mask, it makes a lot more sense to blame it on the unsafe and ineffective face mask you wear on your face all day than to blame it on a cold or flu, something you have had to contend with every year you have been alive and which all humans have had to contend with every year they have been alive.

Did a bioweapon escape from the Wuhan lab? I do not know. You do not know. No one knows without believing some nonsense from two of the most untrustworthy governments in the world — China and the United States.

But if it is that important to you, let us do this:

Why not take off your face mask for a few months, see if the harm you have done to yourself begins to subside, and then let us talk about bat viruses.

Occam's Razor says look at the simplest answer first. Occam's Razor says the unsafe and ineffective, experimental mask is the variable — not a virus. Occam's Razor says the unsafe, ineffective, and experimental Covid shot is the variable, not the virus.

Eliminate the simple explanations from your life and then let us talk about the complex ones.

Logic dictates that approach. Government, media, and medicine suggest you focus on something different, but I know this much — after everyone in the government, the media, and the medical establishment are long gone, some basic reasoning from William of Occam in the thirteenth century will still be with us. Basic logic from Ancient Greece will still be with us. Basic rules of reason and evidence from the sixteenth and seventeenth century underlying the scientific method will still be with us.

Wisdom that has lasted the test of time tells me I cannot take you seriously if you wear an unsafe and ineffective face mask while telling me a bioweapon from Wuhan caused the symptoms that your face mask is known to cause.

Reason 178: The Long-Term Consequences Of Face Mask Wearing Are Likely Far Worse Than We Can Imagine

The long-term consequences of face mask wearing are likely far worse than we can imagine. Baruch Vainshelboim writes in "Face masks in the Covid-19 era: A health hypothesis:"[1]

"Long-term practice of wearing face masks has strong potential for devastating health consequences. Prolonged hypoxic-hypercapnic state compromises normal physiological and psychological balance, deteriorating health and promotes the developing and progression of existing chronic diseases.[2-11] For instance, ischemic heart disease caused by hypoxic damage to the myocardium is the most common form of cardiovascular disease and is a number one cause of death worldwide (44% of all non-communicable diseases) with 17.9 million deaths occurred in 2016.[12] Hypoxia also playing an important role in cancer burden.[13] Cellular hypoxia has strong mechanistic feature in promoting cancer initiation, progression, metastasis, predicting clinical outcomes and usually presents a poorer survival in patients with cancer. Most solid tumors present some degree of hypoxia, which is independent predictor of more aggressive disease, resistance to cancer therapies and poorer clinical outcomes.[14,15] Worth note, cancer is one of the leading causes of death worldwide, with an estimate of more than 18 million new diagnosed cases and 9.6 million cancer-related deaths occurred in 2018.[16]

"With respect to mental health, global estimates showing that Covid-19 will cause a catastrophe due to collateral psychological damage such as quarantine, lockdowns, unemployment, economic collapse, social isolation, violence and suicides.[17-19] Chronic stress along with hypoxic and hypercapnic conditions knocks the body out of balance, and can cause headaches, fatigue, stomach issues, muscle tension, mood disturbances, insomnia and accelerated aging.[20-24] This state suppressing the immune system to protect the body from viruses and bacteria, decreasing cognitive function, promoting the developing and exacerbating the major health issues including hypertension, cardiovascular disease, diabetes, cancer, Alzheimer disease, rising anxiety and depression states, causes social isolation and loneliness and increasing the risk for premature mortality."[25-29]

Though we are beginning to more fully understand the impacts of face masks, the fact that the list of harm caused by a face mask seems to daily grow, indicates we may long be finding new examples of fallout from the face mask debacle of 2020 and 2021.

Reason 179: Face Mask Wearing Creates Symptoms Akin To "Sick Building Syndrome"

We have long known oxygen and carbon dioxide levels of the surrounding environment are important for the wellbeing of a human in that environment.

Kai Kisielinski, in an April 20, 2021 article entitled "Is a Mask That Covers the Mouth and Nose Free from Undesirable Side Effects in Everyday Use and Free of Potential Hazards?" writes:[1]

> "The fact that prolonged exposure to latently elevated CO_2 levels and unfavorable breathing air compositions has disease-promoting effects was recognized early on."

Kisielinski specifically points to a term that many readers will likely recognize — Sick Building Syndrome, and draws parallels between Sick Building Syndrome and mask use:

> "As early as 1983, the WHO described 'Sick Building Syndrome' (SBS) as a condition in which people living indoors experienced acute disease-relevant effects that increased with time of their stay, without specific causes or diseases.[2,3] The syndrome affects people who spend most of their time indoors, often with subliminally elevated CO_2 levels, and are prone to symptoms such as increased heart rate, rise in blood pressure, headaches, fatigue and difficulty concentrating."[3,4]

From headache and fatigue, to more subtle internal changes, face mask wearing and Sick Building Syndrome appear to create similar changes in the body. Kisielinski continues:

> "Some of the complaints described in the mask studies we found are surprisingly similar to those of Sick Building Syndrome.[2] Temperature, carbon dioxide content of the air, headaches, dizziness, drowsiness and itching also play a role in Sick Building Syndrome. On the one hand, masks could themselves be responsible for effects such as those described for Sick Building Syndrome when used for a longer period of time."

Kisielinski takes this a step further and even theorizes that face masks and prolonged indoor conditions may together lead to even more harmful consequences:

"On the other hand, they could additionally intensify these effects when worn in air-conditioned buildings, especially when masks are mandatory indoors. Nevertheless, there was a tendency towards higher systolic blood pressure values in mask wearers in some studies,[5-7] but statistical significance was only found in two studies.[8,9] However, we found more relevant and significant evidence of heart rate increase, headache, fatigue and concentration problems associated with mask wearers indicating the clinical relevance of wearing masks."

The media once spent a great deal of effort sensationalizing Sick Building Syndrome. Today, with the public health threat that face mask mandates pose, the media is woefully silent.

So many media organs have proven untrustworthy through this era. This is up to you, as an individual, and you as a parent or authority figure, to see to it that you do not mask yourself and you never mask the children in your care.

Reason 180: Face Masks Lead To Mask-Induced Exhaustion Syndrome (MIES)

Sick Building Syndrome has similar symptoms to mask wearing. Kisielinski documents those symptoms and distinguishes them from Sick Building Syndrome, because of course they are not caused by being in a building, but by the wearing of a mask. Kisielinski calls it Mask-Induced Exhaustion Syndrome or MIES.

Kai Kisielinski, in an April 20, 2021 article entitled "Is a Mask That Covers the Mouth and Nose Free from Undesirable Side Effects in Everyday Use and Free of Potential Hazards?" describes Mask-Induced Exhaustion Syndrome:[1]

> "Since the symptoms were described in combination in mask wearers and were not observed in isolation in the majority of cases, we refer to them as general Mask-Induced Exhaustion Syndrome (MIES) because of the consistent presentation in numerous papers from different disciplines. These include the following, predominantly statistically significantly ($p < 0.05$) proven pathophysiological changes and subjective complaints, which often occur in combination:
>
> - Increase in dead space volume.[2-5]
>
> - Increase in breathing resistance.[6-9]
>
> - Increase in blood carbon dioxide.[2,3,10-18]
>
> - Decrease in blood oxygen saturation.[6,12,13,17-25]
>
> - Increase in heart rate.[2,7,13,18,21,22]
>
> - Decrease in cardiopulmonary capacity.[6]
>
> - Feeling of exhaustion.[6,7,11,12,18,21,23-26]
>
> - Increase in respiratory rate.[11-13,25]
>
> - Difficulty breathing and shortness of breath.[6,7,11-14,21,25,27-30]
>
> - Headache.[16,18,31-35]
>
> - Dizziness.[13,21]
>
> - Feeling of dampness and heat.[2,6,7,11,21,28,30,36]
>
> - Drowsiness (qualitative neurological deficits).[18,21,23,31,37]
>
> - Decrease in empathy perception.[38]

- Impaired skin barrier function with acne, itching, and skin lesions." [31,39,40]

Here we have a description of Mask-Induced Exhaustion Syndrome. Kisielinski adds words of caution that the above symptoms and pathological consequences are observed in healthy people wearing a mask, which indicates even more pronounced symptoms and pathological consequences for more frail people in a mask. This includes the sick, the elderly, or the young.

"It can be deduced from the results that the effects described in healthy people are all more pronounced in sick people, since their compensatory mechanisms, depending on the severity of the illness, are reduced or even exhausted. Some existing studies on and with patients with measurable pathological effects of the masks support this assumption.[13,14,18,25] In most scientific studies, the exposure time to masks in the context of the measurements/investigations was significantly less (in relation to the total wearing and duration of use) than is expected of the general public under the current pandemic regulations and ordinances. The exposure time limits are little observed or knowingly disregarded in many areas today... The above facts allow the conclusion that the described negative effects of masks, especially in some of our patients and the very elderly, may well be more severe and adverse with prolonged use than presented in some mask studies."

We have here, yet another reason not to mask yourself, anyone around you, and least of all your child.

SUMMARY

Reason 181: Covid Is Hardly More Dangerous Than The Flu, Face Masks Have No Impact On Respiratory Viruses Anyway, And Masks Are Measurably Harmful In The Short-Term, Long-Term, And Cumulatively

To conclude this portion of the book, please allow me to summarize in saying Covid is hardly more dangerous than the flu, masks have no beneficial impact on respiratory viruses anyway, and masks are measurably harmful in the short-term, long-term, and cumulatively.

In an April 20, 2021 article entitled "Is a Mask That Covers the Mouth and Nose Free from Undesirable Side Effects in Everyday Use and Free of Potential Hazards?" Kai Kisielinski writes:[1]

> "On the one hand, the advocacy of an extended mask requirement remains predominantly theoretical and can only be sustained with individual case reports, plausibility arguments based on model calculations and promising in vitro laboratory tests. Moreover, recent studies on Sars-Cov-2 show both a significantly lower infectivity[2] and a significantly lower case mortality than previously assumed, as it could be calculated that the median corrected infection fatality rate (IFR) was 0.10% in locations with a lower than average global Covid-19 population mortality rate.[3] In early October 2020, the WHO also publicly announced that projections show Covid-19 to be fatal for approximately 0.14% of those who become ill — compared to 0.10% for endemic influenza — again a figure far lower than expected."[4]

Covid is hardly more dangerous than the flu. It would have been a big, boring flu season just like every other flu season, if we would have left nature to do its thing. That is not what we did, however. We decided, instead to exacerbate the mistakes. Kisielinski continues:

> "On the other hand, the side effects of masks are clinically relevant. In our work, we focused exclusively on the undesirable and negative side effects that can be produced by masks. Valid significant evidence of combined mask-related changes were objectified (p < 0.05, n ≥ 50%), and we found a clustered and common occurrence of the differ-

ent adverse effects within the respective studies with significantly measured effects. We were able to demonstrate a statistically significant correlation of the observed adverse effect of hypoxia and the symptom of fatigue with $p < 0.05$ in the quantitative evaluation of the primary studies. Our review of the literature shows that both healthy and sick people can experience Mask-Induced Exhaustion Syndrome (MIES), with typical changes and symptoms that are often observed in combination, such as an increase in breathing dead space volume,[5-8] increase in breathing resistance,[9-12] increase in blood carbon dioxide,[5,6,10,13-24] decrease in blood oxygen saturation,[9,16-18,23-25,28-34] increase in heart rate,[10,18,23,24] increase in blood pressure,[10,19] decrease in cardiopulmonary capacity,[9] increase in respiratory rate,[14,17,18,28,29] shortness of breath and difficulty breathing,[9-11,14-19,23,28,30-34] headache,[16,21,23,30,34-38] dizziness,[18,23] feeling hot and clammy,[5,9,10,15,23,30,31,33,39] decreased ability to concentrate,[23] decreased ability to think,[29,40] drowsiness,[16,23,26,29,40] decrease in empathy perception,[41] impaired skin barrier function[40,42,43] with itching,[9,10,30,36,42-46] acne, skin lesions and irritation,[40,42,43] overall perceived fatigue and exhaustion." [9,10,14,16,17,23,26,28,47]

With the above now being made abundantly clear in the pages of this book, I wrote a book, *Face Masks in One Lesson*, that goes in-depth on how to never wear a face mask again. The vow to never wear a face mask again is a vow each self-respecting human should make to himself. For those more interested in accessing that information by video, I also provide high quality videos free of charge to all who sign up at www.RealStevo.com.

Let me close with an abbreviated version of how to never put a mask on yourself or your child again.

CONCLUSION

Now What Do I Do?

I do not care much for mass movements. I do not care much for giant protests. I prefer the power of individual acts of courage.

Big protests tend to be bolstered by strength in numbers. Such masses can easily be manipulated, distracted, and sidetracked, especially when they are cheaply won to a cause — easy come, easy go.

Any day, I will take 10 lions who have stared down a face mask order and never worn a mask, navigating life with calm conversation, over a 10,000 person strong mob that will do anything I ask.

The one will march toward freedom no matter what the person next to him is doing. The latter is fickle, distractable, troublesome, unserious, and of specious ends.

I do not want anyone like that around me, nor should you.

Those tested in battle, resolute about not wearing a mask, grow with every instance of effort invested into them. Water seeds like that, and they will sprout and flourish.

The same may happen with an untested member of the masses, but it is unlikely. It is very likely with the battle-tested individual who has stood against masks.

Just as all that glitters is not gold, the strength of numbers is illusory.

Quality is more important than quantity at moments like these.

That being said, I have nothing against masses of quality people. I will happily attend a protest of 10,000 lions. I will happily encourage 100 million mask-refusing Americans onto the street.

All this is to say: it is all up to you.

Everything comes down to how you live your life.

Do not think too much about a far flung city where you do not spend time. Do not concern yourself with a national retailer you do not visit. Do not even think too much about Washington, D.C., unless you are concretely affected by an individual action taking place there.

Do not do any of that, unless you first have your own life in order and are bored by how easy this process of never wearing a face mask is.

You see, even with health mandates from Washington, D.C., their mask policies require someone else, someone local, to enforce them. That is the person you have to be more concerned about. So much of the huffing and puffing since the Ides of March 2020 is unenforceable nonsense from a bunch of blowhards.

Do not believe the hype, because if you do, it is that much easier to grow demoralized by the hype.

1.   **Find the primary sources.**

Find the policies that affect you, not the articles, or press releases, or emails, or websites *about* the policy. Find the actual policy. "Could you tell me where I could find the PDF of that policy complete with exemptions?" is a useful phrase to get to the five or ten page, sober legal document written by an attorney.

I am not saying I like these policies, or that they should be honored, only that it is good to read these policies so you know exactly what you are dealing with.

Reading this policy is "signal," the important stuff. All other talk about policies should be considered "noise."

2.   **After you have read the policy, put your hacker hat on.**

Look for the loopholes; look for exemptions; look for clever approaches that show this policy to be not applicable to you.

3.   **If they claim to be based on local orders, look at the local orders they claim to be based on.**

All government orders on this topic have exemptions. Such exemptions are required by longstanding federal law.

4.   **It really comes down to human to human conversation**

This involves two things. First, figure out who to ask for something. Ask only those who can give it to you. Second, ask that person in a way that allows that person to say "Yes!" to you. This usually requires thinking of that person first, and considering what he needs from you to be able to say "Yes!"

"I am unable to wear a face mask safely" usually accomplishes that.

Many other methods work. Having a human to human conversation is at the heart of all methods that I find valuable enough to recommend to people. That is what it all comes down to.

How do we, as individuals, return the world around us to a place in which civil conversation is again the preferred method of human interaction?

The simple answer, the tested answer, the effective answer is this: model that behavior in the world around you, and the world around you will tend to return you that favor of interacting with you in a civil, human to human conversation.

5.   **Never ever wear a face mask for any reason.**

If you are going to be successful in this endeavor, you need to resolve to never wear a face mask again — not for any reason. If you can resolve to do that, you will be one of the millions of Americans successfully doing exactly that.

6. Find others who do not wear a face mask.

Get their phone numbers. Call them together in the same physical location, even if just socially. Do this at least once a week.

Before you know it, it will be much more than social — people like us just start to do cool things when we are put in a room with each other together.

Start this routine, even if it is only you and another person initially.

7. Help teach people who want to stop wearing a face mask.

Once you have gone a few days without a face mask, you quickly begin to see how well it all works. Surgeons say "see one, do one, teach one." When they are learning, they often watch a person perform a technique, then they perform the technique successfully, then they teach another that technique. The same works with the face mask technique described here. The more quickly you replicate yourself by teaching this skill, the better it is for you, for others, and for society.

8. Wash. Rinse. Repeat.

Keep doing this, and your one person group of passionate people will be 30, 300, even 3,000, before you know it.

I mean that.

And just like fissile material, you can have one pile on one side of a table doing nothing, another pile on another side of a table doing nothing, but push the two piles together and there will be enough to achieve critical mass and start a chain reaction.

Amazing things can happen when a few special people are brought together. All you need to do is to bring them together.

It is all up to you.

As for this book, I welcome you to use this book as a tool. It is not intended to have all the answers. It is intended to ask a lot of questions, and to bolster your position with a lot of evidence.

My publishing team and I have designed this book to be of a size and weight that allows you to take it with you and wave it around as you speak about the topic of face masks. It has the right amount of heft to thump on a podium or desk as you speak, as a way to emphasize your key points.

While thumping the book on a desk you can ask: "Have you read *Face Masks Hurt Kids* yet?" You can ask that matter-of-factly, as if he would have naturally read it.

Wait for an answer. *Wait for an answer.*

"Do you have any idea what kind of harm these face masks do to kids?"

Wait for an answer. *Wait for an answer.*

"I cannot see how any responsible professional can be mandating them."

Stare at the allegedly responsible professional. Pause for an uncomfortably long period of time as you stare at him. Break the silence dramatically by thumping the book down again.

"Covid is a bad enough illness, and you want to harm them more by putting these face masks on them? It is criminal."

The book is designed as your tool for a moment like that.

It is meant to be easy to access and to have easy to spot main points. It is meant to be a good resource.

I am not a doctor. I write about science. Maybe one day a doctor will be brave enough to write this book. Until then, you have got me. Do not let anyone say to you "Well, it is not written by an MD, is it?"

That does not matter. That is an *ad hominem* fallacy — an attack on the person asking the question rather than an addressing of the question itself. Do not be distracted by such silly and manipulative attempts to distract your well-intentioned interest. If someone wants to criticize this book, make that person interact with the questions raised here and prove to you how wrong these concerns are. That is the proper way to criticize this book or any body of thought. If you insist that person interact with these thoughts in that legitimate way, both you and he will end up closer to the truth, simply because you insisted that legitimate debate take place.

This book exists to make it easy to ask the questions and to not be bullied by anyone in the process.

Is it going to be foolproof?

No.

It all comes down to you. Unless you are superhuman, like each of us, when we try something new, there is a learning curve and a growth process involved.

Be honest. Be sincere. Be strategic.

Do your best. Keep doing your best. Stay encouraged. Fill your reading with the stories of the successful, rather than the stories of anything disheartening. Grow your numbers. Keep doing that over and again and as the saying goes, "The truth always prevails."

Stay focused on that outcome and you will win.

Also, go to www.RealStevo.com right now and sign up. I will happily be part of your emotional life support. I will send you videos on how to do this better. I believe in this stuff and I stand by it. More books are coming and you can always expect encouraging emails from me. I do not send discouraging messages to people. I realize this is psychological warfare and anything that discourages is a bullet fired for the enemy, no matter who it comes from.

Until these health mandates are gone, until we have rolled back tyranny many years into the past, and until we have built a more free world, I am in it to win it.

The ashes of the American empire are all around us.

People like you, me, and our children are needed to build the new America that will prosper long into the future.

Thank you for joining me in that effort.

Allan Stevo
November 17, 2021
Rock Snake Lake
Near Swallow Cliff, California

APPENDIX

Acknowledgements

A lamp is not to be hid under a bushel basket. It is not to be hid under a bed. It is to be allowed to shine before others.

Though I have been a Christian since birth, a more diligent pursuit of the Lord accompanied the writing of this book — through the Bible, through fasting, through prayer. It brought a level of insight and relationship I never imagined possible through my decades of worship. A new chapter has been opened in my life because of my willingness to more obediently pursue the Lord.

Experience has shown that those who have walked that path know these rewards. Experience has also shown, those who have not walked that path and wish not to would not be able to make sense of many words I have to say about that walk.

Wanting that appears to be all the difference. Wanting like you want your next breathe. Wanting to understand God's ways better. Wanting to make faith real. Wanting closeness to God. That deep, long wanting.

It is not just being willing or having "a will" to accomplish something. It goes even further. It becomes a need.

Wanting that, you take some bold leaps of faith that can seem at the same time minutely irrelevant to some in the outside world and also entirely dangerous, harmful, and irrational to others. That wanting drives so many to learn and demand of themselves that which brings them closer to God.

A common characteristic of notable church fathers is that want. I can finally understand what drove Paul to such lengths, what drove early Christians to such lengths, what drove the gaunt saints of the eastern churches to such lengths, what drove the saints of the Roman church to such lengths, what drove men like Jan Hus or Martin Luther to such lengths, perhaps even what drove men like George Washington to such lengths. Men with such a fire are hard for anyone to describe as "reasonable."

The rest of the world would throw around words "fanaticism" or "terrorist" about such men and throw it around loosely, with little interest in understanding what those men have in them. Such men do not have enough of the world in them, and that makes all the difference to the world. It also seems to make all the difference in coming to know God.

In fact, a common characteristic of those who profess to not "get" that discipleship is a lack of want to get it — perhaps a reliance on themselves, or a reliance in their old ways, or a reliance in the bonds of religion.

I once had such characteristics. I once saw myself as reasonable, despite having seen myself as a Christian. I once kept myself from taking that leap of faith that makes all the rest so real. To take that leap of faith makes it nearly impossible to be seen as reasonable to the outside world. I get how weak the excuses can be, excuses I hear so often, and excuses that would so freely leave my own mouth.

There is no perfection that has been reached in this process, in fact, quite the opposite is true. The more I grow, the more I realize how much work I have left. But I have changed my mind and I have resolved to do away with those limitations when I see them.

Those who want to get it, come to get it. Those who do not want to get it, generally fathom such precepts impossible, out of reach, or even not credible.

To say all this is to preface my first thank you in this acknowledgement:

All glory and honor to the Lord for the words contained in this book. This book would not have come into being without constant and clear prompting.

Recognizing that, I give thanks foremost to God for this book.

God encouraged me to write this book. When I stopped writing it, he sent someone to me who barely knew me, who said in prayer she was told this was a book I had put down that needed to be picked up and finished. Her words were "The Lord showed me you have a new book stirring inside of you. Do not delay any longer 'execute' is the word He gave me. Even if that means setting aside what you are working on now. I also want you to know it is very important to spend time in his presence. This is the way you truly get to know anyone, by spending quality time with them. I am sensing Holy Spirit has been telling you this in other ways, and it is time. As you walk in obedience He will write that book through you ..."

Every time I saw that message, I was pushed with greater focus to finish this project.

All thanks, all praise, all glory and honor to God for the writing of this book. All shortcomings in this book are my own.

Face Masks Hurt Kids was finished while reading the book of Luke, the most underrated book of the Bible. It was written appropriately, by a physician.

Luke wrote about influential officials of his day, those in seats of power: "Beware ye of the leaven of the Pharisees, which is hypocrisy." This attack on hypocrisy, this caution around such deceit rings true today.

That is what he had to so poetically say of the earthly power that was so present, involved, tyrannical, and fear-producing in the lives of so many people. It was bolstered by hypocrisy. Its hypocrisy puffed it up, made it look bigger, even made it all so much more palatable. It spread through the air to every corner of the home that it could reach — almost anything. It was almost impossible to contain it was so massively full of hypocrisy and corrupting to all around it. The only way to possibly combat it was to take every morsel that touched the leaven, that touched the hypocrisy, and banish it from the home. That is a fraction of what he had to say about the officials of the day, those who so many people looked up to as righteous examples of authority.

Meanwhile, he wrote about the true authority "Fear not little flock; for it is your Father's good pleasure to give you the kingdom." He wrote to us to fear not, to live in faith. Everything is being established for us. Everything, the entire kingdom is what is being prepared for us. Those are two very different messages about authority, but very compatible — one authority legitimate, one authority illegitimate. Fear not he tenderly writes. Fear not.

As one wise minister counseled me about my thoughts on Luke:

"Absolutely brother Allan, God wants to reveal a whole bunch to you in the book of Luke. These are changing times, these are powerful times to get rid of a whole lot of leaven out of our lives." May this book help you to clear leaven out of your own life, you own home, your own family, your own community, whether that leaven be hypocrisy or some other ill that has spread and needs cleaning out.

My gratitude to the author of that stunningly powerful book.

The Russians have the word "samizdat," to refer to work published outside of approved government channels during time of censorship. This book, more than any I have written, has been that kind of book. As such, virtually everyone in my life who knows about my passion for this subject has turned into a source of research by sending me articles each have come across. Traditional methods of research were not able to suffice for this book. Links from silenced researchers are not able to be found using traditional methods of research. I am grateful to hundreds for helping me to navigate that challenge, not all of whom are mentioned here. Thank you for that help.

Ryan Andersen, Johan Vandertuin, Mitra Vandertuin, Anna Muravitskaya, A.J. Gokcek, Ali Schultz, Alix Mayer, Bishop Gabriel Abdelaziz and Rev. Dorothy Abdelaziz. Ryan & Jezer Delgado, Geoff Brown, Hugh Michael Matheny, Lee Bright, Kenneth Michnay (a victim of the Covid treatment protocol who left us in Thanksgiving 2020), Nick Spanos (one who was briefly treated by doctors for Covid before dismissing the treatment protocol as quackery and survived Thanksgiving 2020), Sheri Nelson, Tara Thornton, Cindy Chaffian, James Jones, Vic Porter, Damon Hyde, Jenny Negron, David Sussman, Beth Greer, Che Coho, Judy Keesecker, Aaron Benda, Karen Roth, Angela Kodicek, Gary Saddlemyer, Robert Katona, Allen Skilicorn, Christina Hildebrand, Milica Tucakovic, Suzy Abbot, Kami Joyce, Mike Hanks, Sydney Powell, Laura Marshall, R.J. Weiss, Tim Engler, Michael Stanchie, Mark Corcoran, Robert Hochberger, Adam Kokesh, Wyatt Bullard, Peter Cioth, Scott Mize, Terri Pope, Rev. Artur Pavlowski, Sevan Kevorkian, Michael Edelstein, Miguel Olivares, Donya Esquerra-Guerrero, Dorota Niewczas, Myles Camack, Doug Pike, Liz Handley, Donald Trowbridge, Meredith McMurray, Anh Coulton, Rev. Michal Misina, John Hochberger, Deborah Michael, Roger Sharp, Alyssa Patrick, David Bullard, Rev. Chase Alderete, Rev. Butch Paugh, Peggy Paul, Deborah McCain, Jeffrey Alan, Aaron Hamilton, Fred Duval, Sheila Heally, Kim Marone, Jared Pascolla, and Liz Buchanan.

My gratitude to Robert Wenzel (1957-2021). In Bob, I had an advocate, someone to bounce ideas off of, a fellow writer, an activist and radical, and someone to plan the unorthodox with. Each time we met, he made sure I was able to recognize the unique contribution that I had to bring to the world around me, through a combination of gifts that he had never before seen in anyone he said. To have such a statement so regularly made from someone my senior, someone so well connected, and someone generally lacking in sentimentality was a considerable encouragement. His presence made the days since the Ides of March 2020 far more tolerable, and perhaps more importantly, made it constantly clear that to whom much is given, much is to be expected.

My appreciation to Rev. Choy, Rev. Rebecca, Prayer Mountain, Shalom Farms, Brickyard Inn, The Nugget, Swallow Cliff, Ron and Marilyn (1940-2021) Blackwood, Cowgirl del Paso, Ben Corona, Bev Henshaw, and Pat Addy, Charlene (1946-2021) & Leslie Dean. Thank you.

Much of my writing on face masks has been a community effort. The greatest online gathering of writers, readers, free men, and activists takes place each day at LewRockwell.com. For this, I am in debt to Mr. Rockwell, who has housed that bold community and given me a place to write for better than a decade.

Without Ron Paul, there is no freedom movement, as we today know it. On December 7, 2007, he became the grandfather of the Tea Party movement when his supporters from Strasbourg, France to Lake Jackson,

Texas organized the first events in the contemporary Tea Party movement. No longer in office, this astute watchdog of government overreach and philosopher, on Tuesday, March 17, 2020, the first day of the San Francisco lockdown penned the syndicated column "The Coronavirus Hoax,"[1] in which he predicts correctly that some will die of corona, so the vulnerable must protect themselves, and that all must remain alert to the authoritarians making Covid an excuse for massive power grabs.

Gary Barnett brought passion. Becky Akers brought standards — from government, to libertarians, to God's servants on earth. Boy was Becky Akers disappointed. When push came to shove, she watched the biggest talkers out there melt into the most compliant on the proving grounds of 2020. She brought friendship to that community as she blogged and reblogged the letters from the trenches.

Pastor Rich Little brought the same and a voice of mainstream Christian wisdom alongside denunciations of his tyrant governor in Michigan. From Bill Sardi to Jon Rappaport, hundreds and thousands of others magnified each other's efforts in a synergy elsewhere unmatched. Truth distilled.

The spirit of the Gadfly Majestic[2] is a most wonderful thing to come out of 2020 and beyond. It has been a gift to live through this year and to be challenged in the way this year has brought challenge. Thousands, too numerous to mention here have brought me untold inspiration by merely being their own free selves and refusing anything but that high standard in life. Though these pages do not allow the space for it, I hope to one day write at length about more of those contributions that the captive media refuses to cover.

The free man of 2020 and 2021 would be the Time Man of the Year in a freer society. That is not the society in which we live, but the remnant thrives strong on the right and somewhat on the left. Any journalist with a dogged determination for the truth from Glenn Greenwald and Matt Taibbi to many others across the spectrum, are writing about the free man and critical of the predictably corrupt writing of our era. In people like that, a torch of decency is kept alive across the political spectrum. It is a joy to walk the earth with such powerful souls such as these mentioned here and to see them so magnificently shine against the dismal backdrop of this era. It is not the backdrop that deserves our attention, with people like this walking the earth. It is the heroes sparkling against that backdrop who deserve our attention.

A pope once wrote "Let us thank God that He makes us live among the present problems. It is no longer permitted to anyone to be mediocre." Each day I see the most magnificent examples of human inspiration.

I am thankful to Tim Scherer, Hector Carmona, Levi & Annette Honaywax, Peter Harrigan, Steven Hertzberg, Henry Ealy, Anthony Koz, Richard Miletic, John Strand, Elma Lindsay, Zack Van Wagoner, Jason T. Reynolds, Julia Pekkala, Lord Timothy McGovern, Peggy Paul, Stanley Swartzentruber, Gary Leland, Michael Hanks, Timothy Engler, Michael McEvoy, Edward Downing Jr., Kevin Young, Scott Mise, Gaynell Riley, Frank and Betsy Grasso, Linda Ikeda, Lee Fernandez, George Joulak, Geoff Brown, Jeshua Richard, Gabrielle Soloma de Cadavid, and Engin Can for their demonstrations of courage.

Thank you to Nick Spanos, Stephen Qwan, Felix Brownstone, Alejandro Pasternak, Walter Block, Robert Wright for introductions and encouragement. I am grateful to Kate Dalley of the *Kate Dalley Show* and Tim Brown of *The Washington Standard*, Ryan McMaken of the *Mises Institute*, Joe Jarvis of *The Daily Bell*, Michael Boldin and Michael Maharrey of the *Tenth Amendment Center*, Kit Knightly of *Off Guardian*, Daniel Ivandjiiski of *Zero Hedge*, Valentin Schmid and Adam Ainsworth of *Epoch Times*, Tom Roten of *The Morning Show*, Jeff Crouere of *Ringside Politics*, Shaun Kraisman and Emma Rechenberg of the *Newsmax TV's National Report*, John Tabacco of the *Liquid Lunch Show*, Adam Kokesh and Marcus Pulis of the *Adam vs The Man*, Bobby Gunther Walsh of the *News Radio 790 WAEB*, Rob Schilling of *The Schilling Show*, Paul Pacelli of *Connecticut Today*, Gary Walk of *700 WLW*, Tom Wood of *The Tom Woods Show*, J.T. Mason of *Birmingham News*, Bill Martinez of *The Bill Martinez Show*, Dan Miller of *In Focus*, Pete Evans of *Evolve with Pete Evans*, Karen Kataline of the *Alan Nathan Show*, Bill Meyer of the *Bill Meyer Show*, Bob Gourley of *Issues Today Radio*, Kim Wade of *The Kim Wade Show*, Steve Noxon of *Talk of the Town*, Nate Thurston of *Good Morning Liberty*, Katie Hess of *The Flowerlounge Podcast*, Lars Larson of *The Lars Larson Show*, Deanna Spingola of the *Deanna Spingola Show*, Vicki McKenna of *The Vicki McKenna Show*, Patrick Smith of *Disenthrall*, Lockwood Phillips of *Viewpoints*, Steve Gruber of the *Steve Gruber Show*, Gareth Icke of *Ikonic*, Diane Jones of *The Diane Jones Show*, Beth Knott of the *MoJo50*, Faune Riggin of *Real Talk with Riggin*, Skyler Collins of *Everything Voluntary*, Michael Schilkman of *The Mike Schilkman Show*, Mike Hayes of *KZIM*, Gary Sadlemeyer of *KFAB's Morning News*, Chuck Wilder of *Talk Back With Chuck Wilder*, Dr. Dan Miller and Joyce Vetere of *In Focus*, Buck Sexton of *Hold the*

Line with Buck Sexton, Jim Mallard of *The Mallard Report*, Bill Zimpfer of *The Talk of Pittsburgh*, Max Schaeffer and Amy Sweet of the *Max & Amy in the Morning Show*, Todd Marino of *Indiana in the Morning*, Bob Sullivan of *San Diego's Morning News*, Tatiana Moroz of *The Tatiana Show*, Craig Dillon of *The Breakfast Club*, Marin County Weston A. Price Foundation, Central Coast Health Coalition, Jason Anderson and Randall Jordan of *the North County Tea Party*, Diane Jones of the *KLPW Morning Show*, Bob Dutko of *The Bob Dutko Show*, Jamie Umphenour of *KPRL*, Doug Pike of *The Doug Pike Show*, Kate Dalley of the *Kate Dalley Show*, Fielden Nolan of the *NoMaskers.org*, Jay LeSeure of the *Morning Meeting*, Janet Meffred of the *Janet Meffred Today*, Chuck Wilder of the *Chuck Wilder Show*, Andy Griffin of the *Morning Rundown*, Todd Walker of *Lima's Morning News*, their producers, their production teams, and many others, for providing additional venues for these ideas.

Thank you to both parents and students such as Irena Stepanova, Jenin Younes, Chris Wark, Alex Gutentag, Mahdyson Stark, and Riley Stark whose work is included in this book.

Many thousands resisted and sent in their notes, notes that were an inspiration to read. Notes from the corona resistance came in from all corners of the world. Among them from:

Robert E. Wright, Bo Andersen, Hoseyn Vosouq, Jeff Berwick, Kellie Hill, Mark Abell, Marc Scott, Pam Buttram, Sharine Borslien, Tazio Zatori, Jose Douglas, Ray Greninger, John Tieber, Geoffrey McKinney, Joyce Smith, Krishna Chandrasekaran, Jean Hodge, Michael F. Denny, Keith Hudson, Karen Stansberry, Elin Carlson, Alex Morris, Ashkan Jafarpisheh, Scott M. Olmsted, Vafa Faez, Judith Sanders, Gerry D. Lebow, Michelle Rice, Anthony Kujawa, Mike Maloney, Pat Goltz, Walter E. Block, Steve Swenson, Mark Higdon, Jim Sheehan, John T. Morzenti, Dave Heng, Larry Moore, David Hathaway, Bruce Bolock, Jeri Dietz, Justin Ptak, John McClain, Thomas Hyland, Walter Dubyna, Becky Akers, Ernest Roberts, Steven Ferry, Kathy Terry, John Howard, William Lensmire, Pat Palmer, Allen Nightingale, Zac Wendroff, Sam Wolanyk, Mary Beth Kaplan, Genevieve Amy Hawkins, Susan Fassanella, Ludvik Kouril, Alex Edwards, Jack Worthington, Bill Spitz, Mark Bombardier, Edward Konecnik, Mark Beck, Mike Falls, Doug Schurman, Ira Katz, Raul De La Garza III, Richard Feibel, Stephen J. Savoie, John Reilly, Charlie Beaird. and DeMar Southard.

Appreciation for an additional show of inspiration is owed to Maureen Block, Alix Mayer, Robert F. Kennedy Jr., Josh Donaldson, J.K. Monagle, Elson Haas, Simone Gold, and Ali Schultz.

Thank you to the many people otherwise involved in this process, such as Louise Taylor, Olha Krasikova, Tara Premenko, Lisa Jackson, Rebecca Raouda-Saviolli, and classicist Mia Forbes. Your efforts have been fantastic thank you. I am most appreciative to Helena Cabell.

My family brought drive, inspiration, and focus by being the people for whom I most wanted to be able to understand this topic and provide leadership. Their generosity and love remind me how well successful families are able to function, even through times of crisis, or perhaps, especially through times of crisis.

I am in debt to the following writers who have preceded me on this subject matter. Jingy Xiao, Boris Borovoy, Kai Kisielinski, Baruch Vainshelboim, Denis Rancourt, Milan Rufus, Alan More, Meredith Wadman, Simon Denyer, Joel Achenbach, Vernon Coleman, Christopher J. Pannucci, Edwin G. Wilkins, Nigel Barlow, Armando Meza, Silke Schwarz, David J. Lewkowicz, Manfred Spitzer, Dina Karvounides, Jonathan Ong, Grace Donnelly, Baskaran Chandrasekaran, Shifra Fernandes, Mayumi Nobuta, Zhang Wanqing, Maximos Fountzas, L. A. Morris, Robert Gearty, C. Raina MacIntyre, Harald Walach, Russel Blaylock, Majid Moshirfar, James H. Bamber and Tracey Christmas.

Baruch Vainshelboim is a perfect example of the work being done on cutting edge Covid research. He is a non-native speaker of English, his work has English language flaws, which I have chosen to leave in place. Such details are part of his style, a style that I have come to greatly appreciate. It is a style that can be worn like a badge of honor, for it says much about him and the times. He is very brave in his willingness to speak out and sees it as his duty to do so even though his English is imperfect and he does not have the massive budget for language editors, that a government or big pharma budget would allow for. Perfection is not the goal of the work being done right now. Big brush strokes are important when society has gone in such a harmful direction. Vainshelboim has done exactly what is needed for times such as these and his work is truly an excellent example of the brave standing up in the face of lies and tyranny pushed upon society by those with the most power.

Vainshelboim is the *samizdat* style truth teller this era demands. Hundreds, thousands, even millions are exactly that — samizdat style truthtellers, navigating life in unofficial channels, telling the truth no matter the cost.

Some choose to focus on the mass of lost sheep seeking a leader — a thought with unlimited downside potential. Some choose to focus on the hyenas of our era looking to take advantage of all around them — another thought with so much downside.

I choose to focus on the brave lions on the prowl, and the brave lions being roused into action. All history depends not on the sheeplike masses, nor on the hyenalike usurpers, interlopers, and malcontents. All history depends on the lions — whether they be steel-spined or slacked-spined, awake or asleep — and I so thank the many lions of this era who are awake and on the prowl. We live in such a special time for the courageous, such a special opportunity, and this book is a product of that time. Thank you fellow lions.

Notes

Reason 1: The CDC Says Face Masks Don't Work

[1] Centers for Disease Control and Prevention. Emerging Infectious Diseases. 2021. Retrieved from https://wwwnc.cdc.gov/eid/

[2] Centers for Disease Control and Prevention. How to Protect Yourself & Others. 2021. Retrieved from https://www.cdc.gov/coronavirus/2019-ncov/prevent-getting-sick/prevention.html

[3] Xiao J, Shiu EYC, Gao H, et al. Nonpharmaceutical Measures for Pandemic Influenza in Nonhealthcare Settings — Personal Protective and Environmental Measures. *Emerging Infectious Diseases*. 2020;26(5):967-975. doi:10.3201/eid 2605.190994

[4] Wong VW, Cowling BJ, Aiello AE. Hand hygiene and risk of influenza virus infections in the community: a systematic review and meta-analysis. Epidemiol Infect. 2014;142:922–32.

[4] Stevo, A. You're Still Exempt. Just Say "I Am Unable to Wear a Face Mask Safely." Nothing More. *LewRockwell*. 2020. Retrieved from https://www.lewrockwell.com/2020/08/allan-stevo/youre-still-exempt-just-say-i-am-unable-to-wear-a-face-mask-safely-nothing-more/

[5] Stevo, A. The 38-Member Blue Ribbon Committee To Protect Society From Itself Has Met And Determined That This Is The Best Way To Lift The Quarantine. *LewRockwell*. 2020. Retrieved from https://www.lewrockwell.com/2020/04/allan-stevo/the-38-member-blue-ribbon-committee-to-protect-society-from-itself-has-met-and-determined-that-this-is-the-best-way-to-lift-the-quarantine/

[6] Stevo, A. Suddenly Everyone Is a Corona Expert. *LewRockwell*. 2020. Retrieved from https://www.lewrockwell.com/2020/03/allan-stevo/suddenly-everyone-is-a-corona-expert/

[7] Stevo, A. COVID-19: The "Experts" Have No Crystal Ball. *Mises Institute*. 2020. Retrieved from https://mises.org/wire/covid-19-experts-have-no-crystal-ball

[8] At the time this book went to press, the paper "Nonpharmaceutical Measures for Pandemic Influenza in Nonhealthcare Settings (https://wwwnc.cdc.gov/eid/article/26/5/19-0994_article#fn1)," the best paper on face masking in 2020, had not been cited 100,000, 10,000 or even 1,000 times. It had been cited a mere 66 times.

Reason 2: CDC & WHO Say Face Masks INCREASE Spread Of Disease

[1] Xiao J, Shiu EYC, Gao H, et al. Nonpharmaceutical Measures for Pandemic Influenza in Nonhealthcare Settings — Personal Protective and Environmental Measures. Emerging Infectious Diseases. 2020;26(5):967-975. doi:10.3201/eid2605.190994

[2] World Health Organization. Advice on the use of masks1 in the community setting in Influenza A (H1N1) outbreaks. 2009. Retrieved from https://www.who.int/csr/resources/publications/Adviceusemaskscommunityrevised.pdf

[3] World Health Organization. Advice on the use of masks1 in the community setting in Influenza A (H1N1) outbreaks. 2009. Retrieved from https://www.who.int/csr/resources/publications/Adviceusemaskscommunityrevised.pdf

[4] World Health Organization. Advice on the use of masks1 in the community setting in Influenza A (H1N1) outbreaks. 2009. Retrieved from https://www.who.int/csr/resources/publications/Adviceusemaskscommunityrevised.pdf

Reason 3: The New England Journal Of Medicine Says Face Masks Do Not Work

[1] Klompas M, Morris CA, Sinclair J, Pearson M, Shenoy ES. Universal Masking in Hospitals in the Covid-19 Era. *New England Journal of Medicine*. 2020;382(21). doi:10.1056/nejmp2006372

[2] Xiao J, Shiu EYC, Gao H, et al. Nonpharmaceutical Measures for Pandemic Influenza in Nonhealthcare Settings — Personal Protective and Environmental Measures. Emerging Infectious Diseases. 2020;26(5):967-975. doi:10.3201/eid2605.190994

Reason 4: The US Food And Drug Administration Says Face Masks Do Not Work

[1] Jennifer Guilfoyle et al v. Austin Beutner et al. 2:21-cv-05009. 37. C.D. Cal. 2021. https://ca.childrens healthdefense.org/wp-content/uploads/complaint_case2.21_vc_05009_06222021.pdf

[2] Quoting this court case, Jennifer Guilfoyle et al v. Austin Beutner et al. 2:21-cv-05009. 37 (C.D. Cal. 2021). https://ca.childrenshealthdefense.org/wp-content/uploads/complaint_case2.21_vc_05009_06222021.pdf

[3] Food and Drug Administration. To: Manufacturers of Face Masks; Health Care Personnel; Hospital Purchasing Departments and Distributors; and Any Other Stakeholders. 2021. Retrieved from https://www.fda.gov/media/137121/download

[4] Food and Drug Administration. Enforcement Policy for Face Masks, Barrier Face Coverings, Face Shields, Surgical Masks, and Respirators During the Coronavirus Disease (COVID-19) Public Health Emergency (Revised). 2021. Retrieved from https://www.fda.gov/media/136449/download

Reason 5: Yes, Data From The Council On Foreign Relations Even Says Face Masks Don't Work

[1] Borovoy B, Huber C, Crisler M. Masks, False Safety And Real Dangers, Part 2: Microbial Challenges From Masks. 2020. Retrieved from https://childrenshealthdefense.org/wp-content/uploads/Masks-false-safety-and-real-dangers-Part-2-Microbial-challenges-from-masks.pdf.

[2] Felter C, Bussemaker N. Which countries are requiring face masks? Council on Foreign Relations. 2020. Retrieved from https://www.cfr.org/in-brief/which-countries-are-requiring-face-masks

[3] COVID Live Update. Worldometer. Retrieved from https://www.worldometers.info/coronavirus/?%3D%3D

Reason 6: Many Other Medical Researchers Say Face Masks Do Not Work

[1] Jefferson T, Mar CBD, Dooley L, et al. Physical interventions to interrupt or reduce the spread of respiratory viruses. *Cochrane Database of Systematic Reviews*. 2011. doi:10.1002/14651858.cd006207.pub4

[2] Jefferson T, Jones M, Al-Ansary L, et al. Physical interventions to interrupt or reduce the spread of respiratory viruses. Part 1 — Face masks, eye protection and person distancing: systematic review and meta-analysis. 2020. doi:10.1101/2020.03.30.20047217

[3] Smith JD, Macdougall CC, Johnstone J, Copes RA, Schwartz B, Garber GE. Effectiveness of N95 respirators versus surgical masks in protecting health care workers from acute respiratory infection: a systematic review and meta-analysis. *Canadian Medical Association Journal*. 2016;188(8):567-574. doi:10.1503/cmaj.150835

[4] Bin-Reza F, Chavarrias VL, Nicoll A, Chamberland ME. The use of masks and respirators to prevent transmission of influenza: a systematic review of the scientific evidence. *Influenza and Other Respiratory Viruses*. 2011;6(4):257-267. doi:10.1111/j.1750-2659.2011.00307.x

[5] Mitchell NJ, Hunt S. Surgical face masks in modern operating rooms — a costly and unnecessary ritual? *Journal of Hospital Infection*. 1991;18(3):239-242. doi:10.1016/0195-6701(91)90148-2

[6] Bae S, Kim M-C, Kim JY, et al. Effectiveness of Surgical and Cotton Masks in Blocking SARS–CoV-2: A Controlled Comparison in 4 Patients. *Annals of Internal Medicine*. 2020;173(1). doi:10.7326/m20-1342

[7] Orr NW. Is a mask necessary in the operating theatre? *Annals of the Royal College of Surgeons of England*. 1981;63(6):390–392.

[8] Tunevall TG. Postoperative wound infections and surgical face masks: A controlled study. *World Journal of Surgery*. 1991;15(3):383-387. doi:10.1007/bf01658736

Reason 7: Countries With Face Mask Mandates Are Not Better Off Than Countries Without Them

[1] Singleton MM. Mask Facts. *Association of American Physicians and Surgeons*. 2021. Retrieved from https://aapsonline.org/mask-facts/

[2] Burrows T. DOUBLE DUTCH Face masks are 'NOT necessary' and could even harm the fight against coronavirus, say Holland's top scientists. *The Sun*. 2020. Retrieved from https://www.thesun.co.uk/news/uknews/12292821/face-masks-not-necessary-say-holland-scientists/

Reason 8: Face Masks Did Not Work In 1918, 1957, 1968, 2002, 2004, And They Do Not Work Now

[1] Kisielinski K, Giboni P, Prescher A, et al. Is a Mask That Covers the Mouth and Nose Free from Undesirable Side Effects in Everyday Use and Free of Potential Hazards? International Journal of Environmental Research and Public Health. 2021;18(8):4344. doi:10.3390/ijerph18084344

[2] Jacobs JL, Ohde S, Takahashi O, Tokuda Y, Omata F, Fukui T. Use of surgical face masks to reduce the incidence of the common cold among health care workers in Japan: A randomized controlled trial. *American Journal of Infection Control*. 2009;37(5):417-419. doi:10.1016/j.ajic.2008.11.002

[3] Macintyre CR, Cauchemez S, Dwyer DE, et al. Face Mask Use and Control of Respiratory Virus Transmission in Households. *Emerging Infectious Diseases*. 2009;15(2):233-241. doi:10.3201/eid1502.081166

[4] Neilson S. The surgical mask is a bad fit for risk reduction. *Canadian Medical Association Journal*. 2016;188(8):606-607. doi:10.1503/cmaj.151236

[5] Belkin NL. The Evolution of the Surgical Mask: Filtering Efficiency versus Effectiveness. *Infection Control and Hospital Epidemiology*. 1997;18(1):49-57. doi:10.1086/647501

[6] Cowling BJ, Chan K-H, Fang VJ, et al. Facemasks and Hand Hygiene to Prevent Influenza Transmission in Households. *Annals of Internal Medicine*. 2009;151(7):437. doi:10.7326/0003-4819-151-7-200910060-00142

[7] Cowling BJ, Zhou Y, Ip DKM, Leung GM, Aiello AE. Face masks to prevent transmission of influenza virus: a systematic review. *Epidemiology and Infection*. 2010;138(4):449-456. doi:10.1017/s0950268809991658

[8] Institute of Medicine (US). Committee on Personal Protective Equipment for Healthcare Personnel to Prevent Transmission of Pandemic Influenza and Other Viral Respiratory Infections: Current Research Issues. In Preventing Transmission of Pandemic Influenza and Other Viral Respiratory Diseases: Personal Protective Equipment for Healthcare Personnel: Update 2010; Larson, E.L., Liverman, C.T., Eds.; National Academies Press (US): Washington, DC, USA, 2011; ISBN 978-0-309-16254-8.

Reason 9: The SARS Hype Is Severely Blown Out Of Proportion

[1] Vainshelboim B. RETRACTED: Facemasks in the COVID-19 era: A health hypothesis. *Medical Hypotheses*. 2021;146. doi:10.1016/j.mehy.2020.110411

[2] Sohrabi C, Alsafi Z, Oneill N, et al. World Health Organization declares global emergency: A review of the 2019 novel coronavirus (COVID-19). *International Journal of Surgery*. 2020;76:71-76. doi:10.1016/j.ijsu.2020.02.034

[3] Worldometer. COVID-19 CORONAVIRUS PANDEMIC. 2020.

[4] Fauci AS, Lane HC, Redfield RR. Covid-19 — Navigating the Uncharted. *New England Journal of Medicine.* 2020;382(13):1268-1269. doi:10.1056/nejme2002387

[5] Shrestha SS, Swerdlow DL, Borse RH, et al. Estimating the Burden of 2009 Pandemic Influenza A (H1N1) in the United States (April 2009-April 2010). *Clinical Infectious Diseases.* 2010;52(Supplement 1). doi:10.1093/cid/ciq012

[6] Thompson WW, Weintraub E, Dhankhar P, et al. Estimates of US influenza-associated deaths made using four different methods. *Influenza and Other Respiratory Viruses.* 2009;3(1):37-49. doi:10.1111/j.1750-2659.2009.00073.x

[7] Centers for Disease Control and Prevention (CDC). Estimates of deaths associated with seasonal influenza — United States, 1976-2007. *MMWR. Morbidity and mortality weekly report*, 2010:59(33):1057–1062.

[8] Richardson S, Hirsch JS, Narasimhan M, et al. Presenting Characteristics, Comorbidities, and Outcomes Among 5700 Patients Hospitalized With COVID-19 in the New York City Area. *Jama.* 2020;323(20):2052. doi:10.1001/jama.2020.6775

[9] Ioannidis JP, Axfors C, Contopoulos-Ioannidis DG. Population-level COVID-19 mortality risk for non-elderly individuals overall and for non-elderly individuals without underlying diseases in pandemic epicenters. *Environmental Research.* 2020;188:109890. doi:10.1016/j.envres.2020.109890

[10] World Health Organization. Advice on the use of masks in the context of COVID-19. Geneva, Switzerland; 2020.

[11] American College of Sports Medicine. Sixth ed. Lippincott Wiliams & Wilkins; Baltimore: 2010. ACSM's Resource Manual for Guidelines for Exercise Testing and Priscription.

[12] Farrell PA, Joyner MJ, Caiozzo VJ. second edition. Lippncott Williams & Wilkins; Baltimore: 2012. ACSM's Advanced Exercise Physiology.

[13] Kenney WL, Wilmore JH, Costill DL. 5th ed. Human Kinetics; Champaign, IL: 2012. Physiology of sport and exercise.

[14] World Health Organization. Advice on the use of masks in the community, during home care and in health care settings in the context of the novel coronavirus (2019-nCoV) outbreak. Geneva, Switzerland; 2020.

[15] Sperlich B, Zinner C, Hauser A, Holmberg HC, Wegrzyk J. The Impact of Hyperoxia on Human Performance and Recovery. Sports Med. 2017;47:429–438.

[16] Wiersinga WJ, Rhodes A, Cheng AC, Peacock SJ, Prescott HC. Pathophysiology, Transmission, Diagnosis, and Treatment of Coronavirus Disease 2019 (COVID-19): A Review. JAMA.

[17] Zhu N, Zhang D, Wang W, Li X, Yang B, Song J. A Novel Coronavirus from Patients with Pneumonia in China, 2019. N Engl J Med. 2020;382:727–733.

[18] Poston JT, Patel BK, Davis AM. Management of Critically Ill Adults With COVID-19. JAMA. 2020.

[19] MacIntyre CR, Seale H, Dung TC, Hien NT, Nga PT, Chughtai A.A. A cluster randomised trial of cloth masks compared with medical masks in healthcare workers. BMJ open. 2015;5.

Reason 10: The Flu Is More Dangerous Than Covid & Neither Of Them Are Stopped By Face Mask Wearing

[1] Pastor Gabe.

[2] Centers for Disease Control and Prevention. Estimated Flu-Related Illnesses, Medical Visits, Hospitalizations, and Deaths in the United States — 2017-2018 Flu Season. 2021. Retrieved from https://www.cdc.gov/flu/about/burden/2017-2018.htm

[3] Centers for Disease Control and Prevention. Estimated Flu-Related Illnesses, Medical visits, Hospitalizations, and Deaths in the United States — 2018-2019 Flu Season. 2021. Retrieved from https://www.cdc.gov/flu/about/burden/2018-2019.html

[4] Centers for Disease Control and Prevention. Estimated Flu-Related Illnesses, Medical visits, Hospitalizations, and Deaths in the United States — 2019-2020 Flu Season. 2021. Retrieved from https://www.cdc.gov/flu/about/burden/2019-2020.html

[5] National Center for Health Statistics. Provisional COVID-19 Deaths: Focus on Ages 0-18 Years. *Centers for Disease Control and Prevention.* 2021. Retrieved from https://data.cdc.gov/NCHS/Provisional-COVID-19-Deaths-Focus-on-Ages-0-18-Yea/nr4s-juj3

[6] Elflein J. COVID-19 deaths reported in the US as of October 20, 2021, by age. Statista. 2021. Retrieved from https://www.statista.com/statistics/1191568/reported-deaths-from-covid-by-age-us/?fbclid=IwAR3FUbyKwzO0f4dH dbagGcNExjZWQa-A10vymnG7KCEJUktBecoBmIDn_dU

[7] National Center for Health Statistics. Provisional COVID-19 Deaths: Focus on Ages 0-18 Years. *Centers for Disease Control and Prevention.* 2021. Retrieved from https://data.cdc.gov/NCHS/Provisional-COVID-19-Deaths-Focus-on-Ages-0-18-Yea/nr4s-juj3

[8] Tsankov BK, Allaire JM, Irvine MA, et al. Severe COVID-19 Infection and Pediatric Comorbidities: A Systematic Review and Meta-Analysis. *International Journal of Infectious Diseases.* 2021;103:246-256. doi:10.1016/j.ijid.2020.11.163

[9] Makary M. The Flimsy Evidence Behind the CDC's Push to Vaccinate Children. *Wall Street Journal.* 2021. Retrieved from https://www.wsj.com/articles/cdc-covid-19-coronavirus-vaccine-side-effects-hospitalization-kids-11626706868

[10] Wark C. Facebook page. Children have a 99.997% COVID-19 survival rate. Accessed August 14, 2021. https://www.facebook.com/chriswark/posts/10159829160569015

[11] Dalley K. Our First Hand ICU Story — What is ACTUALLY Killing People In The Hospital [Video]. Rumble. https://rumble.com/vktdpt-our-first-hand-icu-story-what-is-actually-killing-people-in-the-hospital.html Published August 6, 2021. Accessed August 6, 2021.

Reason 11: If Face Masks Do Not Work, Then Government And Media Are Lying To You — A Very Scary Thought For Some

[1] Rancourt, D.G. Review of scientific reports of harms caused by face masks, up to February 2021. 2021. Retrieved from https://assets.website-files.com/606d3a50c62e44338008303d/6076def5c5421e642472f1ef_5thsciencereview-mask sharm-1.pdf

[2] 2020--Bakhit : "Downsides of face masks and possible mitigation strategies: a systematic review and meta-analysis". Mina Bakhit, Natalia Krzyzaniak, Anna Mae Scott, Justin Clark, Paul Glasziou, Chris Del Mar. medRxiv 2020.06.16.20133207; doi: https://doi.org/10.1101/2020.06.16.20133207. Now accepted for publication in BMJ Open. — https://www.medrxiv.org/content/10.1101/2020.06.16.20133207v1

[3] Elisheva R. Adverse Effects of Prolonged Mask Use among Healthcare Professionals during COVID-19. *Journal of Infectious Diseases and Epidemiology*. 2020;6(3). doi:10.23937/2474-3658/1510130

Reason 12: You Have Been Lied To This Whole Time, Then Vilified If You Ask Too Many Revealing Questions About Those Lies

[1] McNeil Jr DG. How Much Herd Immunity Is Enough?. *The New York Times*. 2020. Retrieved from https://www.nytimes.com/2020/12/24/health/herd-immunity-covid-coronavirus.html

[2] Bai N. Still Confused About Masks? Here's the Science Behind How Face Masks Prevent Coronavirus. University of California San Francisco. 2020. Retrieved from https://www.ucsf.edu/news/2020/06/417906/still-confused-about-masks-heres-science-behind-how-face-masks-prevent

[3] Guerra DD, Guerra DJ. Mask mandate and use efficacy for COVID-19 containment in US States. 2021. doi:10.1101/2021.05.18.21257385

[4] Thompson D. Mask Use by Americans Now Tops 90%, Poll Finds. WebMD. 2020. Retrieved from https://www.webmd.com/lung/news/20201022/mask-use-by-americans-now-tops-90-poll-finds#1

[5] Fisher KA, Tenforde MW, Feldstein LR, et al. Community and Close Contact Exposures Associated with COVID-19 Among Symptomatic Adults ≥18 Years in 11 Outpatient Health Care Facilities. *Morbidity and Mortality Weekly Report*. 2020. Retrieved from https://www.cdc.gov/mmwr/volumes/69/wr/pdfs/mm6936a5-H.pdf#page=4

[6] Bazant MZ, Bush JWM. A guideline to limit indoor airborne transmission of COVID-19. *Proceedings of the National Academy of Sciences*. 2021;118(17). doi:10.1073/pnas.2018995118

[7] National Center for Health Statistics. Weekly Updates by Select Demographic and Geographic Characteristics. *Centers for Disease Control and Prevention*. 2021. Retrieved from https://www.cdc.gov/nchs/nvss/vsrr/covid_weekly/index.htm

[8] Harris C. Autopsy Says George Floyd Tested Positive for Coronavirus, But Death Was Homicide. *People*. 2020. Retrieved from https://people.com/crime/george-floyd-tested-positive-coronavirus-death-homicide/

[9] Swieg, D. New Research Suggests Number of Kids Hospitalized for COVID Is Overcounted. *Intelligencer*. 2021. Retrieved from: https://nymag.com/intelligencer/2021/05/study-number-of-kids-hospitalized-for-covid-is-over counted.html

[10] *Centers for Disease Control and Prevention*. Interim Laboratory Biosafety Guidelines for Handling and Processing Specimens Associated with Coronavirus Disease 2019 (COVID-19) 2021. Retrieved from: https://www.cdc.gov/coronavirus/2019-ncov/lab/lab-biosafety-guidelines.html#

[11] *Centers for Disease Control and Prevention*. COVID-19 Vaccine Effectiveness 2021. Retrieved from: https://www.cdc.gov/coronavirus/2019-ncov/vaccines/effectiveness/index.html?CDC_AA_refVal= https://www.cdc.gov/coronavirus/2019-ncov/vaccines/effectiveness.html

[12] Mandavilli, A. Your Coronavirus Test Is Positive. Maybe It Shouldn't Be. *The New York Times*. 2021. Retrieved by: https://www.nytimes.com/2020/08/29/health/coronavirus-testing.html

[13] Kaplan, J. Workers lost $3.7 trillion in earnings during the pandemic. Women and Gen Z saw the biggest losses. Insider. 2021. Retrieved from: https://www.businessinsider.com/workers-lost-37-trillion-in-earnings-during-the-pandemic-2021-1?IR=T

[14] Kaplan, J. Billionaires made $3.9 trillion during the pandemic — enough to pay for everyone's vaccine. Insider. 2021. Retrieved from: https://www.businessinsider.com/billionaires-made-39-trillion-during-the-pandemic-coronavirus-vaccines-2021-1?IR=T

[15] Peterson-Withorn, C. Nearly 500 People Became Billionaires During The Pandemic Year. Forbes. 2021. Retrieved from: https://www.forbes.com/sites/chasewithorn/2021/04/06/nearly-500-people-have-become-billionaires-during-the-pandemic-year/?sh=6806fef125c0

[16] Mandavilli, A. The Biggest Monster' Is Spreading. And It's Not the Coronavirus. *The New York Times*. 2020. Retrieved from: https://www.nytimes.com/2020/08/03/health/coronavirus-tuberculosis-aids-malaria.html

[17] *BBC News*. Covid-19 disruptions killed 228,000 children in South Asia, says UN report. Retrieved from: https://www.bbc.com/news/world-asia-56425115

[18] Lederer, E.M. UN says 155 million people faced severe hunger last year. *AP News*. 2021. Retrieved from: https://apnews.com/article/united-nations-africa-middle-east-financial-markets-hunger-67eac141dd228d41323b90da7f8b7f3c

[19] Kluger, J. COVID-19 May Lead to a Heart-Disease Surge. *Time*. 2021. Retrieved from: https://time.com/5936029/covid-19-heart-disease-rise/

[20] Eldeib, D. A Crisis of Undiagnosed Cancers Is Emerging in the Pandemic's Second Year. *Propublica*. Retrieved from: https://www.propublica.org/article/a-crisis-of-undiagnosed-cancers-is-emerging-in-the-pandemics-second-year

[21] Bianchi F, Bianchi G, Song D. The Long-Term Impact of the COVID-19 Unemployment Shock on Life Expectancy and Mortality Rates. 2020. doi:10.3386/w28304

[22] *Centers for Disease Control and Prevention*. Overdose Deaths Accelerating During COVID-19. 2020. Retrieved from: https://www.cdc.gov/media/releases/2020/p1218-overdose-deaths-covid-19.html

[23] Miller, A.M. 11% of US adults seriously considered suicide in June, its CDC says. *Business Insider SA*. 2020. Retrieved from: https://www.businessinsider.co.za/cdc-11-percent-us-adults-seriously-considered-suicide-in-june-2020-8

[24] Hodges, L. A Quiet And 'Unsettling' Pandemic Toll: Students Who've Fallen Off The Grid. *NPR*. 2020. Retrieved from: https://www.npr.org/2020/12/29/948866982/a-quiet-and-unsettling-pandemic-toll-students-whove-fallen-off-the-grid

[25] Leeb RT, Bitsko RH, Radhakrishnan L, Martinez P, Njai R, Holland KM. Mental Health–Related Emergency Department Visits Among Children Aged <18 Years During the COVID-19 Pandemic — United States, January 1–October 17, 2020. MMWR Morb Mortal Wkly Rep 2020;69:1675–1680. DOI: http://dx.doi.org/10.15585/mmwr.mm6945a3external icon

Reason 13: If Morality Is Being Argued By Bullies Rather Than Scientific Debate Being Had By Peers, You Know Something Is Wrong

[1] Younes, J. *The Strangely Unscientific Masking of America. American Institute for Economic Research*. 2020. Retrieved from: https://www.aier.org/article/the-strangely-unscientific-masking-of-america/

[2] IHME COVID-19 Forecasting Team. Modeling COVID-19 scenarios for the United States. Nat Med 27, 94–105 (2021). https://doi.org/10.1038/s41591-020-1132-9

[3] Collins, F. Dr. Face Coverings Could Save 130,000 American Lives from COVID-19 by March. *NIH Director's Blog*. 2020. Retrieved from: ps://directorsblog.nih.gov/2020/11/03/face-coverings-could-save-130000-american-lives-by-march/

[4] Mandavilli, A. The Price for Not Wearing Masks: Perhaps 130,000 Lives. *The New York Times*. 2020. Retrieved from: https://www.nytimes.com/2020/10/23/health/covid-deaths.html

[5] Magness, P.W. Case for Mask Mandate Rests on Bad Data. *WSJ Opinion*. Retrieved from: https://www.wsj.com/articles/case-for-mask-mandate-rests-on-bad-data-11605113310?mod=article_inline

[6] As of the time of this writing, the November 3, 2020 election remains a contested election with illegitimate results rooted in the same lack of reliance in reason and evidence. Just as scientism, rather than science, brought us the Covid-19 catastrophe and the anti-scientific fallout, scientism, rather than science, has brought us November 3, 2020, and the anti-scientific fallout. In both scenarios, a rigorous intimacy with the numbers has been ignored in favor of a narrative. The results of such behavior in a free society have been catastrophic.

[7] Acyn @Acyn. President-elect reacts to Scott Atlas. Twitter. 2020. Retrieved from: https://twitter.com/Acyn/status/1328438607770599425

[8] *WSJ Opinion*. Masks Aren't Perfect but Help in Proper Use. Retrieved from: Masks Aren't Perfect but Help in Proper Use.

Reason 14: The Rationale "Comply Or Else" Is Such A Monstrously Bad Rationale, Whenever It Is Used, That It Should Always Trigger A Lack Of Compliance

[1] Borovoy B, Huber C, Crisler M. Masks, false safety and real dangers, Part 2: Microbial challenges from masks. *Primary Doctor Medical Journal*. 2020. Retrieved from https://pdmj.org/papers/masks_false_safety_and_real_dangers_part2/

[2] Huber C. Masks are neither effective nor safe: A summary of the science. Primary Doctor. 2020. Retrieved from https://www.primarydoctor.org/masks-not-effect

[3] Macintyre CR, Seale H, Dung TC, et al. A cluster randomised trial of cloth masks compared with medical masks in healthcare workers. *BMJ Open*. 2015;5(4). doi:10.1136/bmjopen-2014-006577

[4] Kelkar US, Gogate B, Kurpad S, Gogate P, Deshpande M. How effective are face masks in operation theatre? A time frame analysis and recommendations. *International Journal of Infection Control*. 2013;9(1). doi:10.3396/ijic.v9i1.003.13

[5] Kwon JH, Burnham C-AD, Reske KA, et al. Assessment of Healthcare Worker Protocol Deviations and Self-Contamination During Personal Protective Equipment Donning and Doffing. *Infection Control & Hospital Epidemiology*. 2017;38(9):1077-1083. doi:10.1017/ice.2017.121

[6] Orr NWM. Is a mask necessary in the operating theatre? *Annals of the Royal College of Surgeons of England.* 1981;63:390-392. Retrieved from https://muchadoaboutcorona.ca/wp-content/uploads/2020/08/annrcse01509-0009.pdf

[7] Mitchell NJ, Hunt S. Surgical face masks in modern operating rooms — a costly and unnecessary ritual? *Journal of Hospital Infection.* 1991;18(3):239-242. doi:10.1016/0195-6701(91)90148-2

[8] Michigan Medicine, University of Michigan. Estimating the Size of a Burn. 2020. Retrieved from https://www.uofmhealth.org/health-library/sig254759

[9] Mitchell NJ, Hunt S. Surgical face masks in modern operating rooms — a costly and unnecessary ritual? *Journal of Hospital Infection.* 1991;18(3):239-242. doi:10.1016/0195-6701(91)90148-2

[10] Mitchell NJ, Hunt S. Surgical face masks in modern operating rooms — a costly and unnecessary ritual? *Journal of Hospital Infection.* 1991;18(3):239-242. doi:10.1016/0195-6701(91)90148-2

[11] Mclure HA, Talboys CA, Yentis SM, Azadian BS. Surgical face masks and downward dispersal of bacteria. Anaesthesia. 2002;53(7):624-626. doi:10.1046/j.1365-2044.1998.435-az0528.x

Reason 15: "The Precautionary Principal" Has Not Been Followed

[1] The Hippocratic Oath is approximately 2500 years old.

[2] Zimmerman A. The precautionary principle in mask-wearing: when waiting for explicit scientific evidence is unwise. *Voices in Bioethics.* 2020;6. https://doi.org/10.7916/vib.v6i.5896

[3] Rancourt, D.G. Review of scientific reports of harms caused by face masks, up to February 2021. 2021. Retrieved from https://assets.website-files.com/606d3a50c62e44338008303d/6076def5c5421e642472f1ef_5thsciencereview-mask sharm-1.pdf

Reason 16: Mandatory Face Masks Harm 1.5 Billion Students

[1] Rancourt, D.G. Review of scientific reports of harms caused by face masks, up to February 2021. 2021. Retrieved from https://assets.website-files.com/606d3a50c62e44338008303d/6076def5c5421e642472f1ef_5thsciencereview-mask sharm-1.pdf

[2] UNESCO. Education: From Disruption to Recovery. 2020. Retrieved from https://en.unesco.org/covid19/educationresponse

[3] Couzin-Frankel J, Vogel G, Weiland M. Not open and shut. School openings across the globe suggest ways to keep the coronavirus at bay, despite outbreaks. Science. 2020;369:241-245.

[4] Wößmann L. Folgekosten ausbleibenden Lernens: was wir über die Corona-bedingten Schulschließungen aus der Forschung lernen können. Ifo Schnelld. 2020;73

[5] This quote is taken from Couzin-Frankel et al. Not open and shut. School openings across the globe suggest ways to keep the coronavirus at bay, despite outbreaks. Science. 2020;369:241-245., p. 241], who cite an open letter published in June 2020, signed by more than 1500 members of the United Kingdom's Royal College of Paediatrics and Child Health (RCPCH).

[6] Lancet T. Generation coronavirus? *The Lancet.* 2020;395(10242):1949. doi:10.1016/s0140-6736(20)31445-8

[7] Couzin-Frankel J, Vogel G, Weiland M. Not open and shut. School openings across the globe suggest ways to keep the coronavirus at bay, despite outbreaks. Science. 2020;369:241-245.

[8] Spitzer M. Masked education? The benefits and burdens of wearing face masks in schools during the current Corona pandemic. *Trends in Neuroscience and Education.* 2020;20:100138. doi:10.1016/j.tine.2020.100138

Reason 21: You Teach A Child That Reason Does Not Matter

[1] Centers for Disease Control and Prevention. How to Protect Yourself & Others. 2021. Retrieved from https://www.cdc.gov/coronavirus/2019-ncov/prevent-getting-sick/prevention.html

[2] Centers for Disease Control and Prevention. Emerging Infectious Diseases. 2021. Retrieved from https://wwwnc.cdc.gov/eid/

[3] World Health Organization. Advice on the use of masks1 in the community setting in Influenza A (H1N1) outbreaks. 2009. Retrieved from https://www.who.int/csr/resources/publications/Adviceusemaskscommunityrevised.pdf

Reason 31: You Teach Your Child To Misread Romans 13

[1] Library of Congress Exhibitions. Thomas Jefferson Establishing A Federal Republic. n.d. Retrieved from https://www.loc.gov/exhibits/jefferson/jefffed.html#105

Reason 34: Your Child Will Imitate You

[1] Stevo AJ. *In Poems.* CreateSpace Independent Publishing Platform; 2015.

Reason 39: Thank You To The Mother Who Brought Her Son To The Playground

[1] *Goodreads.* Alan Moore. Retrieved from https://www.goodreads.com/quotes/197373-because-while-the-truncheon-may-be-used-in-lieu-of

[2] If I am to paraphrase the boring parental stereotypes that this era repeats. The cartoon character Homer Simpson has somehow become the contemporary American stereotype for a father.

[3] The April 2020 version of me who wrote this chapter would never have imagined the price tag for the corona stupidity to not be in the billions, but in the tens of trillions in the US alone.

Reason 40: Do Not Look At Face Masks For Covid Avoidance, Look At Obesity, Or A Host Of Other Meaningful Comorbidities, But Especially Obesity

[1] List of governor name, state, weight, and height, and estimated body mass index.

[2] Wadman M. Why COVID-19 is more deadly in people with obesity — even if theyre young. *Science.* 2020. doi:10.1126/science.abe7010

[3] Popkin BM, Du S, Green WD, et al. Individuals with obesity and COVID-19: A global perspective on the epidemiology and biological relationships. *Obesity Reviews.* 2020;21(11). doi:10.1111/obr.13128

[4] Chawla D, Rizzo S, Zalocusky K, et al. Descriptive epidemiology of 16,780 hospitalized COVID-19 patients in the United States. 2020. doi:10.1101/2020.07.17.20156265

[5] Matacic C. Blood vessel injury may spur diseases fatal second phase. *Science.* 2020;368(6495):1039-1040. doi:10.1126/science.368.6495.1039

[6] Karlsson EA, Sheridan PA, Beck MA. Diet-Induced Obesity Impairs the T Cell Memory Response to Influenza Virus Infection. *The Journal of Immunology.* 2010;184(6):3127-3133. doi:10.4049/jimmunol.0903220

[7] Neidich SD, Green WD, Rebeles J, et al. Increased risk of influenza among vaccinated adults who are obese. *Int J Obes (Lond).* 2017;41(9):1324-1330. doi:10.1038/ijo.2017.131

Reason 41: Obesity Drives Covid

[1] Denyer S, Achenbach J. Researchers ponder why covid-19 appears deadlier in the US and Europe than in Asia. The Washington Post. 2020. Retrieved from https://www.washingtonpost.com/world/researchers-ponder-why-covid-appears-more-deadly-in-the-us-and-europe-than-in-asia/2020/05/26/81889d06-8a9f-11ea-9759-6d20ba0f2c0e_story.html

Reason 42: Covid-19 Is An IQ Test

[1] Coleman V. Proof That Face Masks Do More Harm Than Good. 2020. Retrieved from https://usercontent.one/wp/www.ooc.one/wp-content/uploads/2020/12/proof-that-masks-do-more-harm-than-good.pdf

Reason 43: You Do Not Want To Wear It, They Do Not Want To Wear It

[1] Genesis 1:27

Reason 44: Ask These Kids What They Think Of Face Masks

[1] 504 plan

Reason 50: The Following List Of Biases

[1] Pannucci CJ, Wilkins EG. Identifying and Avoiding Bias in Research. *Plastic and Reconstructive Surgery.* 2010;126(2):619-625. doi:10.1097/prs.0b013e3181de24bc

[2] Gerhard T. Bias: Considerations for research practice. Am. J. Health. Syst. Pharm. 2008;65:2159-2168.

Reason 52: The Story Of Vioxx

[1] Prakash S, Valentine V. Timeline: The Rise and Fall of Vioxx. *NPR.* 2007. Retrieved from https://www.npr.org/2007/11/10/5470430/timeline-the-rise-and-fall-of-vioxx

Reason 54: Face Masks Hurt Pregnant Women And Their Babies

[1] Tong PS, Kale AS, Ng K, Loke AP, Choolani MA, Lim CL, Chan YH, Chong YS, Tambyah PA, Yong EL. Respiratory consequences of N95-type Mask usage in pregnant healthcare workers-a controlled clinical study. Antimicrob Resist Infect Control. 2015 Nov 16;4:48. doi: 10.1186/s13756-015-0086-z. Erratum in: Antimicrob Resist Infect Control. 2016;5:26. PMID: 26579222; PMCID: PMC4647822.

[2] Jamieson DJ, Honein MA, Rasmussen SA, Williams JL, Swerdlow DL, Biggerstaff MS, et al. H1N1 2009 influenza virus infection during pregnancy in the USA. Lancet. 2009;374:451–8

[3] Bobrowski RA. Pulmonary physiology in pregnancy. Clin Obstet Gynecol. 2010;53:285–300

[4] Murphy VE, Namazy JA, Powell H, Schatz M, Chambers C, Attia J, et al. A meta-analysis of adverse perinatal outcomes in women with asthma. BJOG. 2011;118:1314–23

[5] Fung AM, Wilson DL, Barnes M, Walker SP. Obstructive sleep apnea and pregnancy: the effect on perinatal outcomes. J Perinatol. 2012;32:399–406.

[6] *MedicinePlus.* Preterm Labor. Retrieved from: https://medlineplus.gov/pretermlabor.html

[7] Seeds JW. Impaired fetal growth: definition and clinical diagnosis. Obstet Gynecol. 1984 Sep;64(3):303-10. PMID: 6379528.

[8] *Mayo Clinic.* Preeclampsia. Retrieved from: https://www.mayoclinic.org/diseases-conditions/preeclampsia/symptoms-causes/syc-20355745

454

Reason 55: Face Masks May Cause Mothers To Have Elevated Enough Carbon Dioxide To Prevent Fetuses From Being Able To Clear Their Own Carbon Dioxide

[1] Miller M.T. Thalidomide embryopathy: a model for the study of congenital incomitant horizontal strabismus. US National Library of Medicine Journal. 1991 Retrieved from https://www.ncbi.nlm.nih.gov/pmc/articles/PMC1298636/?page=10

[2] Kisielinski K, Giboni P, Prescher A, et al. Is a Mask That Covers the Mouth and Nose Free from Undesirable Side Effects in Everyday Use and Free of Potential Hazards? International Journal of Environmental Research and Public Health. 2021;18(8):4344. doi:10.3390/ijerph18084344.

[3] Roberge, R.J.; Kim, J.-H.; Powell, J.B. N95 Respirator Use during Advanced Pregnancy. Am. J. Infect. Control 2014, 42, 1097–1100.

[4] Roeckner, J.T.; Krsti´c, N.; Sipe, B.H.; Obi˜can, S.G. N95 Filtering Facepiece Respirator Use during Pregnancy: A Systematic Review. Am. J. Perinatol. 2020, 37, 995–1001.

[5] Tong, P.S.Y.; Kale, A.S.; Ng, K.; Loke, A.P.; Choolani, M.A.; Lim, C.L.; Chan, Y.H.; Chong, Y.S.; Tambyah, P.A.; Yong, E.-L. Respiratory Consequences of N95-Type Mask Usage in Pregnant Healthcare Workers — A Controlled Clinical Study. Antimicrob. Resist. Infect. Control 2015, 4, 48.

Reason 56: Face Masks On Pregnant Women During Exertion Should Be Avoided To Protect The Unborn Child

[1] Kisielinski K, Giboni P, Prescher A, et al. Is a Mask That Covers the Mouth and Nose Free from Undesirable Side Effects in Everyday Use and Free of Potential Hazards? International Journal of Environmental Research and Public Health. 2021;18(8):4344. doi:10.3390/ijerph18084344.

[2] Roeckner, J.T.; Krsti´c, N.; Sipe, B.H.; Obi˜can, S.G. N95 Filtering Facepiece Respirator Use during Pregnancy: A Systematic Review. Am. J. Perinatol. 2020, 37, 995–1001.

[3] Roberge, R.J.; Kim, J.-H.; Powell, J.B. N95 Respirator Use during Advanced Pregnancy. Am. J. Infect. Control 2014, 42, 1097–1100.

[4] Tong, P.S.Y.; Kale, A.S.; Ng, K.; Loke, A.P.; Choolani, M.A.; Lim, C.L.; Chan, Y.H.; Chong, Y.S.; Tambyah, P.A.; Yong, E.-L. Respiratory Consequences of N95-Type Mask Usage in Pregnant Healthcare Workers — A Controlled Clinical Study. Antimicrob. Resist. Infect. Control 2015, 4, 48.

[5] Deoni SC, Beauchemin J, Volpe A, D'Sa V. Impact of the COVID-19 Pandemic on Early Child Cognitive Development: Initial Findings in a Longitudinal Observational Study of Child Health. 2021. doi:10.1101/2021.08.10.21261846

Reason 57: Face Mask Material May Be Teratogenic (They Cause Birth Defects)

[1] Kisielinski K, Giboni P, Prescher A, et al. Is a Mask That Covers the Mouth and Nose Free from Undesirable Side Effects in Everyday Use and Free of Potential Hazards? International Journal of Environmental Research and Public Health. 2021;18(8):4344. doi:10.3390/ijerph18084344.

[2] Roeckner, J.T.; Krsti´c, N.; Sipe, B.H.; Obi˜can, S.G. N95 Filtering Facepiece Respirator Use during Pregnancy: A Systematic Review. Am. J. Perinatol. 2020, 37, 995–1001.

[3] Badri, F.M.A. Surgical Mask Contact Dermatitis and Epidemiology of Contact Dermatitis in Healthcare Workers. Curr. Allergy Clin. Immunol. 2017, 30, 183–188.

Reason 58: Face Masks Are Harmful For Babies

[1] Mayo Clinic. Sudden Infant death syndrome (SIDS). Retrieved from https://www.mayoclinic.org/diseases-conditions/sudden-infant-death-syndrome/symptoms-causes/syc-20352800

[2] Wilkinson, Damon. Doctor warns of suffocation risk from 'cute' baby face masks. *Manchester Evening News*. Aug 2020. Retrieved from https://www.manchestereveningnews.co.uk/news/greater-manchester-news/doctor-warns-suffocation-risk-cute-18715091

Reason 59: Children Are Far More Vulnerable To Harm From Face Masks Than Adults

[1] Kisielinski K, Giboni P, Prescher A, et al. Is a Mask That Covers the Mouth and Nose Free from Undesirable Side Effects in Everyday Use and Free of Potential Hazards? International Journal of Environmental Research and Public Health. 2021;18(8):4344. doi:10.3390/ijerph18084344.

[2] Smart, N.R.; Horwell, C.J.; Smart, T.S.; Galea, K.S. Assessment of the Wearability of Facemasks against Air Pollution in Primary School-Aged Children in London. Int. J. Environ. Res. Public Health 2020, 17, 3935.

[3] Goh, D.Y.T.; Mun, M.W.; Lee, W.L.J.; Teoh, O.H.; Rajgor, D.D. A Randomised Clinical Trial to Evaluate the Safety, Fit, Comfort of a Novel N95 Mask in Children. Sci. Rep. 2019, 9, 18952.

[4] Azuma, K.; Kagi, N.; Yanagi, U.; Osawa, H. Effects of Low-Level Inhalation Exposure to Carbon Dioxide in Indoor Environments: A Short Review on Human Health and Psychomotor Performance. Environ. Int. 2018, 121, 51–56.

Reason 60: Graphene In Face Masks May Pose A Particular Risk

[1] Graphene face masks. *Health Canada*. 2021;(Product Safety). doi:RA-75309 From https://healthycanadians.gc.ca/recall-alert-rappel-avis/hc-sc/2021/75309a-eng.php

455

Reason 61: Inhaled Cotton Fibers Cause Lung Disease

[1] Boris Borovoy, Colleen Huber, Q Makeeta. Masks, false safety and real dangers, Part 1: Friable mask particulate and lung vulnerability. https://childrenshealthdefense.org/the-science-of-masks/ from https://childrenshealthdefense.org/wp-content/uploads/Masks-false-safety-and-real-dangers-Part-1-Friable-mask-particulate-and-lung-vulnerability.pdf

[2] H Kobayashi, S Kanoh, et al. Diffuse lung disease caused by cotton fibre inhalation but distinct from byssinosis. Thorax. Nov 2004. 59 (12). https://thorax.bmj.com/content/59/12/1095

[3] P Lai, D Christiani. Long-Term respiratory health effects in textile workers. Curr Opin Pulm Med. Mar 2013. 19 (2): 152-157. doi: 0.1097/MCP.0b013e32835cee9a https://www.ncbi.nlm.nih.gov/pmc/articles/PMC3725301/

Reason 63: Inhaled Synethetic Fibers Cause Lung Disease

[1] Boris Borovoy, Colleen Huber, Q Makeeta. Masks, false safety and real dangers, Part 1: Friable mask particulate and lung vulnerability. https://childrenshealthdefense.org/the-science-of-masks/ from https://childrenshealthdefense.org/wp-content/uploads/Masks-false-safety-and-real-dangers-Part-1-Friable-mask-particulate-and-lung-vulnerability.pdf

[2] J Cortez Pimentel, R Avila et al. Respiratory disease caused by synthetic fibers: a new occupational disease. Thorax. 1975. 30 (204): 205-19. https://www.ncbi.nlm.nih.gov/pmc/articles/PMC470268/pdf/thorax00140-0084.pdf

Reason 63: Inhaled Fibers Cause Pulmonary Fibrosis

[1] Boris Borovoy, Colleen Huber, Q Makeeta. Masks, false safety and real dangers, Part 1: Friable mask particulate and lung vulnerability. https://childrenshealthdefense.org/the-science-of-masks/ from https://childrenshealthdefense.org/wp-content/uploads/Masks-false-safety-and-real-dangers-Part-1-Friable-mask-particulate-and-lung-vulnerability.pdf

[2] W Wuyts, C Agostini, et al. The pathogenesis of pulmonary fibrosis: a moving target. Eur Rep J. 2013 (41): 1207-1218. DOI: 0.1183/09031936.00073012 https://erj.ersjournals.com/content/41/5/1207

[3] G Oberdorster, E Oberdorster, et al. Nanotoxicology: An emerging discipline evolving from studies of ultrafine particles. Environ Health Perspect. Jul 2005. 113(7): 823-839. doi: 10.1289/ehp.7339 https://www.ncbi.nlm.nih.gov/pmc/articles/PMC1257642/

[4] G Oberdorster, E Oberdorster, et al. Nanotoxicology: An emerging discipline evolving from studies of ultrafine particles. Environ Health Perspect. Jul 2005. 113(7): 823-839. doi: 10.1289/ehp.7339 https://www.ncbi.nlm.nih.gov/pmc/articles/PMC1257642/

[5] J Byrne, J Baugh. The significance of nanoparticles in particle-induced pulmonary fibrosis. McGill J Med. Jan 2008. 11 (1): 43-50. https://www.ncbi.nlm.nih.gov/pmc/articles/PMC2322933/

[6] D Bodian, H Howe. Experimental studies on intraneural spread of poliomyelitis virus. Bull Johns Hopkins Hops. 1941a; 69:248-267. https://www.cabdirect.org/cabdirect/abstract/19422700792

Reason 64: Prolonged Textile Face Mask Use May Lead To Respiratory Illnesses Like Those Experienced By Textile Workers In The Third World

[1] Kisielinski K, Giboni P, Prescher A, et al. Is a Mask That Covers the Mouth and Nose Free from Undesirable Side Effects in Everyday Use and Free of Potential Hazards? International Journal of Environmental Research and Public Health. 2021;18(8):4344. doi:10.3390/ijerph18084344.

[2] World Health Organization. WHO-Advice on the Use of Masks in the Context of COVID-19: Interim Guidance, 5 June 2020; World Health Organization: Geneva, Switzerland, 2020; Available online: https://apps.who.int/iris/handle/10665/332293 (accessed on 7 November 2020

[3] Potluri, P.; Needham, P. Technical Textiles for Protection (Manchester EScholar-The University of Manchester); Woodhead Publishing: Cambridge, UK, 2005.

[4] Klimek, L.; Huppertz, T.; Alali, A.; Spielhaupter, M.; Hörmann, K.; Matthias, C.; Hagemann, J. A New Form of Irritant Rhinitis to Filtering Facepiece Particle (FFP) Masks (FFP2/N95/KN95 Respirators) during COVID-19 Pandemic. World Allergy Organ. J. 2020, 13, 100474.

[5] Lai, P.S.; Christiani, D.C. Long-Term Respiratory Health Effects in Textile Workers. Curr. Opin. Pulm. Med. 2013, 19, 152–157.

[6] Salimi, F.; Morgan, G.; Rolfe, M.; Samoli, E.; Cowie, C.T.; Hanigan, I.; Knibbs, L.; Cope, M.; Johnston, F.H.; Guo, Y.; et al. Long-Term Exposure to Low Concentrations of Air Pollutants and Hospitalisation for Respiratory Diseases: A Prospective Cohort Study in Australia. Environ. Int. 2018, 121, 415–420.

Reason 65: Your Child Inhales Dangerous Chlorine Compounds While Wearing A Face Mask

[1] Singleton MM. Mask Facts. *Association of American Physicians and Surgeons.* 2021. Retrieved from https://aapsonline.org/mask-facts/

[2] *Swiss Policy Research.* Are Face Masks Effective? The Evidence. 2020. Retrieved from https://swprs.org/face-masks-evidence/.

Reason 66: Exhaled Air Contains Over 250 Substances Meant To Be Removed From Your Body And Not Breathed Back In

[1] Kisielinski K, Giboni P, Prescher A, et al. Is a Mask That Covers the Mouth and Nose Free from Undesirable Side Effects in Everyday Use and Free of Potential Hazards? International Journal of Environmental Research and Public Health. 2021;18(8):4344. doi:10.3390/ijerph18084344.

[2] Geer Wallace, M.A.; Pleil, J.D. Evolution of Clinical and Environmental Health Applications of Exhaled Breath Research: Review of Methods: Instrumentation for Gas-Phase, Condensate, and Aerosols. Anal. Chim. Acta 2018, 1024, 18–38.

[3] Salimi, F.; Morgan, G.; Rolfe, M.; Samoli, E.; Cowie, C.T.; Hanigan, I.; Knibbs, L.; Cope, M.; Johnston, F.H.; Guo, Y.; et al. Long-Term Exposure to Low Concentrations of Air Pollutants and Hospitalisation for Respiratory Diseases: A Prospective Cohort Study in Australia. Environ. Int. 2018, 121, 415–420.

[4] Simonton, D.; Spears, M. Human Health Effects from Exposure to Low-Level Concentrations of Hydrogen Sulfide. Occup. Health Saf. (Waco Tex.) 2007, 76, 102–104.

[5] Sukul, P.; Schwartz, J.; Di, Q.; Choirat, C.; Zanobetti, A. Assessing Adverse Health Effects of Long-Term Exposure to Low Levels of Ambient Air Pollution: Phase 1 Research Report; Health Effects Institute: Boston, MA, USA, 2019; pp. 1–51.

[6] Sukul, P.; Schubert, J.K.; Zanaty, K.; Trefz, P.; Sinha, A.; Kamysek, S.; Miekisch, W. Exhaled Breath Compositions under Varying Respiratory Rhythms Reflects Ventilatory Variations: Translating Breathomics towards Respiratory Medicine. Sci. Rep. 2020, 10, 14109.

Reason 67: Eighty-Two Bacterial Colonies And Four Mold Colonies Found On A Child's Face Mask After Eight Hours

[1] Singleton MM. Mask Facts. Association of American Physicians and Surgeons. 2021. Retrieved from https://aaps online.org/mask-facts/

Reason 68: Face Masks Are Breeding Grounds For Bacteria In A Way Our Unmasked Faces Are Not

[1] Borovoy, Boris, Huber Colleen, Crisler Maria. Masks, false safety and real dangers, Part 2: Microbial challenges from masks. Retrieved from https://mask-covid.info/wp-content/uploads/2020/11/Mask_Risks_Part2.pdf#:~:text=Microbial contamination of and from masks Bacteria are,bacterial colonies. Molds and yeasts were also found.

[2] Prussin, A.Garcia, E., et al. Total virus and bacteria concentrations in indoor and outdoor air. Environ Sci Technol Lett. 2015. 2 (4). 84-88. https://dx.doi.org/10.1021%2Facs.estlett.5b00050 https://www.ncbi.nlm.nih.gov/pmc/articles/PMC4515362/

[3] Blick. Your corona mask really is that gruesome. [article in German]. Sep 16, 2020. https://amp.blick.ch/wirtschaft/gebrauchte-exemplare-getestet-so-gruusig-ist-ihre-corona-maske-wirklichid16096358.html?utm_source=twitter&utm_medium=social_user&utm_campaign=blick_amp

[4] Zhiqing, L, et al. Surgical masks as source of bacterial contamination during operative procedures. J Ortho Translation. July 2018. 14. 57-62. https://doi.org/10.1016/j.jot.2018.06.002

[5] Luksamijarulkul. P, Ajempradit N, et al. Microbial contamination on used surgical masks among hospital personnel and microbial air quality in their working wards: A hospital in Bangkok. Oman Med J. Sept 2014. 29 (5). 346-350. https://dx.doi.org/10.5001%2Fomj.2014.92. https://www.ncbi.nlm.nih.

Reason 69: Bacteria On Masks Are Not Benign And Have Been Proven To Be Very Harmful

[1] Borovoy, Boris, Huber Colleen, Crisler Maria. Masks, false safety and real dangers, Part 2: Microbial challenges from masks. Retrieved from https://mask-covid.info/wp-content/uploads/2020/11/Mask_Risks_Part2.pdf#:~:text=Microbial contamination of and from masks Bacteria are,bacterial colonies. Molds and yeasts were also found.

[2] Schnirman, R. Nur, N. et al. A case of legionella pneumonia caused by home use of continuous positive airway pressure. SAGE Open Med Case Rep. 2017; 5: 2050313X17744981. doi:10.1177/2050313X1774498 https://journals.sagepub.com/doi/10.1177/2050313X17744981

[3] Scannapieco. Role of oral bacteria in respiratory infection. J Periodontol. Jul 1999. 70 (7): 793-802. doi: 10.1902/jop.1999.70.7.793. https://pubmed.ncbi.nlm.nih.gov/10440642/

[4] Ortega, O. Clave, P. Oral hygiene, aspiration and aspiration pneumonia: From pathophysiology to therapeutic strategies. Curr Phys Med Rehabil Rep. Oct 2013. 1:292-295. DOI 10.1007/s40141-013-0032-z

[5] Ramondi. Interview with FOX News. 'Mask mouth': Dentists coin new term for smelly side effect of wearing a mask. Aug 7 2020. https://www.foxnews.com/health/mask-mouth-dentists-new-term

[6] Holmer, I. Kuklane, K. et al. Minute volumes and inspiratory flow rates during exhaustive treadmill walking using respirators. Ann Occup Hygiene. 51 (3): 327-335. Apr 2007. https://doi.org/10.1093/annhyg/mem004 https://academic.oup.com/annweh/article/51/3/327/139423

[7] Khair, O.A. Davies, R.J. et al. Bacterial-induced release of inflammatory mediators by bronchial epithelial cells. Eur Resp J. 1996(9): 1913-1922. https://erj.ersjournals.com/content/9/9/1913

[8] Scannapieco, F. Wang, B. et al. Oral bacteria and respiratory infection: Effects on respiratory pathogen adhesion and epithelial cell proinflammatory cytokine production. Ann Periodontol. Dec 1, 2001. https://doi.org/10.1902/annals.2001.6.1.78 https://aap.onlinelibrary.wiley.com/doi/abs/10.1902/annals.2001.6.1.78

[9] Patel, J. Sampson, V. The role of oral bacteria in COVID-19. Lancet. https://doi.org/10.1016/S2666-5247(20)30057-4. https://www.thelancet.com/journals/lanmic/article/PIIS2666-5247(20)30057-4/fulltext

[10] Azarpazhooh, A. Leake, JL. Systematic review of the association between respiratory diseases and oral health. J Periodontol. 2006 (77): 1465-1482. https://pubmed.ncbi.nlm.nih.gov/16945022/

[11] Sjogren, P. Nilsson, E. et al. A systematic review of the preventive effect of oral hygiene on pneumonia and respiratory tract infection in elderly people in hospitals and nursing homes: effect estimates and methodological quality of randomized controlled trials. J Am Geriatr Soc. 2008 (56): 2124-2130. https://pubmed.ncbi.nlm.nih.gov/18795989/

[12] Manger, E. Walshaw, M. et al. Evidence summary: The relationship between oral health and pulmonary disease. Br Dent J. Apr 7 2017. 222 (7): 527-533. doi: 10.1038/sj.bdj.2017.315 https://pubmed.ncbi.nlm.nih.gov/28387268/

[13] Stacy, A. Fleming, D. et al. A commensal bacterium promotes virulence of an opportunistic pathogen via crossrespiration. Am Soc for Microbiol. 7 (3) e00782-16. doi:10.1128/mBio.00782-16 https://mbio.asm.org/content/7/3/e00782-16/article-info

[14] MacIntyre, C. Seale, H. et al. A cluster randomized trial of cloth masks compared with medical masks in healthcare workers. BMJ Open. 2015; 5(4) https://bmjopen.bmj.com/content/5/4/e006577

[15] Xiao, J. Shiu, E. et al. Nonpharmaceutical measures for pandemic influenza in non-healthcare settings — personal protective and environmental measures. Centers for Disease Control. 26(5); 2020 May. https://wwwnc.cdc.gov/eid/article/26/5/19-0994_article

Reason 70: Face Mask Wearing Causes Harmful Bacteria To Proliferate In An Environment Outside The Protection Of The Many PathogenDefenses The Body Has

[1] Kisielinski K, Giboni P, Prescher A, et al. Is a Mask That Covers the Mouth and Nose Free from Undesirable Side Effects in Everyday Use and Free of Potential Hazards? International Journal of Environmental Research and Public Health. 2021;18(8):4344. doi:10.3390/ijerph18084344.

[2] Roberge, R.; Bayer, E.; Powell, J.; Coca, A.; Roberge, M.; Benson, S. Effect of Exhaled Moisture on Breathing Resistance of N95 Filtering Facepiece Respirators. Ann. Occup. Hyg. 2010, 54, 671–677.

[3] MacIntyre, C.R.; Seale, H.; Dung, T.C.; Hien, N.T.; Nga, P.T.; Chughtai, A.A.; Rahman, B.; Dwyer, D.E.; Wang, Q. A Cluster Randomised Trial of Cloth Masks Compared with Medical Masks in Healthcare Workers. BMJ Open 2015, 5, e006577.

[4] MacIntyre, C.R.; Chughtai, A.A. Facemasks for the Prevention of Infection in Healthcare and Community Settings. BMJ 2015, 350, h694.

[5] MacIntyre, C.R.; Wang, Q.; Seale, H.; Yang, P.; Shi, W.; Gao, Z.; Rahman, B.; Zhang, Y.; Wang, X.; Newall, A.T.; et al. A Randomized Clinical Trial of Three Options for N95 Respirators and Medical Masks in Health Workers. Am. J. Respir. Crit. Care Med. 2013, 187, 960–966.

[6] Monalisa, A.C.; Padma, K.B.; Manjunath, K.; Hemavathy, E.; Varsha, D. Microbial Contamination of the Mouth Masks Used by Post-Graduate Students in a Private Dental Institution: An In-Vitro Study. IOSR J. Dent. Med. Sci. 2017, 16, 61–67.

[7] Chughtai, A.A.; Stelzer-Braid, S.; Rawlinson, W.; Pontivivo, G.; Wang, Q.; Pan, Y.; Zhang, D.; Zhang, Y.; Li, L.; MacIntyre, C.R. Contamination by Respiratory Viruses on Outer Surface of Medical Masks Used by Hospital Healthcare Workers. BMC Infect. Dis. 2019, 19, 491.

[8] Luksamijarulkul, P.; Aiempradit, N.; Vatanasomboon, P. Microbial Contamination on Used Surgical Masks among Hospital Personnel and Microbial Air Quality in Their Working Wards: A Hospital in Bangkok. Oman Med. J. 2014, 29, 346–350.

[9] Liu, Z.; Chang, Y.; Chu, W.; Yan, M.; Mao, Y.; Zhu, Z.; Wu, H.; Zhao, J.; Dai, K.; Li, H.; et al. Surgical Masks as Source of Bacterial Contamination during Operative Procedures. J. Orthop. Transl. 2018, 14, 57–62.

[10] Kappstein, I. Mund-Nasen-Schutz in der Öffentlichkeit: Keine Hinweise für eine Wirksamkeit. Krankenh. Up2date 2020, 15, 279–295.

[11] Li, Y.; Tokura, H.; Guo, Y.P.; Wong, A.S.W.; Wong, T.; Chung, J.; Newton, E. Effects of Wearing N95 and Surgical Facemasks on Heart Rate, Thermal Stress and Subjective Sensations. Int. Arch. Occup. Environ. Health 2005, 78, 501–509.

[12] Asadi, S.; Cappa, C.D.; Barreda, S.; Wexler, A.S.; Bouvier, N.M.; Ristenpart, W.D. Efficacy of Masks and Face Coverings in Controlling Outward Aerosol Particle Emission from Expiratory Activities. Sci. Rep. 2020, 10, 15665.

[13] Robert Koch-Institut. Influenza-Monatsbericht; Robert Koch-Institut: Berlin, Germany, 2020.

Reason 72: Face Masks Cause Sore Throats

[1] Bock, H. Infectious disease doctor gives face covering tips to stay healthy. 4 News. 2020. Retrieved from https://cbs4local.com/news/local/infectious-disease-doctor-gives-face-covering-tips-to-stay-healthy

Reason 73: Face Masked People May Be At Greater Risk For Fungal Infections Of Lungs Than Unmasked

[1] Borovoy, B, Huber C, Crisler M. Masks, false safety and real dangers, Part 2: Microbial challenges from masks. Retrieved from https://mask-covid.info/wp-content/uploads/2020/11/Mask_Risks_Part2.pdf#:~:text=Microbial contamination of and from masks Bacteria are,bacterial colonies. Molds and yeasts were also found.

[2] DeSoyza, A. Alberti, S. Bronchiectasis and aspergillosis: How are they linked? Med Mycol Jan 1 2017. 55 (1): 69-81. doi: 10.1093/mmy/myw109. https://pubmed.ncbi.nlm.nih.gov/2779452

[3] Shah, D. jackman, S. et al. Effect of gliotoxin on human polymorphonuclear neutrophils. Infect Dis Obstet Gynecol. 1998. 6 (4). 168-175. https://dx.doi.org/10.1002%2F(SICI)1098-0997(1998)6%3A4%3C168%3A%3AAIDIDOG6%3E3.0.CO% 3B2-Z. https://www.ncbi.nlm.nih.gov/pmc/articles/PMC1784797

Reason 74: Mayo Clinic: Face Mask Wearing Is Leading To An Increase In Staph Infections, As Can Be Expected As They Help Bacteria Access Deeper Quarters Of The Body

[1] Borovoy, B, Huber, C, Crisler, M. Masks, false safety and real dangers, Part 2: Microbial challenges from masks. Retrieved from https://mask-covid.info/wp-content/uploads/2020/11/Mask_Risks_Part2.pdf#:~:text=Microbial contamination of and from masks Bacteria are,bacterial colonies. Molds and yeasts were also found.

[2] Todar, K. The Normal Bacterial Flora of Humans. Online Textbook of Bacteriology. 2020. http://www.textbook ofbacteriology.net/normalflora_3.htm

[3] Glaser, R. Thomas, W. et al. The incidence and pathogenesis of myocarditis in rabbits after group A streptococcal pharyngeal infections. J Exp Med. Jan 1 1956.. 103 (1): 173-188. doi: 10.1084/jem.103.1.173. https://pubmed.ncbi.nlm.nih.gov/13278

[4] Patel, J. Sampson, V. The role of oral bacteria in COVID-19. Lancet. https://doi.org/10.1016/S2666-5247(20)30057-4. https://www.thelancet.com/journals/lanmic/article/PIIS2666-5247(20)30057-4/fulltext

[5] Ramesh, A. Varghese, S. et al. Chronic obstructive pulmonary disease and periodontitis — Unwinding their linking mechanisms. Sept 2015. J Oral Biosci. 58 (1). https://www.researchgate.net/publication/283116707_Chronic_ obstructive_pulmonary_disease_and_periodontit is_-_Unwinding_their_linking_mechanisms

[6] 8 P Heikkila, A But, et al. Periodontitis and cancer mortality: Register-based cohort study of 68,273 adults in 10-year follow-up. Cancer Epidem. Int J Cancer. 142 (11). Jan 11 2018. https://doi.org/10.1002/ijc.31254
https://onlinelibrary.wiley.com/doi/full/10.1002/ijc.31254

[7] Babu, N. Gomes, A. Systemic manifestations of oral diseases. J Oral Maxillofac Pathol. 15 (2); May-Aug 2011. https://dx.doi.org/10.4103%2F0973-029X.84477
https://www.ncbi.nlm.nih.gov/pmc/articles/PMC3329699/

[8] Bingham, C. Moni, M. Periodontal disease and rheumatoid arthritis: the evidence accumulates for complex pathobiologic interactions. Curr Opin Rheumatol. Jul 8 2015. https://dx.doi.org/10.1097%2FBOR.0b013e32835fb8ec
https://www.ncbi.nlm.nih.gov/pmc/articles/PMC4495574/

[9] Feldman, B. The oral microbiome and its links to autoimmunity. The Doctor Weighs In. Aug 26, 2018. https://thedoctorweighsin.com/oral-microbiome-links-autoimmunity/

[10] US Centers for Diseases Control. Erythromycin-resistant Group A Streptococcus. Retrieved from: https://www.cdc.gov/ drugresistance/pdf/threats-report/gas-508.pdf

[11] Dileepan, T. Smith, E. et al. Group A Streptococcus intranasal infection promotes CNS infiltration by streptococcal-specific Th17 cells. J Clin Invest. Jan 2016. 126 (1): 303-317. doi: 10.1172/JCI80792 https://pubmed.ncbi.nlm.nih.gov/26657857/

[12] Mayo Clinic. Staph Infections. [Article is now partially censored.] https://www.mayoclinic.org/diseases-conditions/staph-infections/symptoms-causes/syc-20356221

[13] Terrasse, J. Lere, J. et al. Septicèmie, ostéomyelite, percardite suppurée a staphylocoques; guerison par la pénicilline intraveineuse, intramusculaire, intrapéricardique. [Article in French]. Bull Mem So Med Hop Paris, 1945. 61 (26-31): 400-402. https://pubmed.ncbi.nlm.nih.gov/21021328/

[14] Rubin, R. Moellering, R. Clinical, microbiologic and therapeutic aspects of purulent pericarditis. Am J Med. Jul 1975. 59 (1): 68-78. doi: 10.1016/0002-9343(75)90323-x. https://pubmed.ncbi.nlm.nih.gov/1138554/

[15] Majid, A. Omar, A. Diagnosis and management of purulent pericarditis. Experience with pericardiectomy. J Thorac Cardiovasc Surg. Sept 1991. 102 (3): 413-417. https://pubmed.ncbi.nlm.nih.gov/1881180/

[16] Pankuweit, S. Ristic, A. et al. Bacterial pericarditis: diagnosis and management. Am J Cardiovasc Drugs. 2005. 5 (2): 103-112. doi: 10.2165/00129784-200505020-00004. https://pubmed.ncbi.nlm.nih.gov/15725041/

[17] Taib, R. Penny, P. Infective Endocarditis. In Paediatric Cardiology. (Third Edition). 2010. https://www.science direct.com/book/9780702030642/paediatric-cardiology

[18] Chhatwal, G. Graham, R. Streptococcal diseases. In International Encyclopedia of Public Health (Second Edition). 2017. https://www.sciencedirect.com/referencework/9780128037089/international-encyclopedia-of-public-health

Reason 75: Face Masks Harm A Child's Developing Mind

[1] Rancourt, D.G. Review of scientific reports of harms caused by face masks, up to February 2021. *Children's Health Defence.* 2021. DOI: 10.13140/RG.2.2.14294.37448. Retrieved from https://childrenshealthdefense.org/wp-content/ uploads/5thsciencereview-masksharm-1.pdf

Reason 76: Face Masks Affect A Person's Ability To Think Clearly

[1] Kisielinski K, Giboni P, Prescher A, et al. Is a Mask That Covers the Mouth and Nose Free from Undesirable Side Effects in Everyday Use and Free of Potential Hazards? International Journal of Environmental Research and Public Health. 2021;18(8):4344. doi:10.3390/ijerph18084344.

[2] Rebmann, T.; Carrico, R.; Wang, J. Physiologic and Other Effects and Compliance with Long-Term Respirator Use among Medical Intensive Care Unit Nurses. Am. J. Infect. Control 2013, 41, 1218–1223.

[3] Liu, C.; Li, G.; He, Y.; Zhang, Z.; Ding, Y. Effects of Wearing Masks on Human Health and Comfort during the COVID-19 Pandemic. IOP Conf. Ser. Earth Environ. Sci. 2020, 531, 012034.

[4] Jagim, A.R.; Dominy, T.A.; Camic, C.L.; Wright, G.; Doberstein, S.; Jones, M.T.; Oliver, J.M. Acute Effects of the Elevation Training Mask on Strength Performance in Recreational Weight Lifters. J. Strength Cond. Res. 2018, 32, 482–489.

[5] Drechsler, M.; Morris, J. Carbon Dioxide Narcosis. In StatPearls; StatPearls Publishing: Treasure Island, FL, USA, 2020.

[6] Noble, J.; Jones, J.G.; Davis, E.J. Cognitive Function during Moderate Hypoxaemia. Anaesth. Intensive Care 1993, 21, 180–184.

[7] Fothergill, D.M.; Hedges, D.; Morrison, J.B. Effects of CO_2 and N_2 Partial Pressures on Cognitive and Psychomotor Performance. Undersea Biomed. Res. 1991, 18, 1–19.

[8] Johnson, A.T. Respirator Masks Protect Health but Impact Performance: A Review. J. Biol. Eng. 2016, 10, 4.

[9] Rosner, E. Adverse Effects of Prolonged Mask Use among Healthcare Professionals during COVID-19. J. Infect. Dis. Epidemiol. 2020.

[10] Deutsche Gesetzliche Unfallversicherung. DGUV Grundsätze für Arbeitsmedizinische Vorsorgeuntersuchungen; Alfons, W., Ed.; Gentner Verlag: Stuttgart, Germany, 2010; ISBN 978-3-87247-733-0.

Reason 77: Face Masks Cause Degeneration Of Brains Because Of Lack Of Oxygen

[1] Vernon Dr. Dr. Vernon Coleman: masks and mask wearing: 100 facts you must know. *World Doctors Alliance*. 2021. Retrieved from https://worlddoctorsalliance.com/de/blog/vernon-coleman-more-harm-than-good/

Reason 78: Face Mask Wearing Causes Reduced Attention And Slower Speed In Athletes

[1] Kisielinski K, Giboni P, Prescher A, et al. Is a Mask That Covers the Mouth and Nose Free from Undesirable Side Effects in Everyday Use and Free of Potential Hazards? International Journal of Environmental Research and Public Health. 2021;18(8):4344. doi:10.3390/ijerph18084344.

[2] Cress ML, Forrester K, Probst L, Foster C, Doberstein S, Porcari JP. Effect of Wearing the Elevation Training Mask on Aerobic Capacity, Lung Function, and Hematological Variables. Medicine & Science in Sports & Exercise. 2016;48:1040-1041. doi:10.1249/01.mss.0000488131.38685.16.

[3] Jagim, A.R.; Dominy, T.A.; Camic, C.L.; Wright, G.; Doberstein, S.; Jones, M.T.; Oliver, J.M. Acute Effects of the Elevation Training Mask on Strength Performance in Recreational Weight Lifters. J. Strength Cond. Res. 2018, 32, 482–489.

[4] Smolka, L.; Borkowski, J.; Zaton, M. The Effect of Additional Dead Space on Respiratory Exchange Ratio and Carbon Dioxide Production Due to Training. J. Sports Sci. Med. 2014, 13, 36–43.

[5] Epstein, D.; Korytny, A.; Isenberg, Y.; Marcusohn, E.; Zukermann, R.; Bishop, B.; Minha, S.; Raz, A.; Miller, A. Return to Training in the COVID-19 Era: The Physiological Effects of Face Masks during Exercise. Scand. J. Med. Sci. Sports 2020.

Reason 79: Face Masks Are Disruptive To Basic Human Communication

[1] Kisielinski K, Giboni P, Prescher A, et al. Is a Mask That Covers the Mouth and Nose Free from Undesirable Side Effects in Everyday Use and Free of Potential Hazards? International Journal of Environmental Research and Public Health. 2021;18(8):4344. doi:10.3390/ijerph18084344.

[2] Spitzer M. Masked education? The benefits and burdens of wearing face masks in schools during the current Corona pandemic. *Trends in Neuroscience and Education*. 2020;20:100138. doi:10.1016/j.tine.2020.100138 [CrossRef]

[3] Wong, C.K.M.; Yip, B.H.K.; Mercer, S.; Griffiths, S.; Kung, K.; Wong, M.C.; Chor, J.; Wong, S.Y. Effect of Facemasks on Empathy and Relational Continuity: A Randomised Controlled Trial in Primary Care. BMC Fam. Pract. 2013, 14, 200.

[4] World Health Organization; United Nations Children's Fund. WHO-Advice on the Use of Masks for Children in the Community in the Context of COVID-19: Annex to the Advice on the Use of Masks in the Context of COVID-19, 21 August 2020; World Health Organization: Geneva, Switzerland, 2020.

[5] De Brouwer, C. Wearing a Mask, a Universal Solution against COVID-19 or an Additional Health Risk? 2020. Available online: https://papers.ssrn.com/sol3/papers.cfm?abstract_id=3676885 (accessed on 12 November 2020).

[6] Ewig, S.; Gatermann, S.; Lemmen, S. Die Maskierte Gesellschaft. Pneumologie 2020, 74, 405–408.

[7] Great Barrington Declaration Great Barrington Declaration and Petition. Available online: https://gbdeclaration.org/ (accessed on 9 November 2020).

Reason 81: Babies And Children Especially Read Lips

[1] Rancourt, D.G. Review of scientific reports of harms caused by face masks, up to February 2021. *Children's Health Defence.* 2021. DOI: 10.13140/RG.2.2.14294.37448. Retrieved from https://childrenshealthdefense.org/wp-content/uploads/5thsciencereview-masksharm-1.pdf

Reason 82: Face Masks Act As An Acoustic Filter

[1] Kisielinski K, Giboni P, Prescher A, et al. Is a Mask That Covers the Mouth and Nose Free from Undesirable Side Effects in Everyday Use and Free of Potential Hazards? International Journal of Environmental Research and Public Health. 2021;18(8):4344. doi:10.3390/ijerph18084344.

[2] Heider, C.A.; Álvarez, M.L.; Fuentes-López, E.; González, C.A.; León, N.I.; Verástegui, D.C.; Badía, P.I.; Napolitano, C.A. Prevalence of Voice Disorders in Healthcare Workers in the Universal Masking COVID-19 Era. Laryngoscope 2020.

[3] Asadi, S.; Cappa, C.D.; Barreda, S.; Wexler, A.S.; Bouvier, N.M.; Ristenpart, W.D. Efficacy of Masks and Face Coverings in Controlling Outward Aerosol Particle Emission from Expiratory Activities. Sci. Rep. 2020, 10, 15665.

Reason 83: Face Masks Cause Further Harm To The Mentally Impaired And Hearing Impaired

[1] Kisielinski K, Giboni P, Prescher A, et al. Is a Mask That Covers the Mouth and Nose Free from Undesirable Side Effects in Everyday Use and Free of Potential Hazards? International Journal of Environmental Research and Public Health. 2021;18(8):4344. doi:10.3390/ijerph18084344.

[2] Matuschek, C.; Moll, F.; Fangerau, H.; Fischer, J.C.; Zänker, K.; van Griensven, M.; Schneider, M.; Kindgen-Milles, D.; Knoefel, W.T.; Lichtenberg, A.; et al. Face Masks: Benefits and Risks during the COVID-19 Crisis. Eur. J. Med. Res. 2020, 25, 32.

Reason 84: Face Masks Reduce The Ability For A Child To Bond And Reduce The Ability For A Child To Learn

[1] Rancourt, D.G. Review of scientific reports of harms caused by face masks, up to February 2021. *Children's Health Defence.* 2021. DOI: 10.13140/RG.2.2.14294.37448. Retrieved from https://childrenshealthdefense.org/wp-content/uploads/5thsciencereview-masksharm-1.pdf

Reason 87: Face Masks Block Emotional Signaling Between Students And Teachers, Students And Parents, Students And Students, And Between Students And All Other Humans

[1] Rancourt, D.G. Review of scientific reports of harms caused by face masks, up to February 2021. 2021. Retrieved from https://assets.website-files.com/606d3a50c62e44338008303d/6076def5c5421e642472f1ef_5thsciencereview-masksharm-1.pdf

[2] Spitzer M. Masked education? The benefits and burdens of wearing face masks in schools during the current Corona pandemic. *Trends in Neuroscience and Education.* 2020;20:100138. doi:10.1016/j.tine.2020.100138

Reason 88: Both Face Masks And Face Shields Cause Fear In Children

[1] Kisielinski K, Giboni P, Prescher A, et al. Is a Mask That Covers the Mouth and Nose Free from Undesirable Side Effects in Everyday Use and Free of Potential Hazards? International Journal of Environmental Research and Public Health. 2021;18(8):4344. doi:10.3390/ijerph18084344.

[2] Forgie, S.E.; Reitsma, J.; Spady, D.; Wright, B.; Stobart, K. The "Fear Factor" for Surgical Masks and Face Shields, as Perceived by Children and Their Parents. Pediatrics 2009, 124, e777–e781.

[3] Klompas M, Morris CA, Sinclair J, Pearson M, Shenoy ES. Universal Masking in Hospitals in the Covid-19 Era. New England Journal of Medicine. 2020;382(21). doi:10.1056/nejmp2006372

Reason 89: Face Masks Are Particularly Harmful On A Person's Wellbeing

[1] Kisielinski K, Giboni P, Prescher A, et al. Is a Mask That Covers the Mouth and Nose Free from Undesirable Side Effects in Everyday Use and Free of Potential Hazards? International Journal of Environmental Research and Public Health. 2021;18(8):4344. doi:10.3390/ijerph18084344.

[2] Scarano, A.; Inchingolo, F.; Lorusso, F. Facial Skin Temperature and Discomfort When Wearing Protective Face Masks: Thermal Infrared Imaging Evaluation and Hands Moving the Mask. Int. J. Environ. Res. Public Health 2020, 17, 4624.

[3] Johnson, A.T. Respirator Masks Protect Health but Impact Performance: A Review. J. Biol. Eng. 2016, 10, 4.

[4] Roberge, R.J.; Kim, J.-H.; Coca, A. Protective Facemask Impact on Human Thermoregulation: An Overview. Ann. Occup. Hyg. 2012, 56, 102–112.

Reason 90: Face Masks Help You Raise A Sociopath

[1] Rancourt, D.G. Review of scientific reports of harms caused by face masks, up to February 2021. 2021. Retrieved from https://assets.website-files.com/606d3a50c62e44338008303d/6076def5c5421e642472f1ef_5thsciencereview-masksharm-1.pdf

[2] Spitzer M. Masked education? The benefits and burdens of wearing face masks in schools during the current Corona pandemic. *Trends in Neuroscience and Education.* 2020;20:100138. doi:10.1016/j.tine.2020.100138

Reason 91: Face Mask Peer Pressure Is So Great That Wearing Is Encouraged Far Past The Point Of Harm To The Face Mask Wearer

[1] Kisielinski K, Giboni P, Prescher A, et al. Is a Mask That Covers the Mouth and Nose Free from Undesirable Side Effects in Everyday Use and Free of Potential Hazards? International Journal of Environmental Research and Public Health. 2021;18(8):4344. doi:10.3390/ijerph18084344.

[2] Ryan, R.M.; Deci, E.L. Self-determination theory and the role of basic psychological needs in personality and the organization of behavior. In Handbook of Personality: Theory and Research, 3rd ed.; The Guilford Press: New York, NY, USA, 2008; pp. 654–678. ISBN 978-1-59385-836-0.

[3] Kyung, S.Y.; Kim, Y.; Hwang, H.; Park, J.-W.; Jeong, S.H. Risks of N95 Face Mask Use in Subjects with COPD. Respir. Care 2020, 65, 658–664.

[4] Mo, Y.; Wei, D.; Mai, Q.; Chen, C.; Yu, H.; Jiang, C.; Tan, X. Risk and Impact of Using Mask on COPD Patients with Acute Exacerbation during the COVID-19 Outbreak: A Retrospective Study. Res. Sq. 2020.

Reason 92: Face Masks Are Long Known To Cause Headaches

[1] Kisielinski K, Giboni P, Prescher A, et al. Is a Mask That Covers the Mouth and Nose Free from Undesirable Side Effects in Everyday Use and Free of Potential Hazards? International Journal of Environmental Research and Public Health. 2021;18(8):4344. doi:10.3390/ijerph18084344.

[2] Ong, J.J.Y.; Bharatendu, C.; Goh, Y.; Tang, J.Z.Y.; Sooi, K.W.X.; Tan, Y.L.; Tan, B.Y.Q.; Teoh, H.-L.; Ong, S.T.; Allen, D.M.; et al. Headaches Associated With Personal Protective Equipment-A Cross-Sectional Study among Frontline Healthcare Workers During COVID-19. Headache 2020, 60, 864–877.

[3] Jacobs, J.L.; Ohde, S.; Takahashi, O.; Tokuda, Y.; Omata, F.; Fukui, T. Use of Surgical Face Masks to Reduce the Incidence of the Common Cold among Health Care Workers in Japan: A Randomized Controlled Trial. Am. J. Infect. Control 2009, 37, 417–419.

[4] Ramirez-Moreno, J.M. Mask-Associated de Novo Headache in Healthcare Workers during the Covid-19 Pandemic. medRxiv 2020.

[5] Bharatendu, C.; Ong, J.J.Y.; Goh, Y.; Tan, B.Y.Q.; Chan, A.C.Y.; Tang, J.Z.Y.; Leow, A.S.; Chin, A.; Sooi, K.W.X.; Tan, Y.L.; et al. Powered Air Purifying Respirator (PAPR) Restores the N95 Face Mask Induced Cerebral Hemodynamic Alterations among Healthcare Workers during COVID-19 Outbreak. J. Neurol. Sci. 2020, 417, 117078.

Reason 93: Face Masks Trigger Migraines

[1] Rancourt, D.G. Review of scientific reports of harms caused by face masks, up to February 2021. *Children's Health Defence*. 2021. DOI: 10.13140/RG.2.2.14294.37448. Retrieved from https://childrenshealthdefense.org/wp-content/uploads/5thsciencereview-masksharm-1.pdf

Reason 94: Face Masks Are So Bad For You That The Vast Majority Of Healthy People Get Headaches From Wearing Them

[1] Ong JJY, Bharatendu C, Goh Y, Tang JZY, Sooi KWX, Tan YL, Tan BYQ, Teoh HL, Ong ST, Allen DM, Sharma VK. Headaches Associated With Personal Protective Equipment — A Cross-Sectional Study Among Frontline Healthcare Workers During COVID-19. Headache. 2020 May;60(5):864-877. doi: 10.1111/head.13811. Epub 2020 Apr 12. PMID: 32232837

Reason 95: Face Mask Wearing Causes Neurological Harm And Cognitive Impairment

[1] Kisielinski K, Giboni P, Prescher A, et al. Is a Mask That Covers the Mouth and Nose Free from Undesirable Side Effects in Everyday Use and Free of Potential Hazards? International Journal of Environmental Research and Public Health. 2021;18(8):4344. doi:10.3390/ijerph18084344.

[2] Jamjoom, A.; Nikkar-Esfahani, A.; Fitzgerald, J. Operating Theatre Related Syncope in Medical Students: A Cross Sectional Study. BMC Med. Educ. 2009, 9, 14.

[3] Rosner, E. Adverse Effects of Prolonged Mask Use among Healthcare Professionals during COVID-19. J. Infect. Dis. Epidemiol. 2020.

[4] Rebmann, T.; Carrico, R.; Wang, J. Physiologic and Other Effects and Compliance with Long-Term Respirator Use among Medical Intensive Care Unit Nurses. Am. J. Infect. Control 2013, 41, 1218–1223.

[5] Kyung, S.Y.; Kim, Y.; Hwang, H.; Park, J.-W.; Jeong, S.H. Risks of N95 Face Mask Use in Subjects with COPD. Respir. Care 2020, 65, 658–664.

[6] Liu, C.; Li, G.; He, Y.; Zhang, Z.; Ding, Y. Effects of Wearing Masks on Human Health and Comfort during the COVID-19 Pandemic. IOP Conf. Ser. Earth Environ. Sci. 2020, 531, 012034.

[7] Jagim, A.R.; Dominy, T.A.; Camic, C.L.; Wright, G.; Doberstein, S.; Jones, M.T.; Oliver, J.M. Acute Effects of the Elevation Training Mask on Strength Performance in Recreational Weight Lifters. J. Strength Cond. Res. 2018, 32, 482–489.

[8] Johnson, A.T. Respirator Masks Protect Health but Impact Performance: A Review. J. Biol. Eng. 2016, 10, 4.

[9] Azuma, K.; Kagi, N.; Yanagi, U.; Osawa, H. Effects of Low-Level Inhalation Exposure to Carbon Dioxide in Indoor Environments: A Short Review on Human Health and Psychomotor Performance. Environ. Int. 2018, 121, 51–56.

[10] Drechsler, M.; Morris, J. Carbon Dioxide Narcosis. In StatPearls; StatPearls Publishing: Treasure Island, FL, USA, 2020.

[11] Noble, J.; Jones, J.G.; Davis, E.J. Cognitive Function during Moderate Hypoxaemia. Anaesth. Intensive Care 1993, 21, 180–184.

[12] Fothergill, D.M.; Hedges, D.; Morrison, J.B. Effects of CO_2 and N2 Partial Pressures on Cognitive and Psychomotor Performance. Undersea Biomed. Res. 1991, 18, 1–19.

Reason 96: Face Masks Make Headaches Worse And May Make Other Neurological Pathologies Such As Aneurysms And Tumors Worse

[1] Kisielinski K, Giboni P, Prescher A, et al. Is a Mask That Covers the Mouth and Nose Free from Undesirable Side Effects in Everyday Use and Free of Potential Hazards? International Journal of Environmental Research and Public Health. 2021;18(8):4344. doi:10.3390/ijerph18084344.

[2] Bharatendu, C.; Ong, J.J.Y.; Goh, Y.; Tan, B.Y.Q.; Chan, A.C.Y.; Tang, J.Z.Y.; Leow, A.S.; Chin, A.; Sooi, K.W.X.; Tan, Y.L.; et al. Powered Air Purifying Respirator (PAPR) Restores the N95 Face Mask Induced Cerebral Hemodynamic Alterations among Healthcare Workers during COVID-19 Outbreak. J. Neurol. Sci. 2020, 417, 117078.

[3] Ong, J.J.Y.; Bharatendu, C.; Goh, Y.; Tang, J.Z.Y.; Sooi, K.W.X.; Tan, Y.L.; Tan, B.Y.Q.; Teoh, H.-L.; Ong, S.T.; Allen, D.M.; et al. Headaches Associated With Personal Protective Equipment-A Cross-Sectional Study among Frontline Healthcare Workers During COVID-19. Headache 2020, 60, 864–877.

[4] Jacobs, J.L.; Ohde, S.; Takahashi, O.; Tokuda, Y.; Omata, F.; Fukui, T. Use of Surgical Face Masks to Reduce the Incidence of the Common Cold among Health Care Workers in Japan: A Randomized Controlled Trial. Am. J. Infect. Control 2009, 37, 417–419.

[5] Ramirez-Moreno, J.M. Mask-Associated de Novo Headache in Healthcare Workers during the Covid-19 Pandemic. medRxiv 2020.

[6] van der Kleij, L.A.; De Vis, J.B.; de Bresser, J.; Hendrikse, J.; Siero, J.C.W. Arterial CO_2 Pressure Changes during Hypercapnia Are Associated with Changes in Brain Parenchymal Volume. Eur. Radiol. Exp. 2020, 4, 17.

[7] Butz, U. Rückatmung von Kohlendioxid bei Verwendung von Operationsmasken als hygienischer Mundschutz an medizinischem Fachpersonal. Ph.D. Thesis, Fakultät für Medizin der Technischen Universität München, Munich, Germany, 2005.

[8] Roberge, R.J.; Kim, J.-H.; Benson, S.M. Absence of Consequential Changes in Physiological, Thermal and Subjective Responses from Wearing a Surgical Mask. Respir. Physiol. Neurobiol. 2012, 181, 29–35.

[9] Pifarré, F.; Zabala, D.D.; Grazioli, G.; de Yzaguirre i Maura, I. COVID 19 and Mask in Sports. Apunt. Sports Med. 2020.

[10] Rebmann, T.; Carrico, R.; Wang, J. Physiologic and Other Effects and Compliance with Long-Term Respirator Use among Medical Intensive Care Unit Nurses. Am. J. Infect. Control 2013, 41, 1218–1223.

[11] Roberge, R.J.; Kim, J.-H.; Powell, J.B. N95 Respirator Use during Advanced Pregnancy. Am. J. Infect. Control 2014, 42, 1097–1100.

[12] Kyung, S.Y.; Kim, Y.; Hwang, H.; Park, J.-W.; Jeong, S.H. Risks of N95 Face Mask Use in Subjects with COPD. Respir. Care 2020, 65, 658–664.

[13] Mo, Y.; Wei, D.; Mai, Q.; Chen, C.; Yu, H.; Jiang, C.; Tan, X. Risk and Impact of Using Mask on COPD Patients with Acute Exacerbation during the COVID-19 Outbreak: A Retrospective Study. Res. Sq. 2020.

Reason 97: What They Are Doing To Your Children Makes Them Stupider And Gives Them Learning Disabilities

[1] Deoni SC, Beauchemin J, Volpe A, D'Sa V. Impact of the COVID-19 Pandemic on Early Child Cognitive Development: Initial Findings in a Longitudinal Observational Study of Child Health. 2021. doi:10.1101/2021.08.10.21261846

Reason 98: The Powerful Impact Of Despair

[1] Woolf, S.H. Failing health of the United States. The British Medical Journal. 2018. Retrieved from https://www.bmj.com/content/360/bmj.k496

[2] Donnelly, G. Here's Why Life Expectancy in the US Dropped Again This Year. Fortune. 2018. Retrieved from https://fortune.com/2018/02/09/us-life-expectancy-dropped-again/

[3] Woolf, S.H. Fig 1 Life expectancy at birth in the US and the Organisation for Economic Cooperation and Development, 1995-2015. thebmj. 2018. https://doi.org/10.1136/bmj.k496

[4] OECD. Where: Global reach. Retrieve from: https://www.oecd.org/about/members-and-partners/

[5] Woolf S H, Aron L. Failing health of the United States BMJ 2018; 360 :k496 doi:10.1136/bmj.k496. Retrieved from https://www.bmj.com/content/360/bmj.k496

[6] Haglage, A. US life expectancy has fallen again. Here are three reasons why. Yahoo! News. 2018. Retrieved from https://sg.news.yahoo.com/u-s-life-expectancy-keeps-dropping-alcohol-blame-185004863.html?guccounter=1

[7] Steenhuysen, J. Opioid crisis trims US life expectancy, boosts hepatitis C: CDC. Reuters. 2017. Retrieved from https://www.reuters.com/article/us-usa-healthcare-cdc/opioid-crisis-trims-u-s-life-expectancy-boosts-hepatitis-c-cdc-idUSKBN1EF1TF

[8] Haglage,Abby. US life expectancy has fallen again. Here are three reasons why. Yahoo! News. 2018. Retrieved from https://sg.news.yahoo.com/u-s-life-expectancy-keeps-dropping-alcohol-blame-185004863.html?guccounter=1

[9] *Centers for Disease Control and Prevention*. Understanding the Epidemic. Retrieved from https://www.cdc.gov/opioids/basics/epidemic.html

[10] Ingraham, C. Americans are drinking themselves to death at record rates. *Washington Post*. 2015. Retrieved from https://www.washingtonpost.com/news/wonk/wp/2015/12/22/americans-are-drinking-themselves-to-death-at-record-rates/

[11] Haglage,Abby. US life expectancy has fallen again. Here are three reasons why. Yahoo! News. 2018. Retrieved from https://sg.news.yahoo.com/u-s-life-expectancy-keeps-dropping-alcohol-blame-185004863.html?guccounter=1

[12] Haglage,Abby. US life expectancy has fallen again. Here are three reasons why. Yahoo! News. 2018. Retrieved from https://sg.news.yahoo.com/u-s-life-expectancy-keeps-dropping-alcohol-blame-185004863.html?guccounter=1

[13] Woolf S H, Aron L. Failing health of the United States BMJ 2018; 360 :k496 doi:10.1136/bmj.k496. Retrieved from https://www.bmj.com/content/360/bmj.k496

Reason 99: Face Masks Are Psychologically Harmful For You

[1] Vainshelboim B. Retracted: Facemasks in the COVID-19 era: A health hypothesis [retracted in: Med Hypotheses. 2021 May 12;:110601]. Med Hypotheses. 2021;146:110411. doi:10.1016/j.mehy.2020.110411

[2] Schneiderman N., Ironson G., Siegel S.D. Stress and health: psychological, behavioral, and biological determinants. Annu Rev Clin Psychol. 2005;1:607–628.

[3] Thoits P.A. Stress and health: major findings and policy implications. J Health Soc Behav. 2010;51(Suppl):S41–S53.

[4] Haslam N. Dehumanization: an integrative review. Pers Soc Psychol Rev. 2006;10:252–264.

[5] Cohen S. Social relationships and health. Am Psychol. 2004;59:676–684.

[6] Leigh-Hunt N., Bagguley D., Bash K., Turner V., Turnbull S., Valtorta N. An overview of systematic reviews on the public health consequences of social isolation and loneliness. Public Health. 2017;152:157–171.

[7] Holt-Lunstad J., Smith T.B., Layton J.B. Social relationships and mortality risk: a meta-analytic review. PLoS Med. 2010;7

[8] Shor E., Roelfs D.J. Social contact frequency and all-cause mortality: a meta-analysis and meta-regression. Soc Sci Med. 2015;128:76–86.

[9] American College of Sports Medicine . Sixth ed. Lippincott Wiliams & Wilkins; Baltimore: 2010. ACSM's Resource Manual for Guidelines for Exercise Testing and Prescription.

[10] Farrell P.A., Joyner M.J., Caiozzo V.J. second edition. Lippncott Williams & Wilkins; Baltimore: 2012. ACSM's Advanced Exercise Physiology.

[11] Kenney W.L., Wilmore J.H., Costill D.L. 5th ed. Human Kinetics; Champaign, IL: 2012. Physiology of sport and exercise.

[12] McEwen B.S. Protective and damaging effects of stress mediators. N Engl J Med. 1998;338:171–179.

[13] McEwen B.S. Physiology and neurobiology of stress and adaptation: central role of the brain. Physiol Rev. 2007;87:873–904.

[14] Everly G.S., Lating J.M. 4th ed. NY Springer Nature; New York: 2019. A Clinical Guide to the Treatment of the Human Stress Response.

Reason 100: Face Mask Wearing Is Linked To Substantial Psychological Side Effects

[1] Kisielinski K, Giboni P, Prescher A, et al. Is a Mask That Covers the Mouth and Nose Free from Undesirable Side Effects in Everyday Use and Free of Potential Hazards? International Journal of Environmental Research and Public Health. 2021;18(8):4344. doi:10.3390/ijerph18084344.

[2] Johnson, A.T. Respirator Masks Protect Health but Impact Performance: A Review. J. Biol. Eng. 2016, 10, 4.

[3] Rains, S.A. The Nature of Psychological Reactance Revisited: A Meta-Analytic Review. Hum. Commun. Res. 2013, 39, 47–73.

[4] Matusiak, Ł.; Szepietowska, M.; Krajewski, P.; Białynicki-Birula, R.; Szepietowski, J.C. Inconveniences Due to the Use of Face Masks during the COVID-19 Pandemic: A Survey Study of 876 Young People. Dermatol. Ther. 2020, 33, e13567.

[5] Rosner, E. Adverse Effects of Prolonged Mask Use among Healthcare Professionals during COVID-19. J. Infect. Dis. Epidemiol. 2020.

[6] Drechsler, M.; Morris, J. Carbon Dioxide Narcosis. In StatPearls; StatPearls Publishing: Treasure Island, FL, USA, 2020.

[7] Noble, J.; Jones, J.G.; Davis, E.J. Cognitive Function during Moderate Hypoxaemia. Anaesth. Intensive Care 1993, 21, 180–184.

[8] Fothergill, D.M.; Hedges, D.; Morrison, J.B. Effects of CO_2 and N2 Partial Pressures on Cognitive and Psychomotor Performance. Undersea Biomed. Res. 1991, 18, 1–19.

[9] Rebmann, T.; Carrico, R.; Wang, J. Physiologic and Other Effects and Compliance with Long-Term Respirator Use among Medical Intensive Care Unit Nurses. Am. J. Infect. Control 2013, 41, 1218–1223.

[10] Liu, C.; Li, G.; He, Y.; Zhang, Z.; Ding, Y. Effects of Wearing Masks on Human Health and Comfort during the COVID-19 Pandemic. IOP Conf. Ser. Earth Environ. Sci. 2020, 531, 012034.

[11] Li, Y.; Tokura, H.; Guo, Y.P.; Wong, A.S.W.; Wong, T.; Chung, J.; Newton, E. Effects of Wearing N95 and Surgical Facemasks on Heart Rate, Thermal Stress and Subjective Sensations. Int. Arch. Occup. Environ. Health 2005, 78, 501–509.

[12] Foo, C.C.I.; Goon, A.T.J.; Leow, Y.; Goh, C. Adverse Skin Reactions to Personal Protective Equipment against Severe Acute Respiratory Syndrome–a Descriptive Study in Singapore. Contact Dermat. 2006, 55, 291–294.

[13] Hua, W.; Zuo, Y.; Wan, R.; Xiong, L.; Tang, J.; Zou, L.; Shu, X.; Li, L. Short-Term Skin Reactions Following Use of N95 Respirators and Medical Masks. Contact Dermat. 2020, 83, 115–121.

[14] Prousa, D. Studie zu psychischen und psychovegetativen Beschwerden mit den aktuellen Mund-Nasenschutz-Verordnungen. PsychArchives 2020.

[15] Sell, T.K.; Hosangadi, D.; Trotochaud, M. Misinformation and the US Ebola Communication Crisis: Analyzing the Veracity and Content of Social Media Messages Related to a Fear-Inducing Infectious Disease Outbreak. BMC Public Health 2020, 20, 550.

[16] Ryan, R.M.; Deci, E.L. Self-determination theory and the role of basic psychological needs in personality and the organization of behavior. In Handbook of Personality: Theory and Research, 3rd ed.; The Guilford Press: New York, NY, USA, 2008; pp. 654–678. ISBN 978-1-59385-836-0.

[17] World Health Organization. WHO-Advice on the Use of Masks in the Context of COVID-19: Interim Guidance, 5 June 2020; World Health Organization: Geneva, Switzerland, 2020; Available online: https://apps.who.int/iris/handle/10665/332293 (accessed on 7 November 2020).

Reason 101: Face Mask Wearing Leads To Panic Attacks And Exacerbates Significant Other Psychiatric Conditions

1 Kisielinski K, Giboni P, Prescher A, et al. Is a Mask That Covers the Mouth and Nose Free from Undesirable Side Effects in Everyday Use and Free of Potential Hazards? International Journal of Environmental Research and Public Health. 2021;18(8):4344. doi:10.3390/ijerph18084344.

2 Matuschek, C.; Moll, F.; Fangerau, H.; Fischer, J.C.; Zänker, K.; van Griensven, M.; Schneider, M.; Kindgen-Milles, D.; Knoefel, W.T.; Lichtenberg, A.; et al. Face Masks: Benefits and Risks during the COVID-19 Crisis. Eur. J. Med. Res. 2020, 25, 32.

3 Roberge, R.J.; Coca, A.; Williams, W.J.; Powell, J.B.; Palmiero, A.J. Physiological Impact of the N95 Filtering Facepiece Respirator on Healthcare Workers. Respir. Care 2010, 55, 569–577.

4 Pifarré, F.; Zabala, D.D.; Grazioli, G.; de Yzaguirre i Maura, I. COVID 19 and Mask in Sports. Apunt. Sports Med. 2020.

5 Roeckner, J.T.; Krsti´c, N.; Sipe, B.H.; Obi˜can, S.G. N95 Filtering Facepiece Respirator Use during Pregnancy: A Systematic Review. Am. J. Perinatol. 2020, 37, 995–1001.

6 Butz, U. Rückatmung von Kohlendioxid bei Verwendung von Operationsmasken als hygienischer Mundschutz an medizinischem Fachpersonal. Ph.D. Thesis, Fakultät für Medizin der Technischen Universität München, Munich, Germany, 2005.

7 Roberge, R.J.; Kim, J.-H.; Benson, S.M. Absence of Consequential Changes in Physiological, Thermal and Subjective Responses from Wearing a Surgical Mask. Respir. Physiol. Neurobiol. 2012, 181, 29–35.

8 Roberge, R.J.; Coca, A.; Williams, W.J.; Powell, J.B.; Palmiero, A.J. Physiological Impact of the N95 Filtering Facepiece Respirator on Healthcare Workers. Respir. Care 2010, 55, 569–577.

9 Rebmann, T.; Carrico, R.; Wang, J. Physiologic and Other Effects and Compliance with Long-Term Respirator Use among Medical Intensive Care Unit Nurses. Am. J. Infect. Control 2013, 41, 1218–1223.

[10] Roeckner, J.T.; Krsti´c, N.; Sipe, B.H.; Obi˜can, S.G. N95 Filtering Facepiece Respirator Use during Pregnancy: A Systematic Review. Am. J. Perinatol. 2020, 37, 995–1001.

[11] Georgi, C.; Haase-Fielitz, A.; Meretz, D.; Gäsert, L.; Butter, C. Einfluss gängiger Gesichtsmasken auf physiologische Parameter und Belastungsempfinden unter arbeitstypischer körperlicher Anstrengung. Deutsches Ärzteblatt 2020, 674–675.

[12] Roberge, R.J.; Kim, J.-H.; Powell, J.B. N95 Respirator Use during Advanced Pregnancy. Am. J. Infect. Control 2014, 42, 1097–1100.

[13] Kyung, S.Y.; Kim, Y.; Hwang, H.; Park, J.-W.; Jeong, S.H. Risks of N95 Face Mask Use in Subjects with COPD. Respir. Care 2020, 65, 658–664.

[14] Epstein, D.; Korytny, A.; Isenberg, Y.; Marcusohn, E.; Zukermann, R.; Bishop, B.; Minha, S.; Raz, A.; Miller, A. Return to Training in the COVID-19 Era: The Physiological Effects of Face Masks during Exercise. Scand. J. Med. Sci. Sports 2020.

[15] Mo, Y.; Wei, D.; Mai, Q.; Chen, C.; Yu, H.; Jiang, C.; Tan, X. Risk and Impact of Using Mask on COPD Patients with Acute Exacerbation during the COVID-19 Outbreak: A Retrospective Study. Res. Sq. 2020.

[16] Goh, D.Y.T.; Mun, M.W.; Lee, W.L.J.; Teoh, O.H.; Rajgor, D.D. A Randomised Clinical Trial to Evaluate the Safety, Fit, Comfort of a Novel N95 Mask in Children. Sci. Rep. 2019, 9, 18952.

[17] Bharatendu, C.; Ong, J.J.Y.; Goh, Y.; Tan, B.Y.Q.; Chan, A.C.Y.; Tang, J.Z.Y.; Leow, A.S.; Chin, A.; Sooi, K.W.X.; Tan, Y.L.; et al. Powered Air Purifying Respirator (PAPR) Restores the N95 Face Mask Induced Cerebral Hemodynamic Alterations among Healthcare Workers during COVID-19 Outbreak. J. Neurol. Sci. 2020, 417, 117078.

[18] Tong, P.S.Y.; Kale, A.S.; Ng, K.; Loke, A.P.; Choolani, M.A.; Lim, C.L.; Chan, Y.H.; Chong, Y.S.; Tambyah, P.A.; Yong, E.-L. Respiratory Consequences of N95-Type Mask Usage in Pregnant Healthcare Workers — A Controlled Clinical Study. Antimicrob. Resist. Infect. Control 2015, 4, 48.

[19] Kent, J.M.; Papp, L.A.; Martinez, J.M.; Browne, S.T.; Coplan, J.D.; Klein, D.F.; Gorman, J.M. Specificity of Panic Response to CO(2) Inhalation in Panic Disorder: A Comparison with Major Depression and Premenstrual Dysphoric Disorder. Am. J. Psychiatry 2001, 158, 58–67.

[20]. Morris, L.S.; McCall, J.G.; Charney, D.S.; Murrough, J.W. The Role of the Locus Coeruleus in the Generation of Pathological Anxiety. Brain Neurosci. Adv. 2020, 4.

[21] Gorman, J.M.; Askanazi, J.; Liebowitz, M.R.; Fyer, A.J.; Stein, J.; Kinney, J.M.; Klein, D.F. Response to Hyperventilation in a Group of Patients with Panic Disorder. Am. J. Psychiatry 1984, 141, 857–861.

[22] Roberge, R.J.; Kim, J.-H.; Coca, A. Protective Facemask Impact on Human Thermoregulation: An Overview. Ann. Occup. Hyg. 2012, 56, 102–112.

[23] Tsugawa, A.; Sakurai, S.; Inagawa, Y.; Hirose, D.; Kaneko, Y.; Ogawa, Y.; Serisawa, S.; Takenoshita, N.; Sakurai, H.; Kanetaka, H.; et al. Awareness of the COVID-19 Outbreak and Resultant Depressive Tendencies in Patients with Severe Alzheimer's Disease. JAD 2020, 77, 539–541.

[24] Maguire, P.A.; Reay, R.E.; Looi, J.C. Nothing to Sneeze at-Uptake of Protective Measures against an Influenza Pandemic by People with Schizophrenia: Willingness and Perceived Barriers. Australas. Psychiatry 2019, 27, 171–178.

[25] Jagim, A.R.; Dominy, T.A.; Camic, C.L.; Wright, G.; Doberstein, S.; Jones, M.T.; Oliver, J.M. Acute Effects of the Elevation Training Mask on Strength Performance in Recreational Weight Lifters. J. Strength Cond. Res. 2018, 32, 482–489.

[26] Johnson, A.T. Respirator Masks Protect Health but Impact Performance: A Review. J. Biol. Eng. 2016, 10, 4.

[27] Azuma, K.; Kagi, N.; Yanagi, U.; Osawa, H. Effects of Low-Level Inhalation Exposure to Carbon Dioxide in Indoor Environments: A Short Review on Human Health and Psychomotor Performance. Environ. Int. 2018, 121, 51–56.

[28] Drechsler, M.; Morris, J. Carbon Dioxide Narcosis. In StatPearls; StatPearls Publishing: Treasure Island, FL, USA, 2020.

[29] Noble, J.; Jones, J.G.; Davis, E.J. Cognitive Function during Moderate Hypoxaemia. Anaesth. Intensive Care 1993, 21, 180–184.

[30] Fothergill, D.M.; Hedges, D.; Morrison, J.B. Effects of CO_2 and N2 Partial Pressures on Cognitive and Psychomotor Performance. Undersea Biomed. Res. 1991, 18, 1–19.

[31] COVID-19: Considerations for Wearing Masks|CDC. Available online: https://www.cdc.gov/coronavirus/2019-ncov/preventgetting-sick/cloth-face-cover-guidance.html (accessed on 12 November 2020).

[32] Lim, E.C.H.; Seet, R.C.S.; Lee, K.-H.; Wilder-Smith, E.P.V.; Chuah, B.Y.S.; Ong, B.K.C. Headaches and the N95 Face-mask amongst Healthcare Providers. Acta Neurol. Scand. 2006, 113, 199–202.

Reason 102: Face Masks Have Unstudied Psychological Harm To Children

[1] Rancourt, D.G. Review of scientific reports of harms caused by face masks, up to February 2021. 2021. Retrieved from https://assets.website-files.com/606d3a50c62e44338008303d/6076def5c5421e642472f1ef_5thscicreview-mask sharm-1.pdf

[2] Scheid JL, Lupien SP, Ford GS, West SL. "Commentary: Physiological and Psychological Impact of Face Mask Usage during the COVID-19 Pandemic". Int J Environ Res Public Health. 2020 Sep 12;17(18):6655. doi: 10.3390/ijerph17186655. PMID: 32932652; PMCID: PMC7558090. — https://pubmed.ncbi.nlm.nih.gov/32932652/

Reason 103: CDC And WHO Advise Against Wearing Face Masks During Exercise

[1] Kisielinski K, Giboni P, Prescher A, et al. Is a Mask That Covers the Mouth and Nose Free from Undesirable Side Effects in Everyday Use and Free of Potential Hazards? International Journal of Environmental Research and Public Health. 2021;18(8):4344. doi:10.3390/ijerph18084344.

[2] COVID-19: Considerations for Wearing Masks|CDC. Available online: https://www.cdc.gov/coronavirus/2019-ncov/preventgetting-sick/cloth-face-cover-guidance.html (accessed on 12 November 2020)

[3] COVID-19 Mythbusters–World Health Organization. Available online: https://www.who.int/emergencies/diseases/novelcoronavirus-2019/advice-for-public/myth-busters (accessed on 28 January 2021)

[4] Centers for Disease Control and Prevention. Guidance for Wearing Masks. Retrieved from https://www.cdc.gov/coronavirus/2019-ncov/prevent-getting-sick/cloth-face-cover-guidance.html

Reason 104: Face Masks Are Dangerous When Worn During Exercise

1 Kisielinski K, Giboni P, Prescher A, et al. Is a Mask That Covers the Mouth and Nose Free from Undesirable Side Effects in Everyday Use and Free of Potential Hazards? International Journal of Environmental Research and Public Health. 2021;18(8):4344. doi:10.3390/ijerph18084344.

[2] Pifarré, F.; Zabala, D.D.; Grazioli, G.; de Yzaguirre i Maura, I. COVID 19 and Mask in Sports. Apunt. Sports Med. 2020.

Reason 105: Exercising In A Face Mask Will Hurt You

[1] Chandrasekaran B, Fernandes S. "Exercise with facemask; Are we handling a devil's sword?" — A physiological hypothesis. Med Hypotheses. 2020;144:110002. doi:10.1016/j.mehy.2020.110002

Reason 106: Exercising With A Face Mask May Increase Infection Rates

[1] Chandrasekaran B, Fernandes S. "Exercise with facemask; Are we handling a devil's sword?" — A physiological hypothesis. Med Hypotheses. 2020;144:110002. doi:10.1016/j.mehy.2020.110002

[2] Kempeneers C., Seaton C., Garcia Espinosa B., Chilvers M.A. Ciliary functional analysis: beating a path towards standardization. Pediatr Pulmonol. 2019;54(10):1627–1638.

Reason 107: Even Activity As Simple As Walking Is Made Measurably Harder By A Face Mask, Even Among Healthy People

[1] Kisielinski K, Giboni P, Prescher A, et al. Is a Mask That Covers the Mouth and Nose Free from Undesirable Side Effects in Everyday Use and Free of Potential Hazards? International Journal of Environmental Research and Public Health. 2021;18(8):4344. doi:10.3390/ijerph18084344.

[2] Roberge, R.J.; Kim, J.-H.; Benson, S.M. Absence of Consequential Changes in Physiological, Thermal and Subjective Responses from Wearing a Surgical Mask. Respir. Physiol. Neurobiol. 2012, 181, 29–35.

[3] Fikenzer, S.; Uhe, T.; Lavall, D.; Rudolph, U.; Falz, R.; Busse, M.; Hepp, P.; Laufs, U. Effects of Surgical and FFP2/N95 Face Masks on Cardiopulmonary Exercise Capacity. Clin. Res. Cardiol. 2020, 109, 1522–1530.

Reason 108: Exercising In A Face Mask Harms The Sick

[1] Chandrasekaran B, Fernandes S. "Exercise with facemask; Are we handling a devil's sword?" — A physiological hypothesis. Med Hypotheses. 2020;144:110002. doi:10.1016/j.mehy.2020.110002

[2] Melnikov V.N., Divert V.E., Komlyagina T.G., Consedine N.S. Krivoschekov SG. Baseline values of cardiovascular and respiratory parameters predict response to acute hypoxia in young healthy men. Physiol Res. 2017;66(3):467–479.

Reason 109: N95 Wearing Hurts The Sick

[1] Singleton MM. Mask Facts. Association of American Physicians and Surgeons. 2021. Retrieved from https://aaps online.org/mask-facts/

[2] Kao TW, Huang KC, Huang YL, Tsai TJ, Hsieh BS, Wu MS. The physiological impact of wearing an N95 mask during hemodialysis as a precaution against SARS in patients with end-stage renal disease. J Formos Med Assoc. 2004 Aug;103(8):624-8. PMID: 15340662.)

[3] Kao, Tze-Wah & Huang, Kuo-Chiang & Huang, Yu-Ling & Tsai, Tun-Jun & Hsieh, Bor-Shen & Wu, Ming Shiou. (2004). The physiological impact of wearing an N95 mask during hemodialysis as a precaution against SARS in patients with end-stage renal disease. Journal of the Formosan Medical Association = Taiwan yi zhi. 103. 624-8.

[4] Myers, A. COVID-19 prompts a team of engineers to rethink the humble face mask. Stanford University. 2020. Retrieved from https://engineering.stanford.edu/magazine/article/covid-19-prompts-team-engineers-rethink-humble-face-mask

Reason 110: Simple Activity Is Made Measurably Harder By Mask Wearing In Unwell People

[1] Kisielinski K, Giboni P, Prescher A, et al. Is a Mask That Covers the Mouth and Nose Free from Undesirable Side Effects in Everyday Use and Free of Potential Hazards? International Journal of Environmental Research and Public Health. 2021;18(8):4344. doi:10.3390/ijerph18084344.

[2] Rebmann, T.; Carrico, R.; Wang, J. Physiologic and Other Effects and Compliance with Long-Term Respirator Use among Medical Intensive Care Unit Nurses. Am. J. Infect. Control 2013, 41, 1218–1223.

[3] Kyung, S.Y.; Kim, Y.; Hwang, H.; Park, J.-W.; Jeong, S.H. Risks of N95 Face Mask Use in Subjects with COPD. Respir. Care 2020, 65, 658–664.

[4] Mo, Y.; Wei, D.; Mai, Q.; Chen, C.; Yu, H.; Jiang, C.; Tan, X. Risk and Impact of Using Mask on COPD Patients with Acute Exacerbation during the COVID-19 Outbreak: A Retrospective Study. Res. Sq. 2020.

[5] Kao, T.-W.; Huang, K.-C.; Huang, Y.-L.; Tsai, T.-J.; Hsieh, B.-S.; Wu, M.-S. The Physiological Impact of Wearing an N95 Mask during Hemodialysis as a Precaution against SARS in Patients with End-Stage Renal Disease. J. Formos. Med. Assoc. 2004, 103, 624–628

[6] Matuschek, C.; Moll, F.; Fangerau, H.; Fischer, J.C.; Zänker, K.; van Griensven, M.; Schneider, M.; Kindgen-Milles, D.; Knoefel, W.T.; Lichtenberg, A.; et al. Face Masks: Benefits and Risks during the COVID-19 Crisis. Eur. J. Med. Res. 2020, 25, 32.

Reason 111: The Overweight, Those With COPD, Lung Disease, Cardiac Disease, Pregnant Women, And Stroke Patients Must Be Particularly Cautious Around Face Masks

[1] Kisielinski K, Giboni P, Prescher A, et al. Is a Mask That Covers the Mouth and Nose Free from Undesirable Side Effects in Everyday Use and Free of Potential Hazards? International Journal of Environmental Research and Public Health. 2021;18(8):4344. doi:10.3390/ijerph18084344.

[2] Kyung, S.Y.; Kim, Y.; Hwang, H.; Park, J.-W.; Jeong, S.H. Risks of N95 Face Mask Use in Subjects with COPD. Respir. Care 2020, 65, 658–664.

[3] Rebmann, T.; Carrico, R.; Wang, J. Physiologic and Other Effects and Compliance with Long-Term Respirator Use among Medical Intensive Care Unit Nurses. Am. J. Infect. Control 2013, 41, 1218–1223.

[4] Kao, T.-W.; Huang, K.-C.; Huang, Y.-L.; Tsai, T.-J.; Hsieh, B.-S.; Wu, M.-S. The Physiological Impact of Wearing an N95 Mask during Hemodialysis as a Precaution against SARS in Patients with End-Stage Renal Disease. J. Formos. Med. Assoc. 2004, 103, 624–628.

[5] AAFA Community Services. What People with Asthma Need to Know about Face Masks and Coverings during the COVID-19 Pandemic. Available online: https://community.aafa.org/blog/what-people-with-asthma-need-to-know-about-face-masksand-coverings-during-the-covid-19-pandemic (accessed on 29 January 2021).

[6] Kaw, R.; Hernandez, A.V.; Walker, E.; Aboussouan, L.; Mokhlesi, B. Determinants of Hypercapnia in Obese Patients with Obstructive Sleep Apnea: A Systematic Review and Metaanalysis of Cohort Studies. Chest 2009, 136, 787–796.

[7] Shigemura, M.; Lecuona, E.; Angulo, M.; Homma, T.; Rodríguez, D.A.; Gonzalez-Gonzalez, F.J.; Welch, L.C.; Amarelle, L.; Kim, S.-J.; Kaminski, N.; et al. Hypercapnia Increases Airway Smooth Muscle Contractility via Caspase-7-Mediated MiR-133a-RhoA Signaling. Sci. Transl. Med. 2018, 10, eaat1662.

Reason 112: Japanese Government Warns Face Masks May Cause Heatstroke

[1] The Mainichi. Japan gov't asks people to take off masks outdoors to avoid heatstroke, keep 2m apart. 2020. Retrieved from https://mainichi.jp/english/articles/20200527/p2a/00m/0na/014000c

[2] The Mainichi. Wearing masks in summer can lead to heatstroke; Japan doctors urge self-hydration. 2020. Retrieved from https://mainichi.jp/english/articles/20200519/p2a/00m/0na/016000c

Reason 113: Face Mask Fatalities In Kids

[1] Coleman, V. Dr. Proof That Face Masks Do More Harm Than Good. Freedom of Speech. 2021. Retrieved from https://fos-sa.org/2021/01/06/proof-that-face-masks-do-more-harm-than-good/

Reason 115: Face Mask Wearing Has The Opposite Effect Of The Health-Promoting Deep Breathing Encouraged In Prayer, Meditation, And Holistic Healing

[1] Kisielinski K, Giboni P, Prescher A, et al. Is a Mask That Covers the Mouth and Nose Free from Undesirable Side Effects in Everyday Use and Free of Potential Hazards? International Journal of Environmental Research and Public Health. 2021;18(8):4344. doi:10.3390/ijerph18084344.

[2] Russo, M.A.; Santarelli, D.M.; O'Rourke, D. The Physiological Effects of Slow Breathing in the Healthy Human. Breathe 2017, 13, 298–309.

[3] Nuckowska, M.K.; Gruszecki, M.; Kot, J.; Wolf, J.; Guminski, W.; Frydrychowski, A.F.; Wtorek, J.; Narkiewicz, K.; Winklewski, P.J. Impact of Slow Breathing on the Blood Pressure and Subarachnoid Space Width Oscillations in Humans. Sci. Rep. 2019, 9, 6232.

[4] Melnychuk, M.C.; Dockree, P.M.; O'Connell, R.G.; Murphy, P.R.; Balsters, J.H.; Robertson, I.H. Coupling of Respiration and Attention via the Locus Coeruleus: Effects of Meditation and Pranayama. Psychophysiology 2018, 55, e13091.

[5] Yackle, K.; Schwarz, L.A.; Kam, K.; Sorokin, J.M.; Huguenard, J.R.; Feldman, J.L.; Luo, L.; Krasnow, M.A. Breathing Control Center Neurons That Promote Arousal in Mice. Science 2017, 355, 1411–1415.

[6] Menuet, C.; Connelly, A.A.; Bassi, J.K.; Melo, M.R.; Le, S.; Kamar, J.; Kumar, N.N.; McDougall, S.J.; McMullan, S.; Allen, A.M. PreBötzinger Complex Neurons Drive Respiratory Modulation of Blood Pressure and Heart Rate. eLife 2020, 9, e57288.

[7] Zope, S.A.; Zope, R.A. Sudarshan Kriya Yoga: Breathing for Health. Int. J. Yoga 2013, 6, 4–10.

Reason 116: Surgical Face Masks Were Made For Surgery And Might Not Even Work For That

[1] Vincent M, Edwards P. Disposable surgical face masks for preventing surgical wound infection in clean surgery. Cochrane Database Syst Rev. 2016;4(4):CD002929. Published 2016 Apr 26. doi:10.1002/14651858.CD002929.pub3.

Reason 118: Surgeons, Doctors, And Other Medical Staff In Face Masks May Be More Likely To Harm Patients

[1] Sipherd, R. The third-leading cause of death in US most doctors don't want you to know about. CNBC, 2018. Retrieved from https://www.cnbc.com/2018/02/22/medical-errors-third-leading-cause-of-death-in-america.html. John Hopkins Medicine. Study Suggests Medical Errors Now Third Leading Cause of Death in the US 2016. Retrieved from https://www.hopkinsmedicine.org/news/media/releases/study_suggests_medical_errors_now_third_leading_cause_of_death _in_the_us

[2] Frountzas : M. Frountzas, C. Nikolaou, D. Schizas et al., "Personal protective equipment against COVID-19: Vital for surgeons, harmful for patients?", The American Journal of Surgery. 13 August 2020. https://doi.org/10.1016/j.amjsurg.2020.09.014

Reason 119: The Nebulizer Effect

[1] Miller-Keane Encyclopedia and Dictionary of Medicine, Nursing, and Allied Health, Seventh Edition. S.v. "nebulizer." Retrieved November 4 2021 from https://medical-dictionary.thefreedictionary.com/nebulizer

[2] Kisielinski K, Giboni P, Prescher A, et al. Is a Mask That Covers the Mouth and Nose Free from Undesirable Side Effects in Everyday Use and Free of Potential Hazards? International Journal of Environmental Research and Public Health. 2021;18(8):4344. doi:10.3390/ijerph18084344.

[3] Kappstein, I. Mund-Nasen-Schutz in der Öffentlichkeit: Keine Hinweise für eine Wirksamkeit. Krankenh. Up2date 2020, 15, 279–295.

[4] Asadi, S.; Cappa, C.D.; Barreda, S.; Wexler, A.S.; Bouvier, N.M.; Ristenpart, W.D. Efficacy of Masks and Face Coverings in Controlling Outward Aerosol Particle Emission from Expiratory Activities. Sci. Rep. 2020, 10, 15665.

Reason 120: Face Masks Impair Cognition Among Healthcare Workers

[1] Rancourt, D.G. Review of scientific reports of harms caused by face masks, up to February 2021. 2021. Retrieved from https://assets.website-files.com/606d3a50c62e44338008303d/6076def5c5421e642472f1ef_5thsciencereview-mask sharm-1.pdf

[2] 2020--Rosner : Elisheva Rosner E (2020) "Adverse Effects of Prolonged Mask Use among Healthcare Professionals during COVID-19". Journal of Infectious Disease and Epidemiology 6:130. doi.org/10.23937/2474-3658/1510130 — https://clinmedjournals.org/articles/jide/journal-of-infectious-diseases-and-epidemiology-jide-6-130.php

Reason 121: Face Masks On Medical Workers Hurt Kids

[1] Rancourt, D.G. Review of scientific reports of harms caused by face masks, up to February 2021. Children's Health Defence. 2021. DOI: 10.13140/RG.2.2.14294.37448. Retrieved from https://childrenshealthdefense.org/wp-content/uploads/5thsciencereview-masksharm-1.pdf

[2] Ong JJY, Bharatendu C, Goh Y, et al. Headaches Associated With Personal Protective Equipment — A Cross-Sectional Study Among Frontline Healthcare Workers During COVID-19. Headache. 2020;60(5):864-877. doi:10.1111/head.13811

Reason 122: Face Masks Do Not Bring About Greater "Health" As Defined By The World Health Organization

[1] Kisielinski K, Giboni P, Prescher A, et al. Is a Mask That Covers the Mouth and Nose Free from Undesirable Side Effects in Everyday Use and Free of Potential Hazards? International Journal of Environmental Research and Public Health. 2021;18(8):4344. doi:10.3390/ijerph18084344.

[2] International Health Conference. WHO-Constitution of the World Health Organization. 1946. Bull. World Health Organ. 2002, 80, 983–984.

Reason 123: Reminder: The World Health Organization Even Says Face Masks May Be Dangerous To Your Child

[1] World Health Organization. (2020). Advice on the use of masks in the context of COVID-19: interim guidance, 6 April 2020. World Health Organization. https://apps.who.int/iris/handle/10665/331693. License: CC BY-NC-SA 3.0 IGO

Reason 124: No One Even Uses A Face Mask Correctly

[1] Singleton MM. Mask Facts. Association of American Physicians and Surgeons. 2021. Retrieved from https://aaps online.org/mask-facts/

[2] Walker, M. Study Casts Doubt on N95 Masks for the Public. Medpage Today. 2020. Retrieved from https://www.med pagetoday.com/infectiousdisease/publichealth/86601

Reason 125: Experiments Are Often Done In "Ideal" Settings And Therefore Carry A Bias

[1] Morris LA. Dead Space and Inhaled Carbon Dioxide Levels in Respiratory Protective Equipment. HSE Health & Safety Executive. 1991. Retrieved from https://www.hse.gov.uk/research/crr_pdf/1991/crr91027.

[2] ROTH, 1968. Compendium of human responses to the aerospace environment. Vol.III, Sections 10-16. Albuquerque (NM): Lovelace Foundation for Medical Education and Research. (NASA Contractor Report No. CR-1285 (III)).

[3] JAMES, 1976. Breathing resistance and dead space in respiratory protective devices. Physiological effects of breathing resistance and equipment dead space in respiratory protective devices: status of the problem. Cincinnati (OH): US Department of Health, Education and Welfare. (HEW Publication (NIOSH) 77-161)

Reason 126: Face Masks Are Visibly Misused

[1] Kisielinski K, Giboni P, Prescher A, et al. Is a Mask That Covers the Mouth and Nose Free from Undesirable Side Effects in Everyday Use and Free of Potential Hazards? International Journal of Environmental Research and Public Health. 2021;18(8):4344. doi:10.3390/ijerph18084344.

[2] Belkin, N. The Evolution of the Surgical Mask: Filtering Efficiency versus Effectiveness. Infect. Control Hosp. Epidemiol. 1997, 18, 49–57. [CrossRef]

[3] Matuschek, C.; Moll, F.; Fangerau, H.; Fischer, J.C.; Zänker, K.; van Griensven, M.; Schneider, M.; Kindgen-Milles, D.; Knoefel, W.T.; Lichtenberg, A.; et al. The History and Value of Face Masks. Eur. J. Med. Res. 2020, 25, 23.

[4] Spooner, J.L. History of Surgical Face Masks. AORN J. 1967, 5, 76–80.

[5] Burgess, A.; Horii, M. Risk, Ritual and Health Responsibilisation: Japan's "safety Blanket" of Surgical Face Mask-Wearing. Sociol. Health Illn. 2012, 34, 1184–1198. [CrossRef] [PubMed]

[6] Beck, U. Risk Society, towards a New Modernity; SAGE Publications Ltd: Thousand Oaks, CA, USA, 1992.

[7] Neilson, S. The Surgical Mask Is a Bad Fit for Risk Reduction. CMAJ 2016, 188, 606–607.

[8] Cheng, K.K.; Lam, T.H.; Leung, C.C. Wearing Face Masks in the Community during the COVID-19 Pandemic: Altruism and Solidarity. Lancet 2020.

[9] World Health Organization. WHO-Advice on the Use of Masks in the Context of COVID-19: Interim Guidance, 5 June 2020; World Health Organization: Geneva, Switzerland, 2020; Available online: https://apps.who.int/iris/handle/10665/332293 (accessed on 7 November 2020).

[10] Fisher, K.A.; Tenforde, M.W.; Feldstein, L.R.; Lindsell, C.J.; Shapiro, N.I.; Files, D.C.; Gibbs, K.W.; Erickson, H.L.; Prekker, M.E.; Steingrub, J.S.; et al. Community and Close Contact Exposures Associated with COVID-19 among Symptomatic Adults ≥18 Years in 11 Outpatient Health Care Facilities-United States, July 2020. MMWR Morb. Mortal. Wkly. Rep. 2020, 69, 1258–1264.

[11] Bundgaard, H.; Bundgaard, J.S.; Raaschou-Pedersen, D.E.T.; von Buchwald, C.; Todsen, T.; Norsk, J.B.; Pries-Heje, M.M.; Vissing, C.R.; Nielsen, P.B.; Winsløw, U.C.; et al. Effectiveness of Adding a Mask Recommendation to Other Public Health Measures to Prevent Sars-Cov-2 Infection in Danish Mask Wearers. Ann. Intern. Med. 2020

Reason 127: Mandating Face Mask Wearing Is Unethical

[1] Kisielinski K, Giboni P, Prescher A, et al. Is a Mask That Covers the Mouth and Nose Free from Undesirable Side Effects in Everyday Use and Free of Potential Hazards? International Journal of Environmental Research and Public Health. 2021;18(8):4344. doi:10.3390/ijerph18084344.

[2] World Health Organization. WHO-Advice on the Use of Masks in the Context of COVID-19: Interim Guidance, 5 June 2020; World Health Organization: Geneva, Switzerland, 2020; Available online: https://apps.who.int/iris/handle/10665/332293 (accessed on 7 November 2020)

[3] Jefferson, T.; Jones, M.; Ansari, L.A.A.; Bawazeer, G.; Beller, E.; Clark, J.; Conly, J.; Mar, C.D.; Dooley, E.; Ferroni, E.; et al. Physical Interventions to Interrupt or Reduce the Spread of Respiratory Viruses. Part 1-Face Masks, Eye Protection and Person Distancing: Systematic Review and Meta-Analysis. medRxiv 2020.

[4] Kappstein, I. Mund-Nasen-Schutz in der Öffentlichkeit: Keine Hinweise für eine Wirksamkeit. Krankenh. Up2date 2020, 15, 279–295.

[5] Matuschek, C.; Moll, F.; Fangerau, H.; Fischer, J.C.; Zänker, K.; van Griensven, M.; Schneider, M.; Kindgen-Milles, D.; Knoefel, W.T.; Lichtenberg, A.; et al. Face Masks: Benefits and Risks during the COVID-19 Crisis. Eur. J. Med. Res. 2020, 25, 32.

[6] Xiao, J.; Shiu, E.Y.C.; Gao, H.; Wong, J.Y.; Fong, M.W.; Ryu, S.; Cowling, B.J. Nonpharmaceutical Measures for Pandemic Influenza in Nonhealthcare Settings — Personal Protective and Environmental Measures. Emerg. Infect. Dis. 2020, 26, 967–975.

[7] Bundgaard, H.; Bundgaard, J.S.; Raaschou-Pedersen, D.E.T.; von Buchwald, C.; Todsen, T.; Norsk, J.B.; Pries-Heje, M.M.; Vissing, C.R.; Nielsen, P.B.; Winsløw, U.C.; et al. Effectiveness of Adding a Mask Recommendation to Other Public Health Measures to Prevent Sars-Cov-2 Infection in Danish Mask Wearers. Ann. Intern. Med. 2020

[8] Fisher, K.A.; Tenforde, M.W.; Feldstein, L.R.; Lindsell, C.J.; Shapiro, N.I.; Files, D.C.; Gibbs, K.W.; Erickson, H.L.; Prekker, M.E.; Steingrub, J.S.; et al. Community and Close Contact Exposures Associated with COVID-19 among Symptomatic Adults ≥18 Years in 11 Outpatient Health Care Facilities-United States, July 2020. MMWR Morb. Mortal. Wkly. Rep. 2020, 69, 1258–1264.

[9] Streeck, H.; Schulte, B.; Kuemmerer, B.; Richter, E.; Hoeller, T.; Fuhrmann, C.; Bartok, E.; Dolscheid, R.; Berger, M.; Wessendorf, L.; et al. Infection Fatality Rate of Sars-Cov-2 Infection in a German Community with a Super-Spreading Event. medRxiv 2020.

[10] Ioannidis, J. The Infection Fatality Rate of COVID-19 Inferred from Seroprevalence Data. medRxiv 2020.

[11] Executive Board: Special Session on the COVID-19 Response. Available online: https://www.who.int/newsroom/events/detail/2020/10/05/default-calendar/executive-board-special-session-on-the-covid19-response (accessed on 13 November 2020).

Reason 128: Some Doctors Are Conflicted And Unable To Properly Represent Their Patients' Interests

[1] Kisielinski K, Giboni P, Prescher A, et al. Is a Mask That Covers the Mouth and Nose Free from Undesirable Side Effects in Everyday Use and Free of Potential Hazards? International Journal of Environmental Research and Public Health. 2021;18(8):4344. doi:10.3390/ijerph18084344.

[2] De Brouwer, C. Wearing a Mask, a Universal Solution against COVID-19 or an Additional Health Risk? 2020. Available online: https://papers.ssrn.com/sol3/papers.cfm?abstract_id=3676885 (accessed on 12 November 2020)

[3] Ewig, S.; Gatermann, S.; Lemmen, S. Die Maskierte Gesellschaft. Pneumologie 2020, 74, 405–408.

[4] Great Barrington Declaration Great Barrington Declaration and Petition. Available online: https://gbdeclaration.org/ (accessed on 9 November 2020

[5] WMA-The World Medical Association-WMA Declaration of Geneva. Available online: https://www.wma.net/policies-post/wma-declaration-of-geneva/ (accessed on 7 November 2020

[6] WMA-The World Medical Association-WMA Declaration of Helsinki–Ethical Principles for Medical Research Involving Human Subjects. Available online: https://www.wma.net/policies-post/wma-declaration-of-geneva/ (accessed on 7 November 2020

[7] WMA-The World Medical Association-WMA Declaration of Lisbon on the Rights of the Patient. Available online: https://www.wma.net/policies-post/wma-declaration-of-lisbon-on-the-rights-of-the-patient/ (accessed on 7 November 2020)

Reason 129: Face Masks While Driving Are A Hazard To Your Children

[1] The Law Offices of Michael P Burakoff, P.A. New Jersey Driver Passed Out and Crashed After Wearing N95 Face Mask. 2020. Retrieved from https://www.burakofflaw.com/new-jersey-driver-passed-out-and-crashed-after-wearing-n95-face-mask/

[2] Carrega, C. Driver in crash may have passed out from wearing N95 mask too long: Police. ABC News. 2020. Retrieved from https://abcnews.go.com/US/driver-crash-passed-wearing-n95-mask-long-police/story?id=70346532

[3] Gearty, R. NJ police say 'excessive wearing' of coronavirus mask contributed to driver passing out, crashing car. Fox News. 2020. Retrieved from https://www.foxnews.com/us/nj-police-say-excessive-wearing-of-n95-coronavirus-mask-contributed-to-woman-passing-out-crashing-car

Reason 130: The Face Mask Mandate Was Issued Without A Single Scientific Paper Cited In Support Of Cloth Face Masks Providing Respiratory Protection

[1] Singleton MM. Mask Facts. Association of American Physicians and Surgeons. 2021. Retrieved from https://aapsonline.org/mask-facts/

Reason 131: Wearing Cloth Face Masks Leads To More Flu-Like Illness Than Wearing No Face Mask, Causing Exactly The Opposite Outcome That Mandatory Masking Is Supposed To Prevent

[1] Vainshelboim B. Retracted: Facemasks in the COVID-19 era: A health hypothesis [retracted in: Med Hypotheses. 2021 May 12;:110601]. Med Hypotheses. 2021;146:110411. doi:10.1016/j.mehy.2020.110411

[2] MacIntyre C.R., Seale H., Dung T.C., Hien N.T., Nga P.T., Chughtai A.A. A cluster randomised trial of cloth masks compared with medical masks in healthcare workers. BMJ open. 2015;5

Reason 132: Cloth Face Masks Are Awful

[1] MacIntyre CR, Seale H, Dung TC, et al. A cluster randomised trial of cloth masks compared with medical masks in healthcare workers. BMJ Open. 2015;5(4):e006577. Published 2015 Apr 22. doi:10.1136/bmjopen-2014-006577

Reason 133: Cloth Face Masks Are So Awful That They Should Never Be Recommended To Prevent The Spread Of A Virus

[1] MacIntyre CR, Seale H, Dung TC, et al. A cluster randomised trial of cloth masks compared with medical masks in healthcare workers. BMJ Open. 2015;5(4):e006577. Published 2015 Apr 22. doi:10.1136/bmjopen-2014-006577

[2] Institute of Medicine (IOM). Reusability of Facemasks During an Influenza Pandemic: Facing the Flu — Committee on the Development of Reusable Facemasks for Use During an Influenza Pandemic. National Academy of Sciences, 2006.

[3] Center for Disease Control and Prevention and World Health Organization. Infection control for viral haemorrhagic fevers in the African health care setting. Atlanta: Centers for Disease Control and Prevention, 1998:1–198.

[4] World Health Organization (WHO). Guidelines for the prevention of tuberculosis in health care facilities in resource limited settings, 1999.

Reason 134: Double Masking May Cause Even Higher Risk Of Infection To The Wearer

[1] Singleton MM. Mask Facts. Association of American Physicians and Surgeons. 2021. Retrieved from https://aapsonline.org/mask-facts/

[2] MacIntyre CR, Seale H, Dung TC, et alA cluster randomised trial of cloth masks compared with medical masks in healthcare workers BMJ Open 2015;5:e006577. doi: 10.1136/bmjopen-2014-006577

Reason 135: Years Of Masking Precautions Meant To Benefit The Wearer Were Thrown Out The Window Suddenly In 2020

[1] Kisielinski K, Giboni P, Prescher A, et al. Is a Mask That Covers the Mouth and Nose Free from Undesirable Side Effects in Everyday Use and Free of Potential Hazards? International Journal of Environmental Research and Public Health. 2021;18(8):4344. doi:10.3390/ijerph18084344.

[2] Browse by Country-NATLEX. Available online: https://www.ilo.org/dyn/natlex/natlex4.byCountry?p_lang=en (accessed on 28 January 2021).

[3] BAuA-Sars-Cov-2 FAQ Und Weitere Informationen-Kennzeichnung von Masken Aus USA, Kanada, Australien/Neuseeland, Japan, China Und Korea-Bundesanstalt Für Arbeitsschutz Und Arbeitsmedizin. Available online: https://www.baua.de/DE/Themen/Arbeitsgestaltung-im-Betrieb/Coronavirus/pdf/Kennzeichnung-Masken.html (accessed on 28 January 2021).

[4] Veit, M. Hauptsache Maske!? DAZ.Online. 2020, p. S26. Available online: https://www.deutsche-apotheker-zeitung.de/daz-az/2020/daz-33-2020/hauptsache-maske (accessed on 12 November 2020).

[5] Deutsche Gesetzliche Unfallversicherung. DGUV Grundsätze für Arbeitsmedizinische Vorsorgeuntersuchungen; Alfons, W., Ed.; Gentner Verlag: Stuttgart, Germany, 2010; ISBN 978-3-87247-733-0.

Reason 136: OSHA Considers The MicroEnvironment Of Face Masks As "Not Safe For Workers"

[1] Borovoy, B. Colleen, H. Makeeta, Q. Masks, false safety and real dangers, Part 1: Friable mask particulate and lung vulnerability. https://childrenshealthdefense.org/the-science-of-masks/.from https://childrenshealthdefense.org/wp-content/uploads/Masks-false-safety-and-real-dangers-Part-1-Friable-mask-particulate-and-lung-vulnerability.pdf

[2] Occupational Safety and Health Administration (OSHA), US Department of Labor. Confined or enclosed spaces and other dangerous atmospheres.

https://www.osha.gov/SLTC/etools/shipyard/shiprepair/confinedspace/oxygendeficient.html

[3] Sharma, S. Brown, B. Spirometry and respiratory muscle function during ascent to higher altitudes. Lung. MarApr 2007. 185 (2): 113-21. doi: 10.1007/s00408-006-0108-y https://pubmed.ncbi.nlm.nih.gov/17393241/

[4] Malik, S. Singh, I. Ventilatory capacity among highland Bods: a possible adaptive mechanism at high altitude. Ann Hum Biol. Sep-Oct 1979. 6 (5) 471-6. doi: 10.1080/03014467900003851

https://pubmed.ncbi.nlm.nih.gov/533244/ — Malik SL, Singh IP. Ventilatory capacity among highland Bods: a possible adaptive mechanism at high altitude. Ann Hum Biol. 1979 Sep-Oct;6(5):471-6. doi: 10.1080/03014467900003851. PMID: 533244.

[5] Williams, W. Physiological response to alterations in [O₂] and [CO₂]: relevance to respiratory protective devices. J Int Soc Resp Protection. National Institute for Occupational Safety and Health (NIOSH). 27 (1): 27-51. 2010. https://www.isrp.com/the-isrp-journal/journal-public-abstracts/1154-vol-27-no-1-2010-pp-27-51-wiliams-open-access/file

[6] Holmer, I. Kuklane, K. et al. Minute volumes and inspiratory flow rates during exhaustive treadmill walking using respirators. Ann Occup Hygiene. 51 (3): 327-335. Apr 2007. https://doi.org/10.1093/annhyg/mem004 https://academic.oup.com/annweh/article/51/3/327/139423

[7] 11:40am 26 July 2021, twitter

Reason 137: Increased "Dead Space" Can Be Lethal

[1] Morris LA. Dead Space and Inhaled Carbon Dioxide Levels in Respiratory Protective Equipment. HSE Health & Safety Executive. 1991. Retrieved from https://www.hse.gov.uk/research/crr_pdf/1991/crr91027

[2] LOUHEVAARA (1984). Physiological effects associated with the use of respiratory protective devices. A review. Scandinavian Journal of Work, Environment and Health; 10: 275-281.

[3] COMROE, (1974). Physiology of respiration. An introductory text. 2nd ed. Chicago: Year Book Medical.

[4] JAMES, (1976). Breathing resistance and dead space in respiratory protective devices. Physiological effects of breathing resistance and equipment dead space in respiratory protective devices: status of the problem. Cincinnati (OH): US Department of Health, Education and Welfare. (HEW Publication (NIOSH) 77-161)

[5] DAHLBACK and FALLHAGEN, (1987). A novel method for measuring dead space in respiratory protective equipment. Journal of the International Soc. For Respiratory Protection; 5(1): 12-17.

[6] KLOOS and LAMONICA, (1966). A machine-test method for measuring carbon dioxide in the inspired air of self-contained breathing apparatus. Pittsburgh (PA): US Bureau of Mines. (USBM Report of Investigations 6865).

Reason 138: The Many Details Of Breathing Are Not One-Size-Fits-All, But Highly Individualized And Face Mask Policy Can Therefore Not Be One-Size-Fits-All

[1] Morris LA. Dead Space and Inhaled Carbon Dioxide Levels in Respiratory Protective Equipment. HSE Health & Safety Executive. 1991. Retrieved from https://www.hse.gov.uk/research/crr_pdf/1991/crr91027.pdf

[2] Comte (1972). [The effect of isolating respiratory protective equipment on body functions]. In German. Atemschutz Informationen; 11(3): 55-60.

[3] Leers (1972). Wirkungen des Kohlendioxids beim Benutzen von Atemschutzgeraten. Atemschutz Informationen; 11: 166-235

Reason 139: Too Much Carbon Dioxide

[1] Morris LA. Dead Space and Inhaled Carbon Dioxide Levels in Respiratory Protective Equipment. HSE Health & Safety Executive. 1991. Retrieved from https://www.hse.gov.uk/research/crr_pdf/1991/crr91027

[2] LAMBERTSEN, 1960. Carbon dioxide and respiration in acid-based homeostasis. Anesthesiology; 21: 642-651.

[3] LAMBERTSEN, 1974; NATIONAL INSTITUTE OF OCCUPATIONAL SAFETY AND HEALTH, 1976. Effects of excessive pressures of oxygen, nitrogen, carbon dioxide and carbon monoxide: implications in aerospace, undersea and industrial environments. In: Mountcastle VB, ed. Medical physiology. Vol. 2. 13th ed. St Louis: Mosby: 1563-1597.

[4] MALKIN, 1975. Barometric pressure and gas composition. In: Calvin M, Gazenko OG, eds. Foundations of space biology and medicine. Joint USA/USSR publication in three volumes. Vol. II, Book 1: Ecological and physiological bases of space biology and medicine. Washington (DC): National Aeronautics and Space Administration: 3-64.

[5] LANPHIER and CAMPORESI, 1982. Respiration and exercise. In: Bennett PB, Elliott DH, Eds. The physiology and medicine of diving. 3rd ed. London: Bailliere Tindall: 99-156.

472

[6] BOSTOCK, 1985. An investigation into the performance of positive pressure powered dust hoods and blouses at low flow rates. Annals of Occupational Hygiene; 29: 415-420.

[7] KING, 1949. High concentration — short time exposures and toxicity. Journal of Industrial Hygiene and Toxicology; 31: 365-375.

[8] BROWN, 1930. The physiological effects of high concentrations of carbon dioxide. US Naval Medical Bulletin; 28: 721-734

[9] DRIPPS and COMROE, 1947. The respiratory and circulatory response of normal man to inhalation of 7.6 and 10.4 per cent CO_2 with a comparison of maximal ventilation produced by severe muscular excise, inhalation of CO_2 and maximal voluntary hyperventilation. American Journal of Physiology; 40: 370-377.

[10] EBERSOLE, 1960. The new dimensions of submarine medicine. New England Journal of Medicine; 262: 599-610.

[11] HARRISON and SMITH, 1981. Hazards of enclosed spaces — raised ambient CO_2. Journal of the Royal Naval Medical Services; 67: 138-146.

[12] CHAPIN et al, 1955. Changes in the sensitivity of the respiratory center in man after prolonged exposure to 3% CO_2. In: Rahn H, Fenn WO. Studies in respiratory physiology. 2nd series: Chemistry, mechanics, and circulation of the lung. Ohio: Wright Air Development Center: 250-253. (WADC Technical Report 55-357).

[13] SCHAEFER et al, 1963. Respiratory acclimatization to carbon dioxide. Journal of Applied Physiology; 18: 1071-1078.

[14] Walach H, Weikl R, Prentice J, et al. Experimental Assessment of Carbon Dioxide Content in Inhaled Air With or Without Face Masks in Healthy Children: A Randomized Clinical Trial. JAMA Pediatr. Published online June 30, 2021. doi:10.1001/jamapediatrics.2021.2659

[15] ECRI. Up to 70% of Chinese KN95 Masks Tested by ECRI Don't Meet Minimum Standards. 2020. Retrieved from https://www.ecri.org/press/up-to-70-of-chinese-kn95-masks-tested-by-ecri-dont-meet-minimum-standards

[16] Walach H, Weikl R, Prentice J, et al. Experimental Assessment of Carbon Dioxide Content in Inhaled Air With or Without Face Masks in Healthy Children: A Randomized Clinical Trial. JAMA Pediatr. Published online June 30, 2021. doi:10.1001/jamapediatrics.2021.2659

[17] Schwarz S, Jenetzky E, Krafft H, Maurer T, Martin D. Corona children studies "Co-Ki": first results of a Germany-wide registry on mouth and nose covering (mask) in children. Published 2021. Accessed June 15, 2021. https://www.research square.com/article/rs-124394/v1

[18] Mitteilungen der Ad-hoc-Arbeitsgruppe Innenraumrichtwerte der Innenraumlufthygiene-Kommission des Umweltbundesamtes und der Obersten Landesgesundheitsbehörden. [Health evaluation of carbon dioxide in indoor air]. Bundesgesundheitsblatt Gesundheitsforschung Gesundheitsschutz. 2008;51(11):1358-1369. doi:10.1007/s00103-008-0707-2

[19] Christakis D, Fontanarosa PB. Notice of Retraction. Walach H, et al. Experimental Assessment of Carbon Dioxide Content in Inhaled Air With or Without Face Masks in Healthy Children: A Randomized Clinical Trial. JAMA Pediatr. Published online June 30, 2021. JAMA Pediatr. 2021;175(9):e213252. doi:10.1001/jamapediatrics.2021.3252

[20] Walach H, Klement RJ, Aukema W. The Safety of COVID-19 Vaccinations — We Should Rethink the Policy. Vaccines. 2021; 9(7):693. https://doi.org/10.3390/vaccines9070693

[21] Wadman Meredith. Scientists quit journal board, protesting 'grossly irresponsible' study claiming COVID-19 vaccines kill. Science. 2021. Retrieved from https://www.science.org/content/article/scientists-quit-journal-board-protesting-grossly-irresponsible-study-claiming-covid-19

[22] PUMS. Press statement: COVID-19 Vaccinations. 2021. Retrieved from https://pums.ump.edu.pl/about-pums/news/240-university-statement-regarding-article-by-dr-walach.html

Reason 140: Increases In Exhalation Resistance, Inhalation Resistance, And Temperature May Be Harmful To One Wearing A Face Mask

[1] Morris LA. Dead Space and Inhaled Carbon Dioxide Levels in Respiratory Protective Equipment. HSE Health & Safety Executive. 1991. Retrieved from https://www.hse.gov.uk/research/crr_pdf/1991/crr91027

[2] LOUHEVAARA (1984). Physiological effects associated with the use of respiratory protective devices. A review. Scandinavian Journal of Work, Environment and Health; 10: 275-281.

[3] CHERNIAK and SNIDAL, 1956; The effect of obstruction to breathing on the ventilator response to CO_2. Journal of Clinical Investigation; 35: 1286-12900.

[4] BRODOWSKY et al, 1960. The respiratory response to carbon dioxide in health and in emphysema. Journal of Clinical Investigation; 39: 724-729

[5] CRAIG et al (1970) Exhausting work limited by external resistance and inhalation of carbon dioxide. Journal of Applied Physiology; 29: 847-851

[6] LOVE et al (1979) Tolerance and ventilator response to inhaled CO_2 during exercise and with inspiratory resistive loading. Annals of Occupational Hygiene; 22: 43-53

Reason 141: Face Masks Induce Thermal Stress And Affect Heartrate, Even Among Healthy Adults And Likely Far More Among Children And The Infirm

[1] Fikenzer S. et al. "Effects of surgical and FFP2/N95 face masks on cardiopulmonary exercise capacity," *Clinical Research in Cardiology*, 2020. Retrieved from: https://link.springer.com/article/10.1007/s00392-020-01704-y

[2] Li : Li Y, Tokura H, Guo YP, et al. "Effects of wearing N95 and surgical facemasks on heart rate, thermal stress and subjective sensations". Int Arch Occup Environ Health. 2005;78(6):501-509. doi:10.1007/s00420-004-0584-4 — https://www.ncbi.nlm.nih.gov/pmc/articles/PMC7087880/

[3] Clin Res Cardiol. 2020 Dec;109(12):1522-1530. doi: 10.1007/s00392-020-01704-y. Epub 2020 Jul 6. PMID: 32632523; PMCID: PMC7338098. — https://link.springer.com/article/10.1007/s00392-020-01704-y

[4] Fikenzer: Fikenzer S, Uhe T, Lavall D, Rudolph U, Falz R, Busse M, Hepp P, Laufs U. "Effects of surgical and FFP2/N95 face masks on cardiopulmonary exercise capacity

Reason 142: Hypercapnia

[1] Coleman, V. Dr. Proof That Face Masks Do More Harm Than Good. *Freedom of Speech.* 2021. Retrieved from https://fos-sa.org/2021/01/06/proof-that-face-masks-do-more-harm-than-good/

Reason 143: Face Masks Increase "Dead Space"

[1] Kisielinski K, Giboni P, Prescher A, et al. Is a Mask That Covers the Mouth and Nose Free from Undesirable Side Effects in Everyday Use and Free of Potential Hazards? International Journal of Environmental Research and Public Health. 2021;18(8):4344. doi:10.3390/ijerph18084344.

[2] Butz, U. Rückatmung von Kohlendioxid bei Verwendung von Operationsmasken als hygienischer Mundschutz an medizinischem Fachpersonal. Ph.D. Thesis, Fakultät für Medizin der Technischen Universität München, Munich, Germany, 2005.

[3] Smolka, L.; Borkowski, J.; Zaton, M. The Effect of Additional Dead Space on Respiratory Exchange Ratio and Carbon Dioxide Production Due to Training. J. Sports Sci. Med. 2014, 13, 36–43.

[4] Roberge, R.J.; Kim, J.-H.; Benson, S.M. Absence of Consequential Changes in Physiological, Thermal and Subjective Responses from Wearing a Surgical Mask. Respir. Physiol. Neurobiol. 2012, 181, 29–35

[5] Matuschek, C.; Moll, F.; Fangerau, H.; Fischer, J.C.; Zänker, K.; van Griensven, M.; Schneider, M.; Kindgen-Milles, D.; Knoefel, W.T.; Lichtenberg, A.; et al. Face Masks: Benefits and Risks during the COVID-19 Crisis. Eur. J. Med. Res. 2020, 25, 32.

[6] Roberge, R.J.; Coca, A.; Williams, W.J.; Powell, J.B.; Palmiero, A.J. Physiological Impact of the N95 Filtering Facepiece Respirator on Healthcare Workers. Respir. Care 2010, 55, 569–577.

Reason 144: Face Masks Increase Carbon Dioxide Dangerously And Decrease Oxygen Dangerously

[1] Kisielinski K, Giboni P, Prescher A, et al. Is a Mask That Covers the Mouth and Nose Free from Undesirable Side Effects in Everyday Use and Free of Potential Hazards? International Journal of Environmental Research and Public Health. 2021;18(8):4344. doi:10.3390/ijerph18084344.

[2] Pifarré, F.; Zabala, D.D.; Grazioli, G.; de Yzaguirre i Maura, I. COVID 19 and Mask in Sports. Apunt. Sports Med. 2020. [CrossRef]

[3] Rebmann, T.; Carrico, R.; Wang, J. Physiologic and Other Effects and Compliance with Long-Term Respirator Use among Medical Intensive Care Unit Nurses. Am. J. Infect. Control 2013, 41, 1218–1223.

[4] Roeckner, J.T.; Krsti´c, N.; Sipe, B.H.; Obi˘can, S.G. N95 Filtering Facepiece Respirator Use during Pregnancy: A Systematic Review. Am. J. Perinatol. 2020, 37, 995–1001.

[5] Roberge, R.J.; Kim, J.-H.; Benson, S.M. Absence of Consequential Changes in Physiological, Thermal and Subjective Responses from Wearing a Surgical Mask. Respir. Physiol. Neurobiol. 2012, 181, 29–35.

[6] Roberge, R.J.; Coca, A.; Williams, W.J.; Powell, J.B.; Palmiero, A.J. Physiological Impact of the N95 Filtering Facepiece Respirator on Healthcare Workers. Respir. Care 2010, 55, 569–577.

[7] Georgi, C.; Haase-Fielitz, A.; Meretz, D.; Gäsert, L.; Butter, C. Einfluss gängiger Gesichtsmasken auf physiologische Parameter und Belastungsempfinden unter arbeitstypischer körperlicher Anstrengung. Deutsches Ärzteblatt 2020, 674–675.

[8] Roberge, R.J.; Kim, J.-H.; Powell, J.B. N95 Respirator Use during Advanced Pregnancy. Am. J. Infect. Control 2014, 42, 1097–1100.

[9] Kyung, S.Y.; Kim, Y.; Hwang, H.; Park, J.-W.; Jeong, S.H. Risks of N95 Face Mask Use in Subjects with COPD. Respir. Care 2020, 65, 658–664.

[10] Epstein, D.; Korytny, A.; Isenberg, Y.; Marcusohn, E.; Zukermann, R.; Bishop, B.; Minha, S.; Raz, A.; Miller, A. Return to Training in the COVID-19 Era: The Physiological Effects of Face Masks during Exercise. Scand. J. Med. Sci. Sports 2020.

[11] Mo, Y.; Wei, D.; Mai, Q.; Chen, C.; Yu, H.; Jiang, C.; Tan, X. Risk and Impact of Using Mask on COPD Patients with Acute Exacerbation during the COVID-19 Outbreak: A Retrospective Study. Res. Sq. 2020

[12] Butz, U. Rückatmung von Kohlendioxid bei Verwendung von Operationsmasken als hygienischer Mundschutz an medizinischem Fachpersonal. Ph.D. Thesis, Fakultät für Medizin der Technischen Universität München, Munich, Germany, 2005.

[13] Goh, D.Y.T.; Mun, M.W.; Lee, W.L.J.; Teoh, O.H.; Rajgor, D.D. A Randomised Clinical Trial to Evaluate the Safety, Fit, Comfort of a Novel N95 Mask in Children. Sci. Rep. 2019, 9, 18952.

[14] Bharatendu, C.; Ong, J.J.Y.; Goh, Y.; Tan, B.Y.Q.; Chan, A.C.Y.; Tang, J.Z.Y.; Leow, A.S.; Chin, A.; Sooi, K.W.X.; Tan, Y.L.; et al. Powered Air Purifying Respirator (PAPR) Restores the N95 Face Mask Induced Cerebral Hemodynamic Alterations among Healthcare Workers during COVID-19 Outbreak. J. Neurol. Sci. 2020, 417, 117078.

[15] Tong, P.S.Y.; Kale, A.S.; Ng, K.; Loke, A.P.; Choolani, M.A.; Lim, C.L.; Chan, Y.H.; Chong, Y.S.; Tambyah, P.A.; Yong, E.-L. Respiratory Consequences of N95-Type Mask Usage in Pregnant Healthcare Workers — A Controlled Clinical Study. Antimicrob. Resist. Infect. Control 2015, 4, 48.

[16] Liu, C.; Li, G.; He, Y.; Zhang, Z.; Ding, Y. Effects of Wearing Masks on Human Health and Comfort during the COVID-19 Pandemic. IOP Conf. Ser. Earth Environ. Sci. 2020, 531, 012034. [CrossRef]

[17] Beder, A.; Büyükkoçak, U.; Sabuncuo ̄glu, H.; Keskil, Z.A.; Keskil, S. Preliminary Report on Surgical Mask Induced Deoxygenation during Major Surgery. Neurocirugía 2008, 19, 121–126.

[18] Fikenzer, S.; Uhe, T.; Lavall, D.; Rudolph, U.; Falz, R.; Busse, M.; Hepp, P.; Laufs, U. Effects of Surgical and FFP2/N95 Face Masks on Cardiopulmonary Exercise Capacity. Clin. Res. Cardiol. 2020, 109, 1522–1530. [CrossRef] [PubMed]

[19] Jagim, A.R.; Dominy, T.A.; Camic, C.L.; Wright, G.; Doberstein, S.; Jones, M.T.; Oliver, J.M. Acute Effects of the Elevation Training Mask on Strength Performance in Recreational Weight Lifters. J. Strength Cond. Res. 2018, 32, 482–489. [CrossRef]

[20] Cress ML, Forrester K, Probst L, Foster C, Doberstein S, Porcari JP. Effect of Wearing the Elevation Training Mask on Aerobic Capacity, Lung Function, and Hematological Variables. Medicine & Science in Sports & Exercise. 2016;48:1040-1041. doi:10.1249/01.mss.0000488131.38685.16.

[21] Kao, T.-W.; Huang, K.-C.; Huang, Y.-L.; Tsai, T.-J.; Hsieh, B.-S.; Wu, M.-S. The Physiological Impact of Wearing an N95 Mask during Hemodialysis as a Precaution against SARS in Patients with End-Stage Renal Disease. J. Formos. Med. Assoc. 2004, 103, 624–628.

[22] Li, Y.; Tokura, H.; Guo, Y.P.; Wong, A.S.W.; Wong, T.; Chung, J.; Newton, E. Effects of Wearing N95 and Surgical Facemasks on Heart Rate, Thermal Stress and Subjective Sensations. Int. Arch. Occup. Environ. Health 2005, 78, 501–509.

[23] Johnson, A.T. Respirator Masks Protect Health but Impact Performance: A Review. J. Biol. Eng. 2016, 10, 4.

Reason 145: Face Masks Dangerously Increase The Rebreathing Of Carbon Dioxide

[1] Kisielinski K, Giboni P, Prescher A, et al. Is a Mask That Covers the Mouth and Nose Free from Undesirable Side Effects in Everyday Use and Free of Potential Hazards? International Journal of Environmental Research and Public Health. 2021;18(8):4344. doi:10.3390/ijerph18084344.

[2] Roberge, R.J.; Kim, J.-H.; Benson, S.M. Absence of Consequential Changes in Physiological, Thermal and Subjective Responses from Wearing a Surgical Mask. Respir. Physiol. Neurobiol. 2012, 181, 29–35.

[3] Roberge, R.J.; Coca, A.; Williams, W.J.; Powell, J.B.; Palmiero, A.J. Physiological Impact of the N95 Filtering Facepiece Respirator on Healthcare Workers. Respir. Care 2010, 55, 569–577.

[4] Beder, A.; Büyükkoçak, U.; Sabuncuo ̄glu, H.; Keskil, Z.A.; Keskil, S. Preliminary Report on Surgical Mask Induced Deoxygenation during Major Surgery. Neurocirugía 2008, 19, 121–126.

[5] Kao, T.-W.; Huang, K.-C.; Huang, Y.-L.; Tsai, T.-J.; Hsieh, B.-S.; Wu, M.-S. The Physiological Impact of Wearing an N95 Mask during Hemodialysis as a Precaution against SARS in Patients with End-Stage Renal Disease. J. Formos. Med. Assoc. 2004, 103, 624–628.

[6] Mo, Y.; Wei, D.; Mai, Q.; Chen, C.; Yu, H.; Jiang, C.; Tan, X. Risk and Impact of Using Mask on COPD Patients with Acute Exacerbation during the COVID-19 Outbreak: A Retrospective Study. Res. Sq. 2020

[7] Kyung, S.Y.; Kim, Y.; Hwang, H.; Park, J.-W.; Jeong, S.H. Risks of N95 Face Mask Use in Subjects with COPD. Respir. Care 2020, 65, 658–664.

[8] Johnson, A.T. Respirator Masks Protect Health but Impact Performance: A Review. J. Biol. Eng. 2016, 10, 4.

[9] Rosner, E. Adverse Effects of Prolonged Mask Use among Healthcare Professionals during COVID-19. J. Infect. Dis. Epidemiol.2020.

[10] Azuma, K.; Kagi, N.; Yanagi, U.; Osawa, H. Effects of Low-Level Inhalation Exposure to Carbon Dioxide in Indoor Environments: A Short Review on Human Health and Psychomotor Performance. Environ. Int. 2018, 121, 51–56.

[11] Drechsler, M.; Morris, J. Carbon Dioxide Narcosis. In StatPearls; StatPearls Publishing: Treasure Island, FL, USA, 2020.)

[12] Rebmann, T.; Carrico, R.; Wang, J. Physiologic and Other Effects and Compliance with Long-Term Respirator Use among Medical Intensive Care Unit Nurses. Am. J. Infect. Control 2013, 41, 1218–1223.

[13] Jagim, A.R.; Dominy, T.A.; Camic, C.L.; Wright, G.; Doberstein, S.; Jones, M.T.; Oliver, J.M. Acute Effects of the Elevation Training Mask on Strength Performance in Recreational Weight Lifters. J. Strength Cond. Res. 2018, 32, 482–489.

[14] Noble, J.; Jones, J.G.; Davis, E.J. Cognitive Function during Moderate Hypoxaemia. Anaesth. Intensive Care 1993, 21, 180–184.

[15] Fothergill, D.M.; Hedges, D.; Morrison, J.B. Effects of CO_2 and $N2$ Partial Pressures on Cognitive and Psychomotor Performance. Undersea Biomed. Res. 1991, 18, 1–19.

[16] Liu, C.; Li, G.; He, Y.; Zhang, Z.; Ding, Y. Effects of Wearing Masks on Human Health and Comfort during the COVID-19 Pandemic. IOP Conf. Ser. Earth Environ. Sci. 2020, 531, 012034.

Reason 146: Increased Dead Space Is Significant, And So Is Increased Breathing Resistance

[1] Kisielinski K, Giboni P, Prescher A, et al. Is a Mask That Covers the Mouth and Nose Free from Undesirable Side Effects in Everyday Use and Free of Potential Hazards? International Journal of Environmental Research and Public Health. 2021;18(8):4344. doi:10.3390/ijerph18084344.

[2] Johnson, A.T.; Scott, W.H.; Lausted, C.G.; Coyne, K.M.; Sahota, M.S.; Johnson, M.M. Effect of External Dead Volume on Performance While Wearing a Respirator. AIHAJ-Am. Ind. Hyg. Assoc. 2000, 61, 678–684.

[3] Xu, M.; Lei, Z.; Yang, J. Estimating the Dead Space Volume between a Headform and N95 Filtering Facepiece Respirator Using Microsoft Kinect. J. Occup. Environ. Hyg. 2015, 12, 538–546.

[4] Lee, H.P.; Wang, D.Y. Objective Assessment of Increase in Breathing Resistance of N95 Respirators on Human Subjects. Ann. Occup. Hyg. 2011, 55, 917–921.

[5] Roberge, R.; Bayer, E.; Powell, J.; Coca, A.; Roberge, M.; Benson, S. Effect of Exhaled Moisture on Breathing Resistance of N95 Filtering Facepiece Respirators. Ann. Occup. Hyg. 2010, 54, 671–677.

[6] Johnson, A.T. Respirator Masks Protect Health but Impact Performance: A Review. J. Biol. Eng. 2016, 10, 4.

[7] Kyung, S.Y.; Kim, Y.; Hwang, H.; Park, J.-W.; Jeong, S.H. Risks of N95 Face Mask Use in Subjects with COPD. Respir. Care 2020, 65, 658–664.

Reason 147: Increased Dead Space Increases Breathing Resistance, Leading To Decreased Gas Exchange Of The Respiratory System — And A Cascade Of Other Physiological Side Effects

[1] Kisielinski K, Giboni P, Prescher A, et al. Is a Mask That Covers the Mouth and Nose Free from Undesirable Side Effects in Everyday Use and Free of Potential Hazards? International Journal of Environmental Research and Public Health. 2021;18(8):4344. doi:10.3390/ijerph18084344.

[2] Lee, H.P.; Wang, D.Y. Objective Assessment of Increase in Breathing Resistance of N95 Respirators on Human Subjects. Ann. Occup. Hyg. 2011, 55, 917–921.

[3] Equals averaged inspiration and expiration according to Lee 2011, Lee, H.P.; Wang, D.Y. Objective Assessment of Increase in Breathing Resistance of N95 Respirators on Human Subjects. Ann. Occup. Hyg. 2011, 55, 917–921, including moisture penetration according to Roberge 2010, Roberge, R.; Bayer, E.; Powell, J.; Coca, A.; Roberge, M.; Benson, S. Effect of Exhaled Moisture on Breathing Resistance of N95 Filtering Facepiece Respirators. Ann. Occup. Hyg. 2010, 54, 671–677.

[4] Equals averaged values according to Xu 2015, Xu, M.; Lei, Z.; Yang, J. Estimating the Dead Space Volume between a Headform and N95 Filtering Facepiece Respirator Using Microsoft Kinect. J. Occup. Environ. Hyg. 2015, 12, 538–546

Reason 148: Suprathreshold Stimuli Can Cause Pathological Consequences, But So Can Subthreshold Stimuli

[1] Kisielinski K, Giboni P, Prescher A, et al. Is a Mask That Covers the Mouth and Nose Free from Undesirable Side Effects in Everyday Use and Free of Potential Hazards? International Journal of Environmental Research and Public Health. 2021;18(8):4344. doi:10.3390/ijerph18084344.

[2] Simonton, D.; Spears, M. Human Health Effects from Exposure to Low-Level Concentrations of Hydrogen Sulfide. Occup. Health Saf. (Waco Tex.) 2007, 76, 102–104.

[3] Salimi, F.; Morgan, G.; Rolfe, M.; Samoli, E.; Cowie, C.T.; Hanigan, I.; Knibbs, L.; Cope, M.; Johnston, F.H.; Guo, Y.; et al. Long-Term Exposure to Low Concentrations of Air Pollutants and Hospitalisation for Respiratory Diseases: A Prospective Cohort Study in Australia. Environ. Int. 2018, 121, 415–420.

[4] Dominici, F.; Schwartz, J.; Di, Q.; Braun, D.; Choirat, C.; Zanobetti, A. Assessing Adverse Health Effects of Long-Term Exposure to Low Levels of Ambient Air Pollution: Phase 1 Research Report; Health Effects Institute: Boston, MA, USA, 2019; pp. 1–51.

[5] Alleva, R.; Manzella, N.; Gaetani, S.; Bacchetti, T.; Bracci, M.; Ciarapica, V.; Monaco, F.; Borghi, B.; Amati, M.; Ferretti, G.; et al. Mechanism Underlying the Effect of Long-Term Exposure to Low Dose of Pesticides on DNA Integrity. Environ. Toxicol. 2018, 33, 476–487.

[6] Roh, T.; Lynch, C.F.; Weyer, P.; Wang, K.; Kelly, K.M.; Ludewig, G. Low-Level Arsenic Exposure from Drinking Water Is Associated with Prostate Cancer in Iowa. Environ. Res. 2017, 159, 338–343.

[7] Deering, K.E.; Callan, A.C.; Prince, R.L.; Lim, W.H.; Thompson, P.L.; Lewis, J.R.; Hinwood, A.L.; Devine, A. Low-Level Cadmium Exposure and Cardiovascular Outcomes in Elderly Australian Women: A Cohort Study. Int. J. Hyg. Environ. Health 2018, 221, 347–354.

[8] Kosnett, M. Health Effects of Low Dose Lead Exposure in Adults and Children, and Preventable Risk Posed by the Consumption of Game Meat Harvested with Lead Ammunition. In Ingestion of Lead from Spent Ammunition: Implications for Wildlife and Humans; The Peregrine Fund: Boise, ID, USA, 2009.

[9] Crinnion, W.J. Environmental Medicine, Part Three: Long-Term Effects of Chronic Low-Dose Mercury Exposure. Altern. Med. Rev. 2000, 5, 209–223.

[10] Wu, S.; Han, J.; Vleugels, R.A.; Puett, R.; Laden, F.; Hunter, D.J.; Qureshi, A.A. Cumulative Ultraviolet Radiation Flux in Adulthood and Risk of Incident Skin Cancers in Women. Br. J. Cancer 2014, 110, 1855–1861.

[11] Azuma, K.; Kagi, N.; Yanagi, U.; Osawa, H. Effects of Low-Level Inhalation Exposure to Carbon Dioxide in Indoor Environments: A Short Review on Human Health and Psychomotor Performance. Environ. Int. 2018, 121, 51–56.

[12] Custodis, F.; Schirmer, S.H.; Baumhäkel, M.; Heusch, G.; Böhm, M.; Laufs, U. Vascular Pathophysiology in Response to Increased Heart Rate. J. Am. Coll. Cardiol. 2010, 56, 1973–1983.

[13] Russo, M.A.; Santarelli, D.M.; O'Rourke, D. The Physiological Effects of Slow Breathing in the Healthy Human. Breathe 2017, 13, 298–309.

[14] Nuckowska, M.K.; Gruszecki, M.; Kot, J.; Wolf, J.; Guminski, W.; Frydrychowski, A.F.; Wtorek, J.; Narkiewicz, K.; Winklewski, P.J. Impact of Slow Breathing on the Blood Pressure and Subarachnoid Space Width Oscillations in Humans. Sci. Rep. 2019, 9, 6232.

[15] Pifarré, F.; Zabala, D.D.; Grazioli, G.; de Yzaguirre i Maura, I. COVID 19 and Mask in Sports. Apunt. Sports Med. 2020.

[16] Rebmann, T.; Carrico, R.; Wang, J. Physiologic and Other Effects and Compliance with Long-Term Respirator Use among Medical Intensive Care Unit Nurses. Am. J. Infect. Control 2013, 41, 1218–1223.

[17] Roeckner, J.T.; Krsti´c, N.; Sipe, B.H.; Obi˜can, S.G. N95 Filtering Facepiece Respirator Use during Pregnancy: A Systematic Review. Am. J. Perinatol. 2020, 37, 995–1001.

[18] Georgi, C.; Haase-Fielitz, A.; Meretz, D.; Gäsert, L.; Butter, C. Einfluss gängiger Gesichtsmasken auf physiologische Parameter und Belastungsempfinden unter arbeitstypischer körperlicher Anstrengung. Deutsches Ärzteblatt 2020, 674–675.

[19] Roberge, R.J.; Kim, J.-H.; Powell, J.B. N95 Respirator Use during Advanced Pregnancy. Am. J. Infect. Control 2014, 42, 1097–1100.

[20] Kyung, S.Y.; Kim, Y.; Hwang, H.; Park, J.-W.; Jeong, S.H. Risks of N95 Face Mask Use in Subjects with COPD. Respir. Care 2020, 65, 658–664.

[21] Epstein, D.; Korytny, A.; Isenberg, Y.; Marcusohn, E.; Zukermann, R.; Bishop, B.; Minha, S.; Raz, A.; Miller, A. Return to Training in the COVID-19 Era: The Physiological Effects of Face Masks during Exercise. Scand. J. Med. Sci. Sports 2020.

[22] Mo, Y.; Wei, D.; Mai, Q.; Chen, C.; Yu, H.; Jiang, C.; Tan, X. Risk and Impact of Using Mask on COPD Patients with Acute Exacerbation during the COVID-19 Outbreak: A Retrospective Study. Res. Sq. 2020.

[23] Goh, D.Y.T.; Mun, M.W.; Lee, W.L.J.; Teoh, O.H.; Rajgor, D.D. A Randomised Clinical Trial to Evaluate the Safety, Fit, Comfort of a Novel N95 Mask in Children. Sci. Rep. 2019, 9, 18952.

[24] Bharatendu, C.; Ong, J.J.Y.; Goh, Y.; Tan, B.Y.Q.; Chan, A.C.Y.; Tang, J.Z.Y.; Leow, A.S.; Chin, A.; Sooi, K.W.X.; Tan, Y.L.; et al. Powered Air Purifying Respirator (PAPR) Restores the N95 Face Mask Induced Cerebral Hemodynamic Alterations among Healthcare Workers during COVID-19 Outbreak. J. Neurol. Sci. 2020, 417, 117078.

[25] Tong, P.S.Y.; Kale, A.S.; Ng, K.; Loke, A.P.; Choolani, M.A.; Lim, C.L.; Chan, Y.H.; Chong, Y.S.; Tambyah, P.A.; Yong, E.-L. Respiratory Consequences of N95-Type Mask Usage in Pregnant Healthcare Workers — A Controlled Clinical Study. Antimicrob. Resist. Infect. Control 2015, 4, 48.

[26] Roberge, R.J.; Kim, J.-H.; Benson, S.M. Absence of Consequential Changes in Physiological, Thermal and Subjective Responses from Wearing a Surgical Mask. Respir. Physiol. Neurobiol. 2012, 181, 29–35.

[27] Liu, C.; Li, G.; He, Y.; Zhang, Z.; Ding, Y. Effects of Wearing Masks on Human Health and Comfort during the COVID-19 Pandemic. IOP Conf. Ser. Earth Environ. Sci. 2020, 531, 012034.

[28] Beder, A.; Büyükkoçak, U.; Sabuncuo ˜glu, H.; Keskil, Z.A.; Keskil, S. Preliminary Report on Surgical Mask Induced Deoxygenation during Major Surgery. Neurocirugía 2008, 19, 121–126.

[29] Li, Y.; Tokura, H.; Guo, Y.P.; Wong, A.S.W.; Wong, T.; Chung, J.; Newton, E. Effects of Wearing N95 and Surgical Facemasks on Heart Rate, Thermal Stress and Subjective Sensations. Int. Arch. Occup. Environ. Health 2005, 78, 501–509.

[30] Kao, T.-W.; Huang, K.-C.; Huang, Y.-L.; Tsai, T.-J.; Hsieh, B.-S.; Wu, M.-S. The Physiological Impact of Wearing an N95 Mask during Hemodialysis as a Precaution against SARS in Patients with End-Stage Renal Disease. J. Formos. Med. Assoc. 2004, 103, 624–628

[31] Johnson, A.T. Respirator Masks Protect Health but Impact Performance: A Review. J. Biol. Eng. 2016, 10, 4.

Reason 149: Everyone In A Face Mask Induces A Condition Similar On The Body To Sleep Apnea

[1] Chandrasekaran B, Fernandes S. "Exercise with facemask; Are we handling a devil's sword?" — A physiological hypothesis. Med Hypotheses. 2020;144:110002. doi:10.1016/j.mehy.2020.110002

[2] Cheng Q., Li L., Lin D., Li R., Yue Y., Wei H. Effects of acute hypercapnia on cognitive function in patients undergoing bronchoscope intervention. J Thorac Dis. 2019;11(3):1065–1071.

[3] Stevens D., Jackson B., Carberry J., McLoughlin J., Barr C., Mukherjee S. The impact of obstructive sleep apnoea on balance, gait and falls risk: a narrative review of the literature. J Gerontol A Biol Sci Med Sci. 2020

Reason 150: Exercising In A Face Mask Induces An Artificial Version Of COPD

[1] Chandrasekaran B, Fernandes S. "Exercise with facemask; Are we handling a devil's sword?" — A physiological hypothesis. Med Hypotheses. 2020;144:110002. doi:10.1016/j.mehy.2020.110002

[2] Jacobson T.A., Kler J.S., Hemke M.T., Braun R.K., Meyer K.C., Funk W.E. Direct human health risks of increased atmospheric carbon dioxide. Nat Sustain. 2019;2(8):691–701.

[3] Smith C.L., Whitelaw J.L., Davies B. Carbon dioxide rebreathing in respiratory protective devices: influence of speech and work rate in full-face masks. Ergonomics. 2013;56(5):781–790.

[4] Should Zh.u.W. and how can, exercise be done during a coronavirus outbreak? An interview with Dr. Jeffrey A. Woods. J Sport Health Sci. 2020 Mar;9(2):105–107.

[5] *Centers for Disease Control and Prevention.* Basics About COPD. Retrieved from https://www.cdc.gov/copd/basics-about.html

Reason 151: Face Masks Are Definitely Not Suitable For Epileptics

[1] Kisielinski K, Giboni P, Prescher A, et al. Is a Mask That Covers the Mouth and Nose Free from Undesirable Side Effects in Everyday Use and Free of Potential Hazards? International Journal of Environmental Research and Public Health. 2021;18(8):4344. doi:10.3390/ijerph18084344.

[2] Asadi-Pooya, A.A.; Cross, J.H. Is Wearing a Face Mask Safe for People with Epilepsy? Acta Neurol. Scand. 2020, 142, 314–316.

[3] Guaranha, M.S.B.; Garzon, E.; Buchpiguel, C.A.; Tazima, S.; Yacubian, E.M.T.; Sakamoto, A.C. Hyperventilation Revisited: Physiological Effects and Efficacy on Focal Seizure Activation in the Era o

[4] Centers for Disease Control and Prevention. Epilepsy Prevalence in the United States. 2020. Retrieved from: https://www.cdc.gov/epilepsy/data/index.html

[5] The CDC defines active epilepsy as:

"An adult aged 18 or older has active epilepsy if they report they have a history of doctor-diagnosed epilepsy or seizure disorder and

* Are currently taking medication to control it or

* Had one or more seizures in the past year (or both) (from the National Health Interview Survey, 2015).

A child aged 17 years or younger has active epilepsy if their parent or guardian reports:

* That a doctor or health care provider has ever told them that their child had epilepsy or seizure disorder, and

* Their child currently has epilepsy or seizure disorder (from the National Survey of Children's Health, 2011-2012)."

Centers for Disease Control and Prevention. Epilepsy Prevalence in the United States. 2020. Retrieved from: https://www.cdc.gov/epilepsy/data/index.html

Reason 152: Face Mask Wearing Affects The Central Nervous System And May Increase Sleep Apnea

[1] Kisielinski K, Giboni P, Prescher A, et al. Is a Mask That Covers the Mouth and Nose Free from Undesirable Side Effects in Everyday Use and Free of Potential Hazards? International Journal of Environmental Research and Public Health. 2021;18(8):4344. doi:10.3390/ijerph18084344.

[1] Zoccal, D.B.; Furuya, W.I.; Bassi, M.; Colombari, D.S.A.; Colombari, E. The Nucleus of the Solitary Tract and the Coordination of Respiratory and Sympathetic Activities. Front. Physiol. 2014, 5, 238.

[2] Melnychuk, M.C.; Dockree, P.M.; O'Connell, R.G.; Murphy, P.R.; Balsters, J.H.; Robertson, I.H. Coupling of Respiration and Attention via the Locus Coeruleus: Effects of Meditation and Pranayama. Psychophysiology 2018, 55, e13091.

[3] Xu, M.; Lei, Z.; Yang, J. Estimating the Dead Space Volume between a Headform and N95 Filtering Facepiece Respirator Using Microsoft Kinect. J. Occup. Environ. Hyg. 2015, 12, 538–546.

[4] Lee, H.P.; Wang, D.Y. Objective Assessment of Increase in Breathing Resistance of N95 Respirators on Human Subjects. Ann. Occup. Hyg. 2011, 55, 917–921.

[5] Roberge, R.; Bayer, E.; Powell, J.; Coca, A.; Roberge, M.; Benson, S. Effect of Exhaled Moisture on Breathing Resistance of N95 Filtering Facepiece Respirators. Ann. Occup. Hyg. 2010, 54, 671–677.

[6] Matuschek, C.; Moll, F.; Fangerau, H.; Fischer, J.C.; Zänker, K.; van Griensven, M.; Schneider, M.; Kindgen-Milles, D.; Knoefel, W.T.; Lichtenberg, A.; et al. Face Masks: Benefits and Risks during the COVID-19 Crisis. Eur. J. Med. Res. 2020, 25, 32.

[7] Roberge, R.J.; Coca, A.; Williams, W.J.; Powell, J.B.; Palmiero, A.J. Physiological Impact of the N95 Filtering Facepiece Respirator on Healthcare Workers. Respir. Care 2010, 55, 569–577.

[8] Pifarré, F.; Zabala, D.D.; Grazioli, G.; de Yzaguirre i Maura, I. COVID 19 and Mask in Sports. Apunt. Sports Med. 2020.

[9] Drechsler, M.; Morris, J. Carbon Dioxide Narcosis. In StatPearls; StatPearls Publishing: Treasure Island, FL, USA, 2020.

[10] Lim, E.C.H.; Seet, R.C.S.; Lee, K.-H.; Wilder-Smith, E.P.V.; Chuah, B.Y.S.; Ong, B.K.C. Headaches and the N95 Face-mask amongst Healthcare Providers. Acta Neurol. Scand. 2006, 113, 199–202.

[11] Mo, Y.; Wei, D.; Mai, Q.; Chen, C.; Yu, H.; Jiang, C.; Tan, X. Risk and Impact of Using Mask on COPD Patients with Acute Exacerbation during the COVID-19 Outbreak: A Retrospective Study. Res. Sq. 2020.

[12] Kao, T.-W.; Huang, K.-C.; Huang, Y.-L.; Tsai, T.-J.; Hsieh, B.-S.; Wu, M.-S. The Physiological Impact of Wearing an N95 Mask during Hemodialysis as a Precaution against SARS in Patients with End-Stage Renal Disease. J. Formos. Med. Assoc. 2004, 103, 624–628.

[13] Johnson, A.T.; Scott, W.H.; Lausted, C.G.; Coyne, K.M.; Sahota, M.S.; Johnson, M.M. Effect of External Dead Volume on Performance While Wearing a Respirator. AIHAJ-Am. Ind. Hyg. Assoc. 2000, 61, 678–684.

[14] Georgi, C.; Haase-Fielitz, A.; Meretz, D.; Gäsert, L.; Butter, C. Einfluss gängiger Gesichtsmasken auf physiologische Parameter und Belastungsempfinden unter arbeitstypischer körperlicher Anstrengung. Deutsches Ärzteblatt 2020, 674–675.

[15] Kyung, S.Y.; Kim, Y.; Hwang, H.; Park, J.-W.; Jeong, S.H. Risks of N95 Face Mask Use in Subjects with COPD. Respir. Care 2020, 65, 658–664.

[16] Johnson, A.T. Respirator Masks Protect Health but Impact Performance: A Review. J. Biol. Eng. 2016, 10, 4.

[17] Fikenzer, S.; Uhe, T.; Lavall, D.; Rudolph, U.; Falz, R.; Busse, M.; Hepp, P.; Laufs, U. Effects of Surgical and FFP2/N95 Face Masks on Cardiopulmonary Exercise Capacity. Clin. Res. Cardiol. 2020, 109, 1522–1530.

[18] Tong, P.S.Y.; Kale, A.S.; Ng, K.; Loke, A.P.; Choolani, M.A.; Lim, C.L.; Chan, Y.H.; Chong, Y.S.; Tambyah, P.A.; Yong, E.-L. Respiratory Consequences of N95-Type Mask Usage in Pregnant Healthcare Workers — A Controlled Clinical Study. Antimicrob. Resist. Infect. Control 2015, 4, 48.

[19] Liu, C.; Li, G.; He, Y.; Zhang, Z.; Ding, Y. Effects of Wearing Masks on Human Health and Comfort during the COVID-19 Pandemic. IOP Conf. Ser. Earth Environ. Sci. 2020, 531, 012034.

[20] Beder, A.; Büyükkoçak, U.; Sabuncuo ̄glu, H.; Keskil, Z.A.; Keskil, S. Preliminary Report on Surgical Mask Induced Deoxygenation during Major Surgery. Neurocirugía 2008, 19, 121–126.

[21] Jagim, A.R.; Dominy, T.A.; Camic, C.L.; Wright, G.; Doberstein, S.; Jones, M.T.; Oliver, J.M. Acute Effects of the Elevation Training Mask on Strength Performance in Recreational Weight Lifters. J. Strength Cond. Res. 2018, 32, 482–489.

[22] Butz, U. Rückatmung von Kohlendioxid bei Verwendung von Operationsmasken als hygienischer Mundschutz an medizinischem Fachpersonal. Ph.D. Thesis, Fakultät für Medizin der Technischen Universität München, Munich, Germany, 2005.

[23] Roberge, R.J.; Kim, J.-H.; Benson, S.M. Absence of Consequential Changes in Physiological, Thermal and Subjective Responses from Wearing a Surgical Mask. Respir. Physiol. Neurobiol. 2012, 181, 29–35.

[24] Rebmann, T.; Carrico, R.; Wang, J. Physiologic and Other Effects and Compliance with Long-Term Respirator Use among Medical Intensive Care Unit Nurses. Am. J. Infect. Control 2013, 41, 1218–1223.

[25] Roberge, R.J.; Kim, J.-H.; Powell, J.B. N95 Respirator Use during Advanced Pregnancy. Am. J. Infect. Control 2014, 42, 1097–1100.

[26] Epstein, D.; Korytny, A.; Isenberg, Y.; Marcusohn, E.; Zukermann, R.; Bishop, B.; Minha, S.; Raz, A.; Miller, A. Return to Training in the COVID-19 Era: The Physiological Effects of Face Masks during Exercise. Scand. J. Med. Sci. Sports 2020.

[27] Goh, D.Y.T.; Mun, M.W.; Lee, W.L.J.; Teoh, O.H.; Rajgor, D.D. A Randomised Clinical Trial to Evaluate the Safety, Fit, Comfort of a Novel N95 Mask in Children. Sci. Rep. 2019, 9, 18952.

[28] Bharatendu, C.; Ong, J.J.Y.; Goh, Y.; Tan, B.Y.Q.; Chan, A.C.Y.; Tang, J.Z.Y.; Leow, A.S.; Chin, A.; Sooi, K.W.X.; Tan, Y.L.; et al. Powered Air Purifying Respirator (PAPR) Restores the N95 Face Mask Induced Cerebral Hemodynamic Alterations among Healthcare Workers during COVID-19 Outbreak. J. Neurol. Sci. 2020, 417, 117078.

[29] Liu, C.; Li, G.; He, Y.; Zhang, Z.; Ding, Y. Effects of Wearing Masks on Human Health and Comfort during the COVID-19 Pandemic. IOP Conf. Ser. Earth Environ. Sci. 2020, 531, 012034.

[30] Beder, A.; Büyükkoçak, U.; Sabuncuo ̄glu, H.; Keskil, Z.A.; Keskil, S. Preliminary Report on Surgical Mask Induced Deoxygenation during Major Surgery. Neurocirugía 2008, 19, 121–126.

[31] Li, Y.; Tokura, H.; Guo, Y.P.; Wong, A.S.W.; Wong, T.; Chung, J.; Newton, E. Effects of Wearing N95 and Surgical Facemasks on Heart Rate, Thermal Stress and Subjective Sensations. Int. Arch. Occup. Environ. Health 2005, 78, 501–509.

[32] Morris, L.S.; McCall, J.G.; Charney, D.S.; Murrough, J.W. The Role of the Locus Coeruleus in the Generation of Pathological Anxiety. Brain Neurosci. Adv. 2020, 4.

[33] Gorman, J.M.; Askanazi, J.; Liebowitz, M.R.; Fyer, A.J.; Stein, J.; Kinney, J.M.; Klein, D.F. Response to Hyperventilation in a Group of Patients with Panic Disorder. Am. J. Psychiatry 1984, 141, 857–861.

[34] Andresen, M.C.; Kunze, D.L. Nucleus Tractus Solitarius–Gateway to Neural Circulatory Control. Annu. Rev. Physiol. 1994, 56, 93–116.

[35] Kline, D.D.; Ramirez-Navarro, A.; Kunze, D.L. Adaptive Depression in Synaptic Transmission in the Nucleus of the Solitary Tract after In Vivo Chronic Intermittent Hypoxia: Evidence for Homeostatic Plasticity. J. Neurosci. 2007, 27, 4663–4673.

[36] King, T.L.; Heesch, C.M.; Clark, C.G.; Kline, D.D.; Hasser, E.M. Hypoxia Activates Nucleus Tractus Solitarii Neurons Projecting to the Paraventricular Nucleus of the Hypothalamus. Am. J. Physiol. Regul. Integr. Comp. Physiol. 2012, 302, R1219–R1232.

[37] Russo, M.A.; Santarelli, D.M.; O'Rourke, D. The Physiological Effects of Slow Breathing in the Healthy Human. Breathe 2017, 13, 298–309.

[38] Nuckowska, M.K.; Gruszecki, M.; Kot, J.; Wolf, J.; Guminski, W.; Frydrychowski, A.F.; Wtorek, J.; Narkiewicz, K.; Winklewski, P.J. Impact of Slow Breathing on the Blood Pressure and Subarachnoid Space Width Oscillations in Humans. Sci. Rep. 2019, 9, 6232.

[39] Azuma, K.; Kagi, N.; Yanagi, U.; Osawa, H. Effects of Low-Level Inhalation Exposure to Carbon Dioxide in Indoor Environments: A Short Review on Human Health and Psychomotor Performance. Environ. Int. 2018, 121, 51–56.

[40] Cress ML, Forrester K, Probst L, Foster C, Doberstein S, Porcari JP. Effect of Wearing the Elevation Training Mask on Aerobic Capacity, Lung Function, and Hematological Variables. Medicine & Science in Sports & Exercise. 2016;48:1040-1041. doi:10.1249/01.mss.0000488131.38685.16.

[41] Shenal, B.V.; Radonovich, L.J.; Cheng, J.; Hodgson, M.; Bender, B.S. Discomfort and Exertion Associated with Prolonged Wear of Respiratory Protection in a Health Care Setting. J. Occup. Environ. Hyg. 2011, 9, 59–64.

[42] Kaw, R.; Hernandez, A.V.; Walker, E.; Aboussouan, L.; Mokhlesi, B. Determinants of Hypercapnia in Obese Patients with Obstructive Sleep Apnea: A Systematic Review and Metaanalysis of Cohort Studies. Chest 2009, 136, 787–796.

Reason 153: Face Masks Harm Cancer Patients

[1] Blaylock R, Dr. Blaylock Warns: Face Masks Pose Serious Risks To The Healthy, The Greg Anthony show & His Investigative Journal, 2020. Retrieved from https://greganthonysjournal.wordpress.com/2020/06/23/dr-blaylock-warns-face-masks-pose-serious-risks-to-the-healthy/

[2] Centers for Disease Control and Prevention. Leading Causes of Death. 2019. Retrieved from https://www.cdc.gov/nchs/fastats/leading-causes-of-death.htm. https://www.cdc.gov/nchs/data/nvsr/nvsr70/nvsr70-09-tables-508.pdf

Reason 154: Face Masks Weaken Immunity, And Therefore May Make Children MORE Susceptible To Covid-19

[1] Coleman, V. Dr. Proof That Face Masks Do More Harm Than Good. *Freedom of Speech*. 2021. Retrieved from https://fos-sa.org/2021/01/06/proof-that-face-masks-do-more-harm-than-good/

Reason 155: Face Masks Reduce Healthy Functioning Of The Immune System

[1] Singleton MM. Mask Facts. Association of American Physicians and Surgeons. 2021. Retrieved from https://aapsonline.org/mask-facts/

[2] Self WH, Tenforde MW, Stubblefield WB, et al. Seroprevalence of Sars-Cov-2 Among Frontline Health Care Personnel in a Multistate Hospital Network — 13 Academic Medical Centers, April–June 2020. MMWR Morb Mortal Wkly Rep 2020;69:1221–1226. DOI: http://dx.doi.org/10.15585/mmwr.mm6935e2

Reason 156: Face Mask Wearing Increases Leptin Release

[1] Kisielinski K, Giboni P, Prescher A, et al. Is a Mask That Covers the Mouth and Nose Free from Undesirable Side Effects in Everyday Use and Free of Potential Hazards? International Journal of Environmental Research and Public Health. 2021;18(8):4344. doi:10.3390/ijerph18084344.

[2] Zoccal, D.B.; Furuya, W.I.; Bassi, M.; Colombari, D.S.A.; Colombari, E. The Nucleus of the Solitary Tract and the Coordination of Respiratory and Sympathetic Activities. Front. Physiol. 2014, 5, 238.

Reason 157: Face Mask Wearing May Negatively Influence Metabolism All The Way Down To The Cellular Level

[1] Kisielinski K, Giboni P, Prescher A, et al. Is a Mask That Covers the Mouth and Nose Free from Undesirable Side Effects in Everyday Use and Free of Potential Hazards? International Journal of Environmental Research and Public Health. 2021;18(8):4344. doi:10.3390/ijerph18084344.

[2] Cummins, E.P.; Strowitzki, M.J.; Taylor, C.T. Mechanisms and Consequences of Oxygen and Carbon Dioxide Sensing in Mammals. Physiol. Rev. 2020, 100, 463–488.

Reason 159: Masks Harm Teeth And Gums And Cause A Condition Known As "Mask Mouth"

[1] Vernon Dr. Dr. Vernon coleman: masks and mask wearing: 100 facts you must know. *World Doctors Alliance*. 2021. Retrieved from https://worlddoctorsalliance.com/de/blog/vernon-coleman-more-harm-than-good/

[2] Singleton MM. Mask Facts. Association of American Physicians and Surgeons. 2021. Retrieved from https://aapsonline.org/mask-facts/

[3] Miller, A.M. Dentists say 'mask mouth' can cause serious health complications, including strokes. *Washington Examiner*. 2020. Retrieved from https://www.washingtonexaminer.com/news/mask-mouth-dentists-warn-prolonged-use-of-masks-leading-to-poor-oral-hygiene

[4] Court, A. Dentists declare 'mask mouth' a new phenomenon as they see an explosion in patients suffering from tooth decay and gum disease after wearing face coverings. *Daily Mail*. 2020. Retrieved from https://www.dailymail.co.uk/news/article-8604639/Dentists-says-mask-wearing-causing-tooth-decay-gum-disease.html

[5] Licea, M. 'Mask mouth' is a seriously stinky side effect of wearing masks. New York Post. 2020. Retrieved from https://nypost.com/2020/08/05/mask-mouth-is-a-seriously-stinky-side-effect-of-wearing-masks/

Reason 160: Mask Wearing Causes "Mask Mouth" And Other Harm

[1] Kisielinski K, Giboni P, Prescher A, et al. Is a Mask That Covers the Mouth and Nose Free from Undesirable Side Effects in Everyday Use and Free of Potential Hazards? International Journal of Environmental Research and Public Health. 2021;18(8):4344. doi:10.3390/ijerph18084344.

[2] Muley, P.; 'Mask Mouth'-a Novel Threat to Oral Health in the COVID Era–Dr Pooja Muley. Dental Tribune South Asia 2020. Available online: https://in.dental-tribune.com/news/mask-mouth-a-novel-threat-to-oral-health-in-the-covid-era/ (accessed on 12 November 2020).

[3] Liu, C.; Li, G.; He, Y.; Zhang, Z.; Ding, Y. Effects of Wearing Masks on Human Health and Comfort during the COVID-19 Pandemic. IOP Conf. Ser. Earth Environ. Sci. 2020, 531, 012034.

[4] Lee HP.; Wang DY. Objective Assessment of Increase in Breathing Resistance of N95 Respirators on Human Subjects. Ann.Occup. Hyg. 2011, 55, 917–921.

[5] Roberge, R.; Bayer, E.; Powell, J.; Coca, A.; Roberge, M.; Benson, S. Effect of Exhaled Moisture on Breathing Resistance of N95 Filtering Facepiece Respirators. Ann. Occup. Hyg. 2010, 54, 671–677.

[6] Matusiak, Ł.; Szepietowska, M.; Krajewski, P.; Białynicki-Birula, R.; Szepietowski, J.C. Inconveniences Due to the Use of Face Masks during the COVID-19 Pandemic: A Survey Study of 876 Young People. Dermatol. Ther. 2020, 33, e13567.

[7] Hua, W.; Zuo, Y.; Wan, R.; Xiong, L.; Tang, J.; Zou, L.; Shu, X.; Li, L. Short-Term Skin Reactions Following Use of N95 Respirators and Medical Masks. Contact Dermat. 2020, 83, 115–121.

[8] Scarano, A.; Inchingolo, F.; Lorusso, F. Facial Skin Temperature and Discomfort When Wearing Protective Face Masks: Thermal Infrared Imaging Evaluation and Hands Moving the Mask. Int. J. Environ. Res. Public Health 2020, 17, 4624.

Reason 161: Face Mask Wearing Exacerbates Existing Voice Disorders And May Trigger New Voice Disorders

[1] Kisielinski K, Giboni P, Prescher A, et al. Is a Mask That Covers the Mouth and Nose Free from Undesirable Side Effects in Everyday Use and Free of Potential Hazards? International Journal of Environmental Research and Public Health. 2021;18(8):4344. doi:10.3390/ijerph18084344.

[2] Heider, C.A.; Álvarez, M.L.; Fuentes-López, E.; González, C.A.; León, N.I.; Verástegui, D.C.; Badía, P.I.; Napolitano, C.A. Prevalence of Voice Disorders in Healthcare Workers in the Universal Masking COVID-19 Era. Laryngoscope 2020.

Reason 162: Face Mask Wearing Has Caused A New Condition, A Form Of Face Mask-Induced Rhinitis

[1] Kisielinski K, Giboni P, Prescher A, et al. Is a Mask That Covers the Mouth and Nose Free from Undesirable Side Effects in Everyday Use and Free of Potential Hazards? International Journal of Environmental Research and Public Health. 2021;18(8):4344. doi:10.3390/ijerph18084344.

[2] Klimek, L.; Huppertz, T.; Alali, A.; Spielhaupter, M.; Hörmann, K.; Matthias, C.; Hagemann, J. A New Form of Irritant Rhinitis to Filtering Facepiece Particle (FFP) Masks (FFP2/N95/KN95 Respirators) during COVID-19 Pandemic. World Allergy Organ. J. 2020, 13, 100474.

Reason 163: Face Masks Deform Children's Ears

[1] Rancourt, D.G. Review of scientific reports of harms caused by face masks, up to February 2021. *Children's Health Defence*. 2021. DOI: 10.13140/RG.2.2.14294.37448. Retrieved from https://childrenshealthdefense.org/wp-content/uploads/5thsciencereview-masksharm-1.pdf

[2] 2020--Zanotti : Zanotti, B., Parodi, P.C., Riccio, M. et al. "Can the Elastic of Surgical Face Masks Stimulate Ear Protrusion in Children?". Aesth Plast Surg 44, 1947–1950 (2020). https://doi.org/10.1007/s00266-020-01833-9 — https://link.springer.com/article/10.1007/s00266-020-01833-9

Reason 164: Face Masks Are Bad For Your Face

[1] Vernon Dr. Dr. Vernon coleman: masks and mask wearing: 100 facts you must know. *World Doctors Alliance*. 2021. Retrieved from https://worlddoctorsalliance.com/de/blog/vernon-coleman-more-harm-than-good/

Reason 165: Face Mask Wearing Harms The Skin

[1] Kisielinski K, Giboni P, Prescher A, et al. Is a Mask That Covers the Mouth and Nose Free from Undesirable Side Effects in Everyday Use and Free of Potential Hazards? International Journal of Environmental Research and Public Health. 2021;18(8):4344. doi:10.3390/ijerph18084344.

[2] Roberge, R.J.; Kim, J.-H.; Benson, S.M. Absence of Consequential Changes in Physiological, Thermal and Subjective Responses from Wearing a Surgical Mask. Respir. Physiol. Neurobiol. 2012, 181, 29–35.

481

[3] Roberge, R.J.; Kim, J.-H.; Coca, A. Protective Facemask Impact on Human Thermoregulation: An Overview. Ann. Occup. Hyg. 2012, 56, 102–112.

[4] Scarano, A.; Inchingolo, F.; Lorusso, F. Facial Skin Temperature and Discomfort When Wearing Protective Face Masks: Thermal Infrared Imaging Evaluation and Hands Moving the Mask. Int. J. Environ. Res. Public Health 2020, 17, 4624.

[5] Johnson, A.T. Respirator Masks Protect Health but Impact Performance: A Review. J. Biol. Eng. 2016, 10, 4.

[6] Roberge, R.; Bayer, E.; Powell, J.; Coca, A.; Roberge, M.; Benson, S. Effect of Exhaled Moisture on Breathing Resistance of N95 Filtering Facepiece Respirators. Ann. Occup. Hyg. 2010, 54, 671–677.

[7] COVID-19: Considerations for Wearing Masks CDC. Available online: https://www.cdc.gov/coronavirus/2019-ncov/preventgetting-sick/cloth-face-cover-guidance.html (accessed on 12 November 2020).

[8] Hua, W.; Zuo, Y.; Wan, R.; Xiong, L.; Tang, J.; Zou, L.; Shu, X.; Li, L. Short-Term Skin Reactions Following Use of N95 Respirators and Medical Masks. Contact Dermat. 2020, 83, 115–121.

[9] Luksamijarulkul, P.; Aiempradit, N.; Vatanasomboon, P. Microbial Contamination on Used Surgical Masks among Hospital Personnel and Microbial Air Quality in Their Working Wards: A Hospital in Bangkok. Oman Med. J. 2014, 29, 346–350.

[10] Chughtai, A.A.; Stelzer-Braid, S.; Rawlinson, W.; Pontivivo, G.; Wang, Q.; Pan, Y.; Zhang, D.; Zhang, Y.; Li, L.; MacIntyre, C.R. Contamination by Respiratory Viruses on Outer Surface of Medical Masks Used by Hospital Healthcare Workers. BMC Infect. Dis. 2019, 19, 491.

[11] Monalisa, A.C.; Padma, K.B.; Manjunath, K.; Hemavathy, E.; Varsha, D. Microbial Contamination of the Mouth Masks Used by Post-Graduate Students in a Private Dental Institution: An In-Vitro Study. IOSR J. Dent. Med. Sci. 2017, 16, 61–67.

[12] Liu, Z.; Chang, Y.; Chu, W.; Yan, M.; Mao, Y.; Zhu, Z.; Wu, H.; Zhao, J.; Dai, K.; Li, H.; et al. Surgical Masks as Source of Bacterial Contamination during Operative Procedures. J. Orthop. Transl. 2018, 14, 57–62.

[13] Robert Koch-Institut. Influenza-Monatsbericht; Robert Koch-Institut: Berlin, Germany, 2020.

[14] Techasatian, L.; Lebsing, S.; Uppala, R.; Thaowandee, W.; Chaiyarit, J.; Supakunpinyo, C.; Panombualert, S.; Mairiang, D.; Saengnipanthkul, S.; Wichajarn, K.; et al. The Effects of the Face Mask on the Skin Underneath: A Prospective Survey During the COVID-19 Pandemic. J. Prim. Care Community Health 2020, 11, 2150132720966167.

[15] Lan, J.; Song, Z.; Miao, X.; Li, H.; Li, Y.; Dong, L.; Yang, J.; An, X.; Zhang, Y.; Yang, L.; et al. Skin Damage among Health Care Workers Managing Coronavirus Disease-2019. J. Am. Acad. Dermatol. 2020, 82, 1215–1216.

[16] Rosner, E. Adverse Effects of Prolonged Mask Use among Healthcare Professionals during COVID-19. J. Infect. Dis. Epidemiol. 2020.

[17] Liu, C.; Li, G.; He, Y.; Zhang, Z.; Ding, Y. Effects of Wearing Masks on Human Health and Comfort during the COVID-19 Pandemic. IOP Conf. Ser. Earth Environ. Sci. 2020, 531, 012034.

[18] Foo, C.C.I.; Goon, A.T.J.; Leow, Y.; Goh, C. Adverse Skin Reactions to Personal Protective Equipment against Severe Acute Respiratory Syndrome–a Descriptive Study in Singapore. Contact Dermat. 2006, 55, 291–294.

[19] Szepietowski, J.C.; Matusiak, Ł.; Szepietowska, M.; Krajewski, P.K.; Białynicki-Birula, R. Face Mask-Induced Itch: A SelfQuestionnaire Study of 2,315 Responders during the COVID-19 Pandemic. Acta Derm.-Venereol. 2020, 100, adv00152.

[20] Matusiak, Ł.; Szepietowska, M.; Krajewski, P.; Białynicki-Birula, R.; Szepietowski, J.C. Inconveniences Due to the Use of Face Masks during the COVID-19 Pandemic: A Survey Study of 876 Young People. Dermatol. Ther. 2020, 33, e13567.

[21] Badri, F.M.A. Surgical Mask Contact Dermatitis and Epidemiology of Contact Dermatitis in Healthcare Workers. Curr. Allergy Clin. Immunol. 2017, 30, 183–188.

[22] Darlenski, R.; Tsankov, N. COVID-19 Pandemic and the Skin: What Should Dermatologists Know? Clin. Dermatol. 2020.

Reason 166: Face Mask Use Is Harmful To Eyes

[1] Moshirfar M, West WB Jr, Marx DP. Face Mask-Associated Ocular Irritation and Dryness. Ophthalmol Ther. 2020;9(3):397-400. doi:10.1007/s40123-020-00282-6

Reason 168: Face Masks Are Hard On The Kidneys

[1] Chandrasekaran B, Fernandes S. "Exercise with facemask; Are we handling a devil's sword?" — A physiological hypothesis. Med Hypotheses. 2020;144:110002. doi:10.1016/j.mehy.2020.110002

[2] Voulgaris A., Marrone O., Bonsignore M.R., Steiropoulos P. Chronic kidney disease in patients with obstructive sleep apnea. A narrative review. Sleep Med Rev. 2019;10(47):74–89

[3] Huang Y.S., Guilleminault C., Hwang F.M., Cheng C., Lin C.H., Li H.Y. Inflammatory cytokines in pediatric obstructive sleep apnea. Medicine (Baltimore) 2016;95(41)

Reason 169: N95 Respirators Are Bad For Your Kidneys As Well

[1] Vainshelboim B. Retracted: Facemasks in the COVID-19 era: A health hypothesis [retracted in: Med Hypotheses. 2021 May 12;:110601]. Med Hypotheses. 2021;146:110411. doi:10.1016/j.mehy.2020.110411

[2] Kao T.W., Huang K.C., Huang Y.L., Tsai T.J., Hsieh B.S., Wu M.S. The physiological impact of wearing an N95 mask during hemodialysis as a precaution against SARS in patients with end-stage renal disease. J Formos Med Assoc. 2004;103:624–628.

[3] United States Department of Labor. Occupational Safety and Health Administration. Respiratory Protection Standard, 29 CFR 1910.134; 2007.

[4] Zheng G.Q., Wang Y., Wang X.T. Chronic hypoxia-hypercapnia influences cognitive function: a possible new model of cognitive dysfunction in chronic obstructive pulmonary disease. Med Hypotheses. 2008;71:111–113.

Reason 170: You Need To Breathe, Everyone Needs To Breathe, Your Child Even Needs To Breathe

[1] Vainshelboim B. Retracted: Facemasks in the COVID-19 era: A health hypothesis [retracted in: Med Hypotheses. 2021 May 12;:110601]. Med Hypotheses. 2021;146:110411. doi:10.1016/j.mehy.2020.110411

[2] Farrell P.A., Joyner M.J., Caiozzo V.J. second edition. Lippncott Williams & Wilkins; Baltimore: 2012. ACSM's Advanced Exercise Physiology.

[3] Kenney W.L., Wilmore J.H., Costill D.L. 5th ed. Human Kinetics; Champaign, IL: 2012. Physiology of sport and exercise.

[4] American College of Sports Medicine . Sixth ed. Lippincott Wiliams & Wilkins; Baltimore: 2010. ACSM's Resource Manual for Guidelines for Exercise Testing and Priscription.

[5] (Patil K.D., Halperin H.R., Becker L.B. Cardiac arrest: resuscitation and reperfusion. Circ Res. 2015;116:2041–2049.

[6] Hazinski M.F., Nolan J.P., Billi J.E., Bottiger B.W., Bossaert L., de Caen A.R. Part 1: Executive summary: 2010 International Consensus on Cardiopulmonary Resuscitation and Emergency Cardiovascular Care Science With Treatment Recommendations. Circulation. 2010;122:S250–S275.

[7] Kleinman M.E., Goldberger Z.D., Rea T., Swor R.A., Bobrow B.J., Brennan E.E. American Heart Association Focused Update on Adult Basic Life Support and Cardiopulmonary Resuscitation Quality: An Update to the American Heart Association Guidelines for Cardiopulmonary Resuscitation and Emergency Cardiovascular Care. Circulation. 2018;137:e7–e13.

[8] Patil K.D., Halperin H.R., Becker L.B. Cardiac arrest: resuscitation and reperfusion. Circ Res. 2015;116:2041–2049.

[9] Hazinski M.F., Nolan J.P., Billi J.E., Bottiger B.W., Bossaert L., de Caen A.R. Part 1: Executive summary: 2010 International Consensus on Cardiopulmonary Resuscitation and Emergency Cardiovascular Care Science With Treatment Recommendations. Circulation. 2010;122:S250–S275.

[10] Kleinman M.E., Goldberger Z.D., Rea T., Swor R.A., Bobrow B.J., Brennan E.E. American Heart Association Focused Update on Adult Basic Life Support and Cardiopulmonary Resuscitation Quality: An Update to the American Heart Association Guidelines for Cardiopulmonary Resuscitation and Emergency Cardiovascular Care. Circulation. 2018;137:e7–e13.

[11] Lurie K.G., Nemergut E.C., Yannopoulos D., Sweeney M. The Physiology of Cardiopulmonary Resuscitation. Anesth Analg. 2016;122:767–783.

[12] Chandrasekaran B., Fernandes S. "Exercise with facemask; Are we handling a devil's sword?" — A physiological hypothesis. Med Hypotheses. 2020;144

[13] American College of Sports Medicine . Sixth ed. Lippincott Wiliams & Wilkins; Baltimore: 2010. ACSM's Resource Manual for Guidelines for Exercise Testing and Priscription.

[14] Farrell P.A., Joyner M.J., Caiozzo V.J. second edition. Lippncott Williams & Wilkins; Baltimore: 2012. ACSM's Advanced Exercise Physiology.

[15] Kenney W.L., Wilmore J.H., Costill D.L. 5th ed. Human Kinetics; Champaign, IL: 2012. Physiology of sport and exercise.

[16] Farrell P.A., Joyner M.J., Caiozzo V.J. second edition. Lippncott Williams & Wilkins; Baltimore: 2012. ACSM's Advanced Exercise Physiology.

[17] Kenney W.L., Wilmore J.H., Costill D.L. 5th ed. Human Kinetics; Champaign, IL: 2012. Physiology of sport and exercise.

[18] Laveneziana P., Albuquerque A., Aliverti A., Babb T., Barreiro E., Dres M. ERS statement on respiratory muscle testing at rest and during exercise. Eur Respir J. 2019;53

[19] American Thoracic Society/European Respiratory, S ATS/ERS Statement on respiratory muscle testing. Am J Respir Crit Care Med. 2002;166:518–624.

[20] American College of Sports Medicine . Sixth ed. Lippincott Wiliams & Wilkins; Baltimore: 2010. ACSM's Resource Manual for Guidelines for Exercise Testing and Priscription.

[21] Farrell P.A., Joyner M.J., Caiozzo V.J. second edition. Lippncott Williams & Wilkins; Baltimore: 2012. ACSM's Advanced Exercise Physiology.

[22] Kenney W.L., Wilmore J.H., Costill D.L. 5th ed. Human Kinetics; Champaign, IL: 2012. Physiology of sport and exercise.

[23] Kao T.W., Huang K.C., Huang Y.L., Tsai T.J., Hsieh B.S., Wu M.S. The physiological impact of wearing an N95 mask during hemodialysis as a precaution against SARS in patients with end-stage renal disease. J Formos Med Assoc. 2004;103:624–628.

[24] United States Department of Labor. Occupational Safety and Health Administration. Respiratory Protection Standard, 29 CFR 1910.134; 2007.

[25] American College of Sports Medicine . Sixth ed. Lippincott Wiliams & Wilkins; Baltimore: 2010. ACSM's Resource Manual for Guidelines for Exercise Testing and Priscription.

[26] Farrell P.A., Joyner M.J., Caiozzo V.J. second edition. Lippncott Williams & Wilkins; Baltimore: 2012. ACSM's Advanced Exercise Physiology.

[27] Kenney W.L., Wilmore J.H., Costill D.L. 5th ed. Human Kinetics; Champaign, IL: 2012. Physiology of sport and exercise.

[28] ATS/ACCP Statement on cardiopulmonary exercise testing Am J Respir Crit Care Med. 2003;167:211–277.

[29] American College of Sports Medicine . 9th ed. Wolters Kluwer/Lippincott Williams & Wilkins Health; Philadelphia: 2014. ACSM's guidelines for exercise testing and prescription.

[30] Balady G.J., Arena R., Sietsema K., Myers J., Coke L., Fletcher G.F. Clinician's Guide to cardiopulmonary exercise testing in adults: a scientific statement from the American Heart Association. Circulation. 2010;122:191–225.

[31] Ferrazza A.M., Martolini D., Valli G., Palange P. Cardiopulmonary exercise testing in the functional and prognostic evaluation of patients with pulmonary diseases. Respiration. 2009;77:3–17.

[32] Fletcher G.F., Ades P.A., Kligfield P., Arena R., Balady G.J., Bittner V.A. Exercise standards for testing and training: a scientific statement from the American Heart Association. Circulation. 2013;128:873–934.

[33] Guazzi M., Adams V., Conraads V., Halle M., Mezzani A., Vanhees L. EACPR/AHA Scientific Statement. Clinical recommendations for cardiopulmonary exercise testing data assessment in specific patient populations. Circulation. 2012;126:2261–2274.

[34] Naeije R., Dedobbeleer C. Pulmonary hypertension and the right ventricle in hypoxia. Exp Physiol. 2013;98:1247–1256.

[35] ATS/ACCP Statement on cardiopulmonary exercise testing Am J Respir Crit Care Med. 2003;167:211–277.

[36] American College of Sports Medicine . 9th ed. Wolters Kluwer/Lippincott Williams & Wilkins Health; Philadelphia: 2014. ACSM's guidelines for exercise testing and prescription.

[37] Balady G.J., Arena R., Sietsema K., Myers J., Coke L., Fletcher G.F. Clinician's Guide to cardiopulmonary exercise testing in adults: a scientific statement from the American Heart Association. Circulation. 2010;122:191–225.

[38] Ferrazza A.M., Martolini D., Valli G., Palange P. Cardiopulmonary exercise testing in the functional and prognostic evaluation of patients with pulmonary diseases. Respiration. 2009;77:3–17.

[39] Fletcher G.F., Ades P.A., Kligfield P., Arena R., Balady G.J., Bittner V.A. Exercise standards for testing and training: a scientific statement from the American Heart Association. Circulation. 2013;128:873–934.

[40] Guazzi M., Adams V., Conraads V., Halle M., Mezzani A., Vanhees L. EACPR/AHA Scientific Statement. Clinical recommendations for cardiopulmonary exercise testing data assessment in specific patient populations. Circulation. 2012;126:2261–2274.

[41] Fisher E.M., Noti J.D., Lindsley W.G., Blachere F.M., Shaffer R.E. Validation and application of models to predict facemask influenza contamination in healthcare settings. Risk Anal. 2014;34:1423–1434.

[42] World Health Organization. Advice on the use of masks in the context of COVID-19. Geneva, Switzerland; 2020.

[43] MacIntyre C.R., Seale H., Dung T.C., Hien N.T., Nga P.T., Chughtai A.A. A cluster randomised trial of cloth masks compared with medical masks in healthcare workers. BMJ open. 2015;5

[44] Leung N.H.L., Chu D.K.W., Shiu E.Y.C., Chan K.H., McDevitt J.J., Hau B.J.P. Respiratory virus shedding in exhaled breath and efficacy of face masks. Nat Med. 2020;26:676–680.

[45] Kao T.W., Huang K.C., Huang Y.L., Tsai T.J., Hsieh B.S., Wu M.S. The physiological impact of wearing an N95 mask during hemodialysis as a precaution against SARS in patients with end-stage renal disease. J Formos Med Assoc. 2004;103:624–628.

[46] United States Department of Labor. Occupational Safety and Health Administration. Respiratory Protection Standard, 29 CFR 1910.134; 2007.

[47] Fisher E.M., Noti J.D., Lindsley W.G., Blachere F.M., Shaffer R.E. Validation and application of models to predict facemask influenza contamination in healthcare settings. Risk Anal. 2014;34:1423–1434.

[48] Fisher E.M., Noti J.D., Lindsley W.G., Blachere F.M., Shaffer R.E. Validation and application of models to predict facemask influenza contamination in healthcare settings. Risk Anal. 2014;34:1423–1434.

[49] World Health Organization. Advice on the use of masks in the context of COVID-19. Geneva, Switzerland; 2020.

[50] MacIntyre C.R., Seale H., Dung T.C., Hien N.T., Nga P.T., Chughtai A.A. A cluster randomised trial of cloth masks compared with medical masks in healthcare workers. BMJ open. 2015;5

[51] Leung N.H.L., Chu D.K.W., Shiu E.Y.C., Chan K.H., McDevitt J.J., Hau B.J.P. Respiratory virus shedding in exhaled breath and efficacy of face masks. Nat Med. 2020;26:676–680.

[52] Kao T.W., Huang K.C., Huang Y.L., Tsai T.J., Hsieh B.S., Wu M.S. The physiological impact of wearing an N95 mask during hemodialysis as a precaution against SARS in patients with end-stage renal disease. J Formos Med Assoc. 2004;103:624–628.

[53] United States Department of Labor. Occupational Safety and Health Administration. Respiratory Protection Standard, 29 CFR 1910.134; 2007.

[54] Beder A., Buyukkocak U., Sabuncuoglu H., Keskil Z.A., Keskil S. Preliminary report on surgical mask induced deoxygenation during major surgery. Neurocirugia (Astur) 2008;19:121–126.

[55] Ong J.J.Y., Bharatendu C., Goh Y., Tang J.Z.Y., Sooi K.W.X., Tan Y.L. Headaches Associated With Personal Protective Equipment — A Cross-Sectional Study Among Frontline Healthcare Workers During COVID-19. Headache. 2020;60: 864–877.

Reason 171: Face Masks Affect The Heart

[1] Rancourt, D.G. Review of scientific reports of harms caused by face masks, up to February 2021. *Children's Health Defence.* 2021. DOI: 10.13140/RG.2.2.14294.37448. Retrieved from https://childrenshealthdefense.org/wp-content/uploads/5thsciencereview-masksharm-1.pdf

Reason 172: Face Masks Lead To Exhaustion And An Increased Stress On The Heart

[1] Kisielinski K, Giboni P, Prescher A, et al. Is a Mask That Covers the Mouth and Nose Free from Undesirable Side Effects in Everyday Use and Free of Potential Hazards? International Journal of Environmental Research and Public Health. 2021;18(8):4344. doi:10.3390/ijerph18084344.

[2] Li, Y.; Tokura, H.; Guo, Y.P.; Wong, A.S.W.; Wong, T.; Chung, J.; Newton, E. Effects of Wearing N95 and Surgical Facemasks on Heart Rate, Thermal Stress and Subjective Sensations. Int. Arch. Occup. Environ. Health 2005, 78, 501–509.

Reason 174: Face Mask Wearing Comes With Environmental Effects

[1] Kisielinski K, Giboni P, Prescher A, et al. Is a Mask That Covers the Mouth and Nose Free from Undesirable Side Effects in Everyday Use and Free of Potential Hazards? International Journal of Environmental Research and Public Health. 2021;18(8):4344. doi:10.3390/ijerph18084344.

[2] Fadare, O.O.; Okoffo, E.D. Covid-19 Face Masks: A Potential Source of Microplastic Fibers in the Environment. Sci. Total Environ. 2020, 737, 140279.

[3] Potluri, P.; Needham, P. Technical Textiles for Protection (Manchester EScholar-The University of Manchester); Woodhead Publishing: Cambridge, UK, 2005.

[4] Schnurr, R.E.J.; Alboiu, V.; Chaudhary, M.; Corbett, R.A.; Quanz, M.E.; Sankar, K.; Srain, H.S.; Thavarajah, V.; Xanthos, D.; Walker, T.R. Reducing Marine Pollution from Single-Use Plastics (SUPs): A Review. Mar. Pollut. Bull. 2018, 137, 157–171.

[5] Luksamijarulkul, P.; Aiempradit, N.; Vatanasomboon, P. Microbial Contamination on Used Surgical Masks among Hospital Personnel and Microbial Air Quality in Their Working Wards: A Hospital in Bangkok. Oman Med. J. 2014, 29, 346–350.

[6] Chughtai, A.A.; Stelzer-Braid, S.; Rawlinson, W.; Pontivivo, G.; Wang, Q.; Pan, Y.; Zhang, D.; Zhang, Y.; Li, L.; MacIntyre, C.R. Contamination by Respiratory Viruses on Outer Surface of Medical Masks Used by Hospital Healthcare Workers. BMC Infect. Dis. 2019, 19, 491.

[7] Monalisa, A.C.; Padma, K.B.; Manjunath, K.; Hemavathy, E.; Varsha, D. Microbial Contamination of the Mouth Masks Used by Post-Graduate Students in a Private Dental Institution: An In-Vitro Study. IOSR J. Dent. Med. Sci. 2017, 16, 61–67.

[8] Liu, Z.; Chang, Y.; Chu, W.; Yan, M.; Mao, Y.; Zhu, Z.; Wu, H.; Zhao, J.; Dai, K.; Li, H.; et al. Surgical Masks as Source of Bacterial Contamination during Operative Procedures. J. Orthop. Transl. 2018, 14, 57–62.

[9] Reid, A.J.; Carlson, A.K.; Creed, I.F.; Eliason, E.J.; Gell, P.A.; Johnson, P.T.J.; Kidd, K.A.; MacCormack, T.J.; Olden, J.D.; Ormerod, S.J.; et al. Emerging Threats and Persistent Conservation Challenges for Freshwater Biodiversity. Biol. Rev. Camb. Philos. Soc. 2019, 94, 849–873.

Reason 175: The Great Pacific Face Mask Patch

[1] Thomala LL. Daily production volume of medical face masks in China as of April 30, 2020, by type. 2021. Statista. Retrieved from: https://www.statista.com/statistics/1094428/china-medical-mask-daily-production-volume-by-type/

[2] Lu Marcus.1.6 Billion Disposable Masks Entered Our Oceans in 2020. *Visual Capitalist.* 2021. Retrieved from https://www.visualcapitalist.com/1-6-billion-disposable-masks-entered-our-oceans-in-2020/

[3] *Oceans Asia.* COVID-19 Facemasks & Marine Plastic Pollution. Retrieved from https://oceansasia.org/covid-19-facemasks/

Reason 176: Kids Are Not A Biohazard — Dirty Face Masks On The Ground Are The True Biohazard

[1] Bamber J H, Christmas T. Covid-19: Each discarded face mask is a potential biohazard BMJ 2020; 369 :m2012 doi:10.1136/bmj.m2012

[2] Javid B, Weekes MP, Matheson NJ. Covid-19: should the public wear face masks?BMJ2020;369:m1442. doi:10.1136/bmj.m1442 pmid:32273278FREE Full TextGoogle Scholar

[3] Chughtai AA, Stelzer-Braid S, Rawlinson W, et al. Contamination by respiratory viruses on outer surface of medical masks used by hospital healthcare workers. BMC Infect Dis2019;19:491. doi:10.1186/s12879-019-4109-x pmid:31159777CrossRefPubMedGoogle Scholar

[4] Shenal BV, Radonovich LJ Jr., Cheng J, Hodgson M, Bender BS. Discomfort and exertion associated with prolonged wear of respiratory protection in a health care setting. J Occup Environ Hyg2012;9:59-64. doi:10.1080/15459624.2012.635133 pmid:22168256CrossRefPubMedGoogle Scholar"

Reason 178: The Long-Term Consequences Of Face Mask Wearing Are Likely Far Worse Than We Can Imagine

[1] Vainshelboim B. Retracted: Facemasks in the COVID-19 era: A health hypothesis [retracted in: Med Hypotheses. 2021 May 12;:110601]. Med Hypotheses. 2021;146:110411. doi:10.1016/j.mehy.2020.110411

[2] Lurie K.G., Nemergut E.C., Yannopoulos D., Sweeney M. The Physiology of Cardiopulmonary Resuscitation. Anesth Analg. 2016;122:767–783.

[3] American College of Sports Medicine . 9th ed. Wolters Kluwer/Lippincott Williams & Wilkins Health; Philadelphia: 2014. ACSM's guidelines for exercise testing and prescription.

[4] Balady G.J., Arena R., Sietsema K., Myers J., Coke L., Fletcher G.F. Clinician's Guide to cardiopulmonary exercise testing in adults: a scientific statement from the American Heart Association. Circulation. 2010;122:191–225.

[5] Naeije R., Dedobbeleer C. Pulmonary hypertension and the right ventricle in hypoxia. Exp Physiol. 2013;98: 1247–1256.

[6] Schneiderman N., Ironson G., Siegel S.D. Stress and health: psychological, behavioral, and biological determinants. Annu Rev Clin Psychol. 2005;1:607–628.

[7] Thoits P.A. Stress and health: major findings and policy implications. J Health Soc Behav. 2010;51(Suppl):S41–S53.

[8] World Health Organization. World health statistics 2018: monitoring health for the SDGs, sustainable development goals Geneva, Switzerland; 2018.

[9] American College of Sports Medicine . Sixth ed. Lippincott Wiliams & Wilkins; Baltimore: 2010. ACSM's Resource Manual for Guidelines for Exercise Testing and Priscription.

[10] Farrell P.A., Joyner M.J., Caiozzo V.J. second edition. Lippncott Williams & Wilkins; Baltimore: 2012. ACSM's Advanced Exercise Physiology.

[11] Kenney W.L., Wilmore J.H., Costill D.L. 5th ed. Human Kinetics; Champaign, IL: 2012. Physiology of sport and exercise.

[12] World Health Organization. World health statistics 2018: monitoring health for the SDGs, sustainable development goals Geneva, Switzerland; 2018.

[13] World Health Organization. World Cancer Report 2014. Lyon; 2014.

[14] Wiggins J.M., Opoku-Acheampong A.B., Baumfalk D.R., Siemann D.W., Behnke B.J. Exercise and the Tumor Microenvironment: Potential Therapeutic Implications. Exerc Sport Sci Rev. 2018;46:56–64.

[15] Ashcraft K.A., Warner A.B., Jones L.W., Dewhirst M.W. Exercise as Adjunct Therapy in Cancer. Semin Radiat Oncol. 2019;29:16–24.

[16] Bray F., Ferlay J., Soerjomataram I., Siegel R.L., Torre L.A., Jemal A. Global Cancer Statistics 2018: GLOBOCAN Estimates of Incidence and Mortality Worldwide for 36 Cancers in 185 Countries. CA Cancer J Clin. 2018

[17] Brooks S.K., Webster R.K., Smith L.E., Woodland L., Wessely S., Greenberg N. The psychological impact of quarantine and how to reduce it: rapid review of the evidence. Lancet. 2020;395:912–920.

[18] Galea S., Merchant R.M., Lurie N. The Mental Health Consequences of COVID-19 and Physical Distancing: The Need for Prevention and Early Intervention. JAMA Intern Med. 2020;180:817–818.

[19] Izaguirre-Torres D., Siche R. Covid-19 disease will cause a global catastrophe in terms of mental health: A hypothesis. Med Hypotheses. 2020;143

[20] Schneiderman N., Ironson G., Siegel S.D. Stress and health: psychological, behavioral, and biological determinants. Annu Rev Clin Psychol. 2005;1:607–628.

[21] Thoits P.A. Stress and health: major findings and policy implications. J Health Soc Behav. 2010;51(Suppl):S41–S53.

[22] Kudielka B.M., Wust S. Human models in acute and chronic stress: assessing determinants of individual hypothalamus-pituitary-adrenal axis activity and reactivity. Stress. 2010;13:1–14.

[23] Morey J.N., Boggero I.A., Scott A.B., Segerstrom S.C. Current Directions in Stress and Human Immune Function. Curr Opin Psychol. 2015;5:13–17.

[24] Sapolsky R.M., Romero L.M., Munck A.U. How do glucocorticoids influence stress responses? Integrating permissive, suppressive, stimulatory, and preparative actions. Endocr Rev. 2000;21:55–89.

[25] Schneiderman N., Ironson G., Siegel S.D. Stress and health: psychological, behavioral, and biological determinants. Annu Rev Clin Psychol. 2005;1:607–628.

[26] Thoits P.A. Stress and health: major findings and policy implications. J Health Soc Behav. 2010;51(Suppl):S41–S53.

[27] Leigh-Hunt N., Bagguley D., Bash K., Turner V., Turnbull S., Valtorta N. An overview of systematic reviews on the public health consequences of social isolation and loneliness. Public Health. 2017;152:157–171.

[28] Everly G.S., Lating J.M. 4th ed. NY Springer Nature; New York: 2019. A Clinical Guide to the Treatment of the Human Stress Response.

[29] Morey J.N., Boggero I.A., Scott A.B., Segerstrom S.C. Current Directions in Stress and Human Immune Function. Curr Opin Psychol. 2015;5:13–17.

Reason 179: Face Mask Wearing Creates Symptoms Akin To "Sick Building Syndrome"

[1] Kisielinski K, Giboni P, Prescher A, et al. Is a Mask That Covers the Mouth and Nose Free from Undesirable Side Effects in Everyday Use and Free of Potential Hazards? International Journal of Environmental Research and Public Health. 2021;18(8):4344. doi:10.3390/ijerph18084344.

[2] Jafari, M.J.; Khajevandi, A.A.; Mousavi Najarkola, S.A.; Yekaninejad, M.S.; Pourhoseingholi, M.A.; Omidi, L.; Kalantary, S. Association of Sick Building Syndrome with Indoor Air Parameters. Tanaffos 2015, 14, 55–62.

[3] Redlich, C.A.; Sparer, J.; Cullen, M.R. Sick-Building Syndrome. Lancet 1997, 349, 1013–1016.

[4] Azuma, K.; Kagi, N.; Yanagi, U.; Osawa, H. Effects of Low-Level Inhalation Exposure to Carbon Dioxide in Indoor Environments: A Short Review on Human Health and Psychomotor Performance. Environ. Int. 2018, 121, 51–56.

[5] Georgi, C.; Haase-Fielitz, A.; Meretz, D.; Gäsert, L.; Butter, C. Einfluss gängiger Gesichtsmasken auf physiologische Parameter und Belastungsempfinden unter arbeitstypischer körperlicher Anstrengung. Deutsches Ärzteblatt 2020, 674–675.

[6] Fikenzer, S.; Uhe, T.; Lavall, D.; Rudolph, U.; Falz, R.; Busse, M.; Hepp, P.; Laufs, U. Effects of Surgical and FFP2/N95 Face Masks on Cardiopulmonary Exercise Capacity. Clin. Res. Cardiol. 2020, 109, 1522–1530.

[7] Kao, T.-W.; Huang, K.-C.; Huang, Y.-L.; Tsai, T.-J.; Hsieh, B.-S.; Wu, M.-S. The Physiological Impact of Wearing an N95 Mask during Hemodialysis as a Precaution against SARS in Patients with End-Stage Renal Disease. J. Formos. Med. Assoc. 2004, 103, 624–628.

[8] Mo, Y.; Wei, D.; Mai, Q.; Chen, C.; Yu, H.; Jiang, C.; Tan, X. Risk and Impact of Using Mask on COPD Patients with Acute Exacerbation during the COVID-19 Outbreak: A Retrospective Study. Res. Sq. 2020.

[9] Li, Y.; Tokura, H.; Guo, Y.P.; Wong, A.S.W.; Wong, T.; Chung, J.; Newton, E. Effects of Wearing N95 and Surgical Facemasks on Heart Rate, Thermal Stress and Subjective Sensations. Int. Arch. Occup. Environ. Health 2005, 78, 501–509.

Reason 180: Face Masks Lead To Mask-Induced Exhaustion Syndrome (MIES)

[1] Kisielinski K, Giboni P, Prescher A, et al. Is a Mask That Covers the Mouth and Nose Free from Undesirable Side Effects in Everyday Use and Free of Potential Hazards? International Journal of Environmental Research and Public Health. 2021;18(8):4344. doi:10.3390/ijerph18084344.

[2] Roberge, R.J.; Kim, J.-H.; Powell, J.B. N95 Respirator Use during Advanced Pregnancy. Am. J. Infect. Control 2014, 42, 1097–1100.

[3] Epstein, D.; Korytny, A.; Isenberg, Y.; Marcusohn, E.; Zukermann, R.; Bishop, B.; Minha, S.; Raz, A.; Miller, A. Return to Training in the COVID-19 Era: The Physiological Effects of Face Masks during Exercise. Scand. J. Med. Sci. Sports 2020.

[4] Johnson, A.T.; Scott, W.H.; Lausted, C.G.; Coyne, K.M.; Sahota, M.S.; Johnson, M.M. Effect of External Dead Volume on Performance While Wearing a Respirator. AIHAJ-Am. Ind. Hyg. Assoc. 2000, 61, 678–684.

[5] Xu, M.; Lei, Z.; Yang, J. Estimating the Dead Space Volume between a Headform and N95 Filtering Facepiece Respirator Using Microsoft Kinect. J. Occup. Environ. Hyg. 2015, 12, 538–546.

[6] Fikenzer, S.; Uhe, T.; Lavall, D.; Rudolph, U.; Falz, R.; Busse, M.; Hepp, P.; Laufs, U. Effects of Surgical and FFP2/N95 Face Masks on Cardiopulmonary Exercise Capacity. Clin. Res. Cardiol. 2020, 109, 1522–1530.

[7] Li, Y.; Tokura, H.; Guo, Y.P.; Wong, A.S.W.; Wong, T.; Chung, J.; Newton, E. Effects of Wearing N95 and Surgical Facemasks on Heart Rate, Thermal Stress and Subjective Sensations. Int. Arch. Occup. Environ. Health 2005, 78, 501–509.

[8] Roberge, R.; Bayer, E.; Powell, J.; Coca, A.; Roberge, M.; Benson, S. Effect of Exhaled Moisture on Breathing Resistance of N95 Filtering Facepiece Respirators. Ann. Occup. Hyg. 2010, 54, 671–677.

[9] Lee, S.-A.; Grinshpun, S.A.; Reponen, T. Respiratory Performance Offered by N95 Respirators and Surgical Masks: Human Subject Evaluation with NaCl Aerosol Representing Bacterial and Viral Particle Size Range. Ann. Occup. Hyg. 2008, 52, 177–185.

[10] Butz, U. Rückatmung von Kohlendioxid bei Verwendung von Operationsmasken als hygienischer Mundschutz an medizinischem Fachpersonal. Ph.D. Thesis, Fakultät für Medizin der Technischen Universität München, Munich, Germany, 2005.

[11] Roberge, R.J.; Kim, J.-H.; Benson, S.M. Absence of Consequential Changes in Physiological, Thermal and Subjective Responses from Wearing a Surgical Mask. Respir. Physiol. Neurobiol. 2012, 181, 29–35.

[12] Georgi, C.; Haase-Fielitz, A.; Meretz, D.; Gäsert, L.; Butter, C. Einfluss gängiger Gesichtsmasken auf physiologische Parameter und Belastungsempfinden unter arbeitstypischer körperlicher Anstrengung. Deutsches Ärzteblatt 2020, 674–675.

[13] Kyung, S.Y.; Kim, Y.; Hwang, H.; Park, J.-W.; Jeong, S.H. Risks of N95 Face Mask Use in Subjects with COPD. Respir. Care 2020, 65, 658–664.

[14] Mo, Y.; Wei, D.; Mai, Q.; Chen, C.; Yu, H.; Jiang, C.; Tan, X. Risk and Impact of Using Mask on COPD Patients with Acute Exacerbation during the COVID-19 Outbreak: A Retrospective Study. Res. Sq. 2020.

[15] Goh, D.Y.T.; Mun, M.W.; Lee, W.L.J.; Teoh, O.H.; Rajgor, D.D. A Randomised Clinical Trial to Evaluate the Safety, Fit, Comfort of a Novel N95 Mask in Children. Sci. Rep. 2019, 9, 18952.

[16] Bharatendu, C.; Ong, J.J.Y.; Goh, Y.; Tan, B.Y.Q.; Chan, A.C.Y.; Tang, J.Z.Y.; Leow, A.S.; Chin, A.; Sooi, K.W.X.; Tan, Y.L.; et al. Powered Air Purifying Respirator (PAPR) Restores the N95 Face Mask Induced Cerebral Hemodynamic Alterations among Healthcare Workers during COVID-19 Outbreak. J. Neurol. Sci. 2020, 417, 117078.

[17] Tong, P.S.Y.; Kale, A.S.; Ng, K.; Loke, A.P.; Choolani, M.A.; Lim, C.L.; Chan, Y.H.; Chong, Y.S.; Tambyah, P.A.; Yong, E.-L. Respiratory Consequences of N95-Type Mask Usage in Pregnant Healthcare Workers — A Controlled Clinical Study. Antimicrob. Resist. Infect. Control 2015, 4, 48.

[18] Rebmann, T.; Carrico, R.; Wang, J. Physiologic and Other Effects and Compliance with Long-Term Respirator Use among Medical Intensive Care Unit Nurses. Am. J. Infect. Control 2013, 41, 1218–1223.

[19] Pifarré, F.; Zabala, D.D.; Grazioli, G.; de Yzaguirre i Maura, I. COVID 19 and Mask in Sports. Apunt. Sports Med. 2020.

[20] Tong, P.S.Y.; Kale, A.S.; Ng, K.; Loke, A.P.; Choolani, M.A.; Lim, C.L.; Chan, Y.H.; Chong, Y.S.; Tambyah, P.A.; Yong, E.-L. Respiratory Consequences of N95-Type Mask Usage in Pregnant Healthcare Workers — A Controlled Clinical Study. Antimicrob. Resist. Infect. Control 2015, 4, 48.

[21] Liu, C.; Li, G.; He, Y.; Zhang, Z.; Ding, Y. Effects of Wearing Masks on Human Health and Comfort during the COVID-19 Pandemic. IOP Conf. Ser. Earth Environ. Sci. 2020, 531, 012034.

[22] Beder, A.; Büyükkoçak, U.; Sabuncuo ̆glu, H.; Keskil, Z.A.; Keskil, S. Preliminary Report on Surgical Mask Induced Deoxygenation during Major Surgery. Neurocirugía 2008, 19, 121–126.

[23] Jagim, A.R.; Dominy, T.A.; Camic, C.L.; Wright, G.; Doberstein, S.; Jones, M.T.; Oliver, J.M. Acute Effects of the Elevation Training Mask on Strength Performance in Recreational Weight Lifters. J. Strength Cond. Res. 2018, 32, 482–489.

[24] Cress ML, Forrester K, Probst L, Foster C, Doberstein S, Porcari JP. Effect of Wearing the Elevation Training Mask on Aerobic Capacity, Lung Function, and Hematological Variables. Medicine & Science in Sports & Exercise. 2016;48:1040-1041. doi:10.1249/01.mss.0000488131.38685.16.

[25] Kao, T.-W.; Huang, K.-C.; Huang, Y.-L.; Tsai, T.-J.; Hsieh, B.-S.; Wu, M.-S. The Physiological Impact of Wearing an N95 Mask during Hemodialysis as a Precaution against SARS in Patients with End-Stage Renal Disease. J. Formos. Med. Assoc. 2004, 103, 624–628.

[26] Shenal, B.V.; Radonovich, L.J.; Cheng, J.; Hodgson, M.; Bender, B.S. Discomfort and Exertion Associated with Prolonged Wear of Respiratory Protection in a Health Care Setting. J. Occup. Environ. Hyg. 2011, 9, 59–64.

[27] Matusiak, Ł.; Szepietowska, M.; Krajewski, P.; Białynicki-Birula, R.; Szepietowski, J.C. Inconveniences Due to the Use of Face Masks during the COVID-19 Pandemic: A Survey Study of 876 Young People. Dermatol. Ther. 2020, 33, e13567.

[28] Scarano, A.; Inchingolo, F.; Lorusso, F. Facial Skin Temperature and Discomfort When Wearing Protective Face Masks: Thermal Infrared Imaging Evaluation and Hands Moving the Mask. Int. J. Environ. Res. Public Health 2020, 17, 4624.

[29] Person, E.; Lemercier, C.; Royer, A.; Reychler, G. Effet du port d'un masque de soins lors d'un test de marche de six minutes chez des sujets sains. Rev. Mal. Respir. 2018, 35, 264–268.

[30] Smart, N.R.; Horwell, C.J.; Smart, T.S.; Galea, K.S. Assessment of the Wearability of Facemasks against Air Pollution in Primary School-Aged Children in London. Int. J. Environ. Res. Public Health 2020, 17, 3935.

[31] Rosner, E. Adverse Effects of Prolonged Mask Use among Healthcare Professionals during COVID-19. J. Infect. Dis. Epidemiol. 2020.

[32] Ong, J.J.Y.; Bharatendu, C.; Goh, Y.; Tang, J.Z.Y.; Sooi, K.W.X.; Tan, Y.L.; Tan, B.Y.Q.; Teoh, H.-L.; Ong, S.T.; Allen, D.M.; et al. Headaches Associated With Personal Protective Equipment-A Cross-Sectional Study among Frontline Healthcare Workers During COVID-19. Headache 2020, 60, 864–877.

[33] Jacobs, J.L.; Ohde, S.; Takahashi, O.; Tokuda, Y.; Omata, F.; Fukui, T. Use of Surgical Face Masks to Reduce the Incidence of the Common Cold among Health Care Workers in Japan: A Randomized Controlled Trial. Am. J. Infect. Control 2009, 37, 417–419.

[34] Ramirez-Moreno, J.M. Mask-Associated de Novo Headache in Healthcare Workers during the Covid-19 Pandemic. medRxiv 2020.

[35] Lim, E.C.H.; Seet, R.C.S.; Lee, K.-H.; Wilder-Smith, E.P.V.; Chuah, B.Y.S.; Ong, B.K.C. Headaches and the N95 Face-mask amongst Healthcare Providers. Acta Neurol. Scand. 2006, 113, 199–202.

[36] Matuschek, C.; Moll, F.; Fangerau, H.; Fischer, J.C.; Zänker, K.; van Griensven, M.; Schneider, M.; Kindgen-Milles, D.; Knoefel, W.T.; Lichtenberg, A.; et al. Face Masks: Benefits and Risks during the COVID-19 Crisis. Eur. J. Med. Res. 2020, 25, 32.

[37] Johnson, A.T. Respirator Masks Protect Health but Impact Performance: A Review. J. Biol. Eng. 2016, 10, 4.

[38] Wong, C.K.M.; Yip, B.H.K.; Mercer, S.; Griffiths, S.; Kung, K.; Wong, M.C.; Chor, J.; Wong, S.Y. Effect of Facemasks on Empathy and Relational Continuity: A Randomised Controlled Trial in Primary Care. BMC Fam. Pract. 2013, 14, 200.

[39] Foo, C.C.I.; Goon, A.T.J.; Leow, Y.; Goh, C. Adverse Skin Reactions to Personal Protective Equipment against Severe Acute Respiratory Syndrome–a Descriptive Study in Singapore. Contact Dermat. 2006, 55, 291–294.

[40] Hua, W.; Zuo, Y.; Wan, R.; Xiong, L.; Tang, J.; Zou, L.; Shu, X.; Li, L. Short-Term Skin Reactions Following Use of N95 Respirators and Medical Masks. Contact Dermat. 2020, 83, 115–121.

Reason 181: Covid Is Hardly More Dangerous Than The Flu, Face Masks Have No Impact On Respiratory Viruses Anyway, And Masks Are Measurably Harmful In The Short-Term, Long-Term, And Cumulatively

[1] Kisielinski K, Giboni P, Prescher A, et al. Is a Mask That Covers the Mouth and Nose Free from Undesirable Side Effects in Everyday Use and Free of Potential Hazards? International Journal of Environmental Research and Public Health. 2021;18(8):4344. doi:10.3390/ijerph18084344.

[2] Streeck, H.; Schulte, B.; Kuemmerer, B.; Richter, E.; Hoeller, T.; Fuhrmann, C.; Bartok, E.; Dolscheid, R.; Berger, M.; Wessendorf, L.; et al. Infection Fatality Rate of Sars-Cov-2 Infection in a German Community with a Super-Spreading Event. medRxiv 2020.

[3] Ioannidis, J. The Infection Fatality Rate of COVID-19 Inferred from Seroprevalence Data. medRxiv 2020.

[4] Executive Board: Special Session on the COVID-19 Response. Available online: https://www.who.int/news-room/events/detail/2020/10/05/default-calendar/executive-board-special-session-on-the-covid19-response (accessed on 13 November 2020).

[5] Roberge, R.J.; Kim, J.-H.; Powell, J.B. N95 Respirator Use during Advanced Pregnancy. Am. J. Infect. Control 2014, 42, 1097–1100.

[6] Epstein, D.; Korytny, A.; Isenberg, Y.; Marcusohn, E.; Zukermann, R.; Bishop, B.; Minha, S.; Raz, A.; Miller, A. Return to Training in the COVID-19 Era: The Physiological Effects of Face Masks during Exercise. Scand. J. Med. Sci. Sports 2020.

[7] Johnson, A.T.; Scott, W.H.; Lausted, C.G.; Coyne, K.M.; Sahota, M.S.; Johnson, M.M. Effect of External Dead Volume on Performance While Wearing a Respirator. AIHAJ-Am. Ind. Hyg. Assoc. 2000, 61, 678–684.

[8] Xu, M.; Lei, Z.; Yang, J. Estimating the Dead Space Volume between a Headform and N95 Filtering Facepiece Respirator Using Microsoft Kinect. J. Occup. Environ. Hyg. 2015, 12, 538–546.

[9] Fikenzer, S.; Uhe, T.; Lavall, D.; Rudolph, U.; Falz, R.; Busse, M.; Hepp, P.; Laufs, U. Effects of Surgical and FFP2/N95 Face Masks on Cardiopulmonary Exercise Capacity. Clin. Res. Cardiol. 2020, 109, 1522–1530.

[10] Li, Y.; Tokura, H.; Guo, Y.P.; Wong, A.S.W.; Wong, T.; Chung, J.; Newton, E. Effects of Wearing N95 and Surgical Facemasks on Heart Rate, Thermal Stress and Subjective Sensations. Int. Arch. Occup. Environ. Health 2005, 78, 501–509.

[11] Lee HP.; Wang DY. Objective Assessment of Increase in Breathing Resistance of N95 Respirators on Human Subjects. Ann Occup. Hyg. 2011, 55, 917–921.

[12] Roberge, R.; Bayer, E.; Powell, J.; Coca, A.; Roberge, M.; Benson, S. Effect of Exhaled Moisture on Breathing Resistance of N95 Filtering Facepiece Respirators. Ann. Occup. Hyg. 2010, 54, 671–677. Particle Size Range. Ann. Occup. Hyg. 2008, 52, 177–185.

[13] Butz, U. Rückatmung von Kohlendioxid bei Verwendung von Operationsmasken als hygienischer Mundschutz an medizinischem Fachpersonal. Ph.D. Thesis, Fakultät für Medizin der Technischen Universität München, Munich, Germany, 2005.

[14] Roberge, R.J.; Kim, J.-H.; Benson, S.M. Absence of Consequential Changes in Physiological, Thermal and Subjective Responses from Wearing a Surgical Mask. Respir. Physiol. Neurobiol. 2012, 181, 29–35.

[15] Roberge, R.J.; Coca, A.; Williams, W.J.; Powell, J.B.; Palmiero, A.J. Physiological Impact of the N95 Filtering Facepiece Respirator on Healthcare Workers. Respir. Care 2010, 55, 569–577.

[16] Rebmann, T.; Carrico, R.; Wang, J. Physiologic and Other Effects and Compliance with Long-Term Respirator Use among Medical Intensive Care Unit Nurses. Am. J. Infect. Control 2013, 41, 1218–1223

[17] Georgi, C.; Haase-Fielitz, A.; Meretz, D.; Gäsert, L.; Butter, C. Einfluss gängiger Gesichtsmasken auf physiologische Parameter und Belastungsempfinden unter arbeitstypischer körperlicher Anstrengung. Deutsches Ärzteblatt 2020, 674–675.

489

[18] Kyung, S.Y.; Kim, Y.; Hwang, H.; Park, J.-W.; Jeong, S.H. Risks of N95 Face Mask Use in Subjects with COPD. Respir. Care 2020, 65, 658–664.

[19] Mo, Y.; Wei, D.; Mai, Q.; Chen, C.; Yu, H.; Jiang, C.; Tan, X. Risk and Impact of Using Mask on COPD Patients with Acute Exacerbation during the COVID-19 Outbreak: A Retrospective Study. Res. Sq. 2020.

[20] Goh, D.Y.T.; Mun, M.W.; Lee, W.L.J.; Teoh, O.H.; Rajgor, D.D. A Randomised Clinical Trial to Evaluate the Safety, Fit, Comfort of a Novel N95 Mask in Children. Sci. Rep. 2019, 9, 18952.

[21] Bharatendu, C.; Ong, J.J.Y.; Goh, Y.; Tan, B.Y.Q.; Chan, A.C.Y.; Tang, J.Z.Y.; Leow, A.S.; Chin, A.; Sooi, K.W.X.; Tan, Y.L.; et al. Powered Air Purifying Respirator (PAPR) Restores the N95 Face Mask Induced Cerebral Hemodynamic Alterations among Healthcare Workers during COVID-19 Outbreak. J. Neurol. Sci. 2020, 417, 117078.

[22] Tong, P.S.Y.; Kale, A.S.; Ng, K.; Loke, A.P.; Choolani, M.A.; Lim, C.L.; Chan, Y.H.; Chong, Y.S.; Tambyah, P.A.; Yong, E.-L. Respiratory Consequences of N95-Type Mask Usage in Pregnant Healthcare Workers — A Controlled Clinical Study. Antimicrob. Resist. Infect. Control 2015, 4, 48.

[23] Liu, C.; Li, G.; He, Y.; Zhang, Z.; Ding, Y. Effects of Wearing Masks on Human Health and Comfort during the COVID-19 Pandemic. IOP Conf. Ser. Earth Environ. Sci. 2020, 531, 012034.

[24] Beder, A.; Büyükkoçak, U.; Sabuncuo ̄glu, H.; Keskil, Z.A.; Keskil, S. Preliminary Report on Surgical Mask Induced Deoxygenation during Major Surgery. Neurocirugía 2008, 19, 121–126.

[25] Pifarré, F.; Zabala, D.D.; Grazioli, G.; de Yzaguirre i Maura, I. COVID 19 and Mask in Sports. Apunt. Sports Med. 2020.

[26] Jagim, A.R.; Dominy, T.A.; Camic, C.L.; Wright, G.; Doberstein, S.; Jones, M.T.; Oliver, J.M. Acute Effects of the Elevation Training Mask on Strength Performance in Recreational Weight Lifters. J. Strength Cond. Res. 2018, 32, 482–489.

[27] Cress ML, Forrester K, Probst L, Foster C, Doberstein S, Porcari JP. Effect of Wearing the Elevation Training Mask on Aerobic Capacity, Lung Function, and Hematological Variables. Medicine & Science in Sports & Exercise. 2016;48:1040-1041. doi:10.1249/01.mss.0000488131.38685.16.

[28] Kao, T.-W.; Huang, K.-C.; Huang, Y.-L.; Tsai, T.-J.; Hsieh, B.-S.; Wu, M.-S. The Physiological Impact of Wearing an N95 Mask during Hemodialysis as a Precaution against SARS in Patients with End-Stage Renal Disease. J. Formos. Med. Assoc. 2004, 103, 624–628.

[29] Johnson, A.T. Respirator Masks Protect Health but Impact Performance: A Review. J. Biol. Eng. 2016, 10, 4.

[30] Matusiak, Ł.; Szepietowska, M.; Krajewski, P.; Białynicki-Birula, R.; Szepietowski, J.C. Inconveniences Due to the Use of Face Masks during the COVID-19 Pandemic: A Survey Study of 876 Young People. Dermatol. Ther. 2020, 33, e13567.

[31] Scarano, A.; Inchingolo, F.; Lorusso, F. Facial Skin Temperature and Discomfort When Wearing Protective Face Masks: Thermal Infrared Imaging Evaluation and Hands Moving the Mask. Int. J. Environ. Res. Public Health 2020, 17, 4624.

[32] Person, E.; Lemercier, C.; Royer, A.; Reychler, G. Effet du port d'un masque de soins lors d'un test de marche de six minutes chez des sujets sains. Rev. Mal. Respir. 2018, 35, 264–268.

[33] Smart, N.R.; Horwell, C.J.; Smart, T.S.; Galea, K.S. Assessment of the Wearability of Facemasks against Air Pollution in Primary School-Aged Children in London. Int. J. Environ. Res. Public Health 2020, 17, 3935.

[34] Rosner, E. Adverse Effects of Prolonged Mask Use among Healthcare Professionals during COVID-19. J. Infect. Dis. Epidemiol. 2020.

[35] Ong, J.J.Y.; Bharatendu, C.; Goh, Y.; Tang, J.Z.Y.; Sooi, K.W.X.; Tan, Y.L.; Tan, B.Y.Q.; Teoh, H.-L.; Ong, S.T.; Allen, D.M.; et al. Headaches Associated With Personal Protective Equipment-A Cross-Sectional Study among Frontline Healthcare Workers During COVID-19. Headache 2020, 60, 864–877.

[36] Jacobs, J.L.; Ohde, S.; Takahashi, O.; Tokuda, Y.; Omata, F.; Fukui, T. Use of Surgical Face Masks to Reduce the Incidence of the Common Cold among Health Care Workers in Japan: A Randomized Controlled Trial. Am. J. Infect. Control 2009, 37, 417–419.

[37] Ramirez-Moreno, J.M. Mask-Associated de Novo Headache in Healthcare Workers during the Covid-19 Pandemic. medRxiv 2020.

[38] Lim, E.C.H.; Seet, R.C.S.; Lee, K.-H.; Wilder-Smith, E.P.V.; Chuah, B.Y.S.; Ong, B.K.C. Headaches and the N95 Face-mask amongst Healthcare Providers. Acta Neurol. Scand. 2006, 113, 199–202.

[39] Roberge, R.J.; Kim, J.-H.; Coca, A. Protective Facemask Impact on Human Thermoregulation: An Overview. Ann. Occup. Hyg. 2012, 56, 102–112.

[40] Rosner, E. Adverse Effects of Prolonged Mask Use among Healthcare Professionals during COVID-19. J. Infect. Dis. Epidemiol. 2020.

[41] Wong, C.K.M.; Yip, B.H.K.; Mercer, S.; Griffiths, S.; Kung, K.; Wong, M.C.; Chor, J.; Wong, S.Y. Effect of Facemasks on Empathy and Relational Continuity: A Randomised Controlled Trial in Primary Care. BMC Fam. Pract. 2013, 14, 200.

[42] Foo, C.C.I.; Goon, A.T.J.; Leow, Y.; Goh, C. Adverse Skin Reactions to Personal Protective Equipment against Severe Acute Respiratory Syndrome-a Descriptive Study in Singapore. Contact Dermat. 2006, 55, 291–294.

[43] Hua, W.; Zuo, Y.; Wan, R.; Xiong, L.; Tang, J.; Zou, L.; Shu, X.; Li, L. Short-Term Skin Reactions Following Use of N95 Respirators and Medical Masks. Contact Dermat. 2020, 83, 115–121.

[44] Techasatian, L.; Lebsing, S.; Uppala, R.; Thaowandee, W.; Chaiyarit, J.; Supakunpinyo, C.; Panombualert, S.; Mairiang, D.; Saengnipanthkul, S.; Wichajarn, K.; et al. The Effects of the Face Mask on the Skin Underneath: A Prospective Survey During the COVID-19 Pandemic. J. Prim. Care Community Health 2020, 11, 2150132720966167.

[45] Lan, J.; Song, Z.; Miao, X.; Li, H.; Li, Y.; Dong, L.; Yang, J.; An, X.; Zhang, Y.; Yang, L.; et al. Skin Damage among Health Care Workers Managing Coronavirus Disease-2019. J. Am. Acad. Dermatol. 2020, 82, 1215–1216.

[46] Szepietowski, J.C.; Matusiak, Ł.; Szepietowska, M.; Krajewski, P.K.; Białynicki-Birula, R. Face Mask-Induced Itch: A SelfQuestionnaire Study of 2,315 Responders during the COVID-19 Pandemic. Acta Derm.-Venereol. 2020, 100, adv00152.

[47] Shenal, B.V.; Radonovich, L.J.; Cheng, J.; Hodgson, M.; Bender, B.S. Discomfort and Exertion Associated with Prolonged Wear of Respiratory Protection in a Health Care Setting. J. Occup. Environ. Hyg. 2011, 9, 59–64.

Acknowledgements

[1] Paul, R. The Coronavirus Hoax. *LewRockwell.com.* 2020. Retrieved from https://www.lewrockwell.com/2020/03/ron-paul/the-coronavirus-hoax/.

[2] Allen, S. The Fear Mask and the "I Surrender" Pose. *LewRockwell.com.* 2020. Retrieved from https://www.lewrockwell.com/2020/04/allan-stevo/the-fear-mask-and-the-i-surrender-pose/

Index

#

1918, 31, 54, 201
1948 Geneva Declaration, 301
1957, 31
1968, 31
2002, 31
2009, 31, 50, 70
2014 Ebola epidemic, 254
77% of Americans are overweight or obese, 106
81% (128 workers) developed new headaches during their work shifts, 400

A

a careful risk–benefit analysis is becoming increasingly relevant for patients and their practitioners regarding the potential long-term effects of masks, 302
abscesses, 188
abscesses in lung tissue, 198
absence of recycling and disposal strategies, 408
accelerated aging process, 399
accelerated heart rate, 394
accumulation of carbon dioxide, 256
acetone, 179
acidic environment, 266, 267, 350
acidosis, 325, 399
acne, 40, 41, 144, 253, 291, 295, 381, 382, 383, 384, 424, 428
acoustic filter, 220, 374
acoustical treatment, 217
actions speak louder than words, 80
activation of the "fight or flight" stress response, 399
acute (sudden) hypercapnia, 334
acute hypercapnia, 349
adenovirus, 191
adrenalin, 251
Aerodynamic Particle Sizer, 192
aerosols, 191
aggregatibacteria actinomycetemcomitans, 188
air exchange, 54, 174, 175, 263
air pollution, 343
airflow, 104, 389
airtight, 50, 350
airway inflammation, 187
airway resistance, 156, 268, 341
alcohol, 155, 247, 304
alcohol abuse, 248
allopathic medicine, 282
allyl methyl sulfide, 179
altered gait velocities and falls, 349
altered skin flora, 373
altruism, 299
alveolitis, 172
Alzheimer disease, 399, 420
ambient carbon dioxide, 318
ambient oxygen, 318
American Asthma and Allergy Society, 275
Americans, 43, 44, 51, 52, 58, 106, 131, 132, 217, 247, 248, 350, 352, 357, 393, 417, 431
amino acids, 349
anaerobic metabolism, 266
ancient Greece, 418
Andersen, Catherine, 105
anesthesia, 257
aneurysms, 242
angular cheilitis, 381
angulation of the outer ear, 379

antibacterial, 169
antibiotic therapy, 200
antibodies, 187, 190, 198, 363
anti-bootlicker reading of Romans 13, 88
Antistreptolysin O test, 198
antiviral, 169
anxiety, 19, 20, 113, 165, 251, 254, 256, 257, 287, 288, 293, 299, 399, 420
anxiety and psychovegetative stress reactions in children, 254
anxiety states in panic disorders, 256
anxiety-reduced freedom of movement, 299
April 3, 2020 and the implementation of the CDC mask, 11, 19, 39, 44, 75, 216, 322, 417
Arizona, 1
arterial CO2 concentrations, 350
arteriosclerosis, 344
artificial inducement of COPD (Chronic obstructive pulmonary), 334
asbestos dust, 170
asbestosis, 170
Asian countries, 107
aspergillomas, 196
aspergillosis, 196
Aspergillus, 185, 191, 196
aspirated, 187, 188
Assange, Julian, 49
asthma, 156, 165, 171, 172, 295, 343, 344
Atlas Mountains of Morroco, 371
atopic predisposition (allergy tendency), 384
Australia, 24, 25
authority, 29, 49, 62, 63, 64, 75, 78, 82, 83, 87, 88, 89, 92, 94, 99, 114, 118, 122, 280, 286, 329, 422
auto-antibodies, 199
auto-immune diseases, 198
auto-immune encephalitis, 199
autonomic dysfunction, 393
average life expectancy for Americans, 247
average wearing time of mask, 205
avoidable errors, 207
avoidance of pain, 64
axons, 175

B

bacteremia, 142, 200
bacteria, 54, 55, 56, 149, 184, 185, 186, 187, 188, 189, 190, 191, 194, 195, 198, 199, 200, 201, 361, 367, 371, 372, 381, 382, 409, 419
bacterial colonies, 140, 183, 184
bacterial colonization, 187
bacterial droplet contamination, 299
bacterial optimization, 383
bacterial-induced chronic airway inflammation, 140
bag boy, 1
barbaric past, xiv
basal ganglia encephalitis, 144, 199
basic human-to-human connectivity, 250
because
    I am a coward, 70
    I love you, 70
    I will not stand up to evil, even if it, 70
    it is good for you, 70
    it is safer, 70
    those are the rules, 77
    we are told to, 70
Beck, Melinda, 105
behavioral norms, 225
behavioralism, 65
biofilm, 187

biohazard, 183, 186, 223, 409, 413, 414
black lung, 170
block emotional signaling between teacher and learner, 59
block emotional signaling between teachers
and students, 222
blood and treasure, 56
blood brain barrier, 199
blood carbon dioxide, 158, 211, 235, 242, 256, 337, 354, 356, 423, 428
blood gases, 275, 335, 338, 355
blood gas-related volume shifts, 243
blood oxygen saturation, 337, 338, 423, 428
blood pressure, 138, 140, 141, 143, 156, 165, 252, 270, 272, 273, 344, 355, 356, 421, 422, 428
blood pressure increase, 355
blood pressure values, 273, 422
blood vessels, 104, 140, 141, 142, 143, 144, 242, 251, 344, 384
boardroom, 63
bocavirus, 191
bonding between teachers and learners, 222, 230
bone, 105, 175, 200
bone marrow, 105, 175
Borg Rating Scale, 339
Borg scale, 269
Borovoy, Boris, 23, 54, 56, 170, 172, 174, 184, 186, 191, 196, 198, 318, 445
both face masks and face shields cause fear
in children, 227
boundaries, 4, 91, 94, 101
boy in the bubble, the, 101
bradycardia, 165
brain
        brain centers, 282, 365
        brain metabolism, 349
        brain volume shifts, 143, 242
        brainstem, 256, 355
        brainwashing, 115
Brazil, 23, 25
break a child, 78
break a horse, 78
breath provocation tests, 256
breathing
        air with O2 concentration below 19.5% is
        considered oxygen-deficiency, 394
        difficulties during the exercise, 338
        problems, 165, 295, 384
        resistance, 138, 158, 324, 330, 331, 335, 340, 341, 342, 354, 373, 423, 428
        through the open mouth, 373
        zone carbon dioxide concentrations, 323
breathlessness, 138, 273, 331, 341
breeding ground for various pathogens, 190
bronchi, 140, 276, 335
bronchiectasis, 140, 172, 196
bronchitis, 140, 165, 172
bronchopulmonary diseases, 140, 172
bullies bully, 49
bullying begets bullying, 73
byssinosis, 170, 171, 177

C

Caesar, 87, 88
Canadian Government, 169
canaries, 164, 367
cancer, 36, 46, 147, 198, 251, 343, 357, 365, 399, 419, 420
cancer patients, 357
cancer therapies, 419
candida, 146, 191, 196, 373
Candida albicans, 146, 373
candidiasis, 146, 373
capillary action, 191

carbon dioxide, 137, 138, 139, 141, 158, 159, 208, 211, 235, 240, 242, 256, 265, 266, 268, 269, 272, 273, 298, 304, 320, 321, 322, 323, 325, 326, 327, 328, 330, 331, 334, 335, 336, 337, 338, 340, 344, 349, 354, 355, 357, 393, 397, 421
        in the inhaled air, 344
        levels, 138, 141, 235, 240, 265, 298, 320, 321, 322, 323, 325, 326, 330, 339, 354, 421
        partial pressure, 273, 335, 340, 354
        retention, 141, 330, 331
cardiac, 141, 142, 266, 268, 270, 275, 281, 344, 397
        compensation of the pulmonary, 268
        disease, 275
        dysfunction, 142, 344
        overload, 141, 266, 270
        patients, 275
cardiopulmonary, 138, 141, 165, 268, 273, 275, 332, 398, 423, 428
        and neurological complications, 398
        capacity, 138, 141, 268, 423, 428
        disease, 165
        exercise capacity, 332
        lifestyle diseases, 356
cardiovascular, 142, 165, 175, 198, 201, 210, 251, 344, 357, 399, 419, 420
        consequences, 344
        disease, 142, 198, 201, 399, 419, 420
        impairment, 165
        optimization, 210
        system, 175
carotid bodies, 318
cartilage, 145, 379
cascade of other physiological side effects, 342
CD4+T - lymphocyte, 361
CDC (Centers for Disease Control and Prevention), 11, 12, 13, 14, 15, 17, 19, 20, 36, 37, 39, 43, 44, 188, 247, 257, 258, 263, 264, 309, 327, 352, 363
cellular hypoxia, 419
cellular oxygen supply, 365
Centers for Disease Control and Prevention (CDC), 258, 263, 311
central nervous system, 143, 175, 242, 354, 355
cerebral cortex (homunculus), 229, 254
cerebral ischemia, 143, 349
cerebral metabolism, 349
cerebral perfusion, 143, 349
changes in blood gas parameters (O2 and CO2), 339
checks and balances
        between branches, 86
        between individuals and federal, 86
        between local and federal, 86
        between state and federal, 86
cheilitis, 146, 373
chemoreceptors, 355
chest cavity, 104
chest discomfort, 138, 271, 394
child abuse, xiv, 59
childhood is the training ground for adulthood, 81
China, 24, 25, 279, 311, 411, 417
Christian, 44, 86, 438, 439, 442
chronic, 34, 35, 104, 105, 137, 139, 140, 156, 172, 179, 187, 196, 199, 208, 252, 266, 270, 272, 295, 343, 355, 365, 389, 393, 394, 397, 419
        airway infection syndrome, 196
        bronchitis, 140, 172
        inflammation, 104, 105, 139, 149, 188, 397
        inflammatory changes, 199
        mild or moderate hypoxemia and
        hypercapnia, 397
        obstructive pulmonary disease (COPD), 139, 272, 350, 394
        pneumonia, 140, 172

respiratory or breathing problems, 295
    stress condition, 399
    subthreshold intake of arsenic, 343
churches did not behave pro-actively enough to trigger
Romans 13, they merely treated press releases as
Gospel, 88
cigarettes, 155
circular reasoning, 52
civic participation, 86, 87
Clason, George, 68
claustrophobia, 165
cleaning, 12, 13, 150, 253, 440
clear carbon dioxide from the blood, 334
clearly dangerous public health approaches, 133
clinically relevant fungal, bacterial or viral infections, 382
clinically relevant fungal, bacterial, and viral
infections, 139
clinically relevant psychological and neurological
effects, 339
cloth face coverings, 309
cloth face mask efficacy, 311
cloth mask, 188, 310, 311, 312, 319
cloth masks, 55, 268, 309, 310, 311, 312, 313
cloth masks are awful, 311
cloth masks are even worse for you, 310
cloth masks carry disease, 311
CNS (Central Nervous System), 164
coaches, 75
coal dust, 170
coal miner pneumoconiosis, 170
coal miners, 164, 170
Coca-Cola, 95
cognition, 32, 40, 41, 149, 150, 210, 235, 237, 240, 250,
291, 292, 304, 305
cognitive function, 419
cognitive impairment, 149, 240, 292, 295
collagen fibers, 172
collapse of airways, 104
collateral psychological damage, 419
collective fear mongering, 299
community masks, 177, 190, 268, 317, 384
comorbidities, 29, 103, 106, 322
compensatory increased respiratory rate, 273
compliance is the last thing a free thinking person wants to
teach a child, 66
comply or else, 54, 56
components, 167, 170, 179, 244, 257, 399
compost, 196
compromised cognitive performance, 149, 399
computer screen use, 237
concentration problems, 207, 339, 422
conditioning, 64, 65
confirmation bias, 52, 122
conflicted doctors, 283
conformity, 61, 101, 116, 117, 122, 254
confusion, 151, 240, 257, 339
congenital heart disease, 165
conscious awareness, 225
Consultation Empathy Care Measury, 215
contact dermatitis, 381, 385
contact eczema, 384
contagion, 222, 230
continuous and adequate oxygen (O2) supply to
all organs, 397
continuous monitoring, 258
continuous positive airway pressure (CPAP), 186
contributes to increased aerosol production, 220
control centers of the affected brain, 355
convection currents, 191
COPD (Chronic obstructive pulmonary disease), 139, 171,
188, 229, 272, 273, 275, 334, 350, 356
COPD patients, 273
coronary heart disease, 142, 344
coronaviruses, 55, 184, 417

cortisol, 148, 251, 399
coughing, 11, 192, 194, 343
counselors, 75
courage, xv, 1, 2, 3, 4, 41, 93, 101, 102, 431, 443
covering the lower half of the face reduces the ability to
communicate, 222, 230
Covid injections, 56
Covid-19, 11, 13, 17, 18, 19, 20, 22, 23, 24, 25, 26, 29, 33,
34, 35, 36, 37, 38, 39, 40, 41, 43, 44, 45, 58, 86, 88, 100,
103, 104, 105, 106, 107, 108, 122, 123, 137, 169, 188,
192, 193, 198, 238, 239, 244, 250, 257, 264, 273, 275,
279, 288, 291, 292, 293, 294, 309, 310, 318, 328, 329,
361, 367, 383, 394, 397, 400, 413, 417, 419, 427, 521
Covid-19 hoax is an IQ test, 108
Cowan, Thomas, 68
cowardice, 1, 2, 3, 4, 67, 80
cowardly Christian, 86
cracking and sores at the corners of the mouth, 381
cranial health, 371
craniofacial deformities, 166
cribriform plate, 199
crucible, 98, 99
crush their spirit, 61
Cupertino, California, 371
cycleway, 413
cystic fibrosis, 165
cytokine production, 188
cytokines, 105, 199

D

damage to blood vessels supplying the brain, 344
damage to children's brains, 209
dangling from a rearview mirror for 6 months, 297
de novo PPE-associated headaches, 143, 238
Dead Poet's Society, 61, 62
dead space, 139, 158, 160, 179, 180, 200, 210, 211, 256,
320, 321, 323, 324, 326, 327, 330, 335, 338, 340, 342,
354, 423, 428
dead space volume, 158, 179, 180, 210, 256, 321, 335,
338, 340, 342, 354, 423, 428
dead space volume that is almost doubled by wearing
a mask, 354
deaf and hard of hearing, 147, 217
debate, 48, 49, 120, 123, 124, 248, 311, 329, 335, 434
decaying leaves, 196
decaying teeth, 187, 372
decline in pH levels, 399
decomposition, 409
decrease in blood oxygen saturation, 423, 428
decrease in cardiopulmonary capacity, 423, 428
decrease in Cerebrospinal fluid (CSF) spaces, 242
decrease in empathy perception, 215, 423, 428
decrease in oxygen saturation (SpO2), 211, 272,
273, 337, 339
decrease in pH levels, 397
decrease in psychomotoric abilities, 339
decreased gas exchange, 342
deep breathing, 139, 282
deeper tissue, 146, 187, 189, 198, 201
deform children's ears, 379
dehumanizing movements, 250
dehydration, 148, 237, 277, 373
deliver babies, 157
dementia, 150, 209, 257
dendrites, 175
Denmark, 23, 24, 26, 59
dental caries, 145, 187
dental procedure, 198, 201
dentists, 40, 187, 371
depression, 251, 399, 420
depressive self-experience, 151, 254
dermatoses, 288

devalue your own parental authority, 75
developing children, 205
diabetes, 149, 165, 198, 248, 399, 420
dialysis, 271, 393, 394
diaphragmatic splinting, 156
difficulty
    breathing, 263, 384, 428
    breathing and shortness of breath, 423
    in concentration, 208
diffusion of CO2 from the fetal blood, 158
dirty face masks, 413
dirty face masks on the ground, 413
discarded hypodermic needles and syringes, 413
discomfort, 147, 150, 172, 229, 253, 288, 293, 295, 331, 332, 350, 383, 403, 414
discouragement, 150, 221
disease-causing bacteria, 191
disease-promoting effects, 421
disease-relevant consequences, 165, 343, 344
disorientation, 240, 257
disrupt social interaction, 146, 215
disruption of doctor-patient relationship, 147, 215
disruption of non-verbal communication, 221
disruption of respiratory physiology, 138, 165
distraction, 102, 150, 207, 253
disturbance of skin function, 384
disturbed barrier function of the skin, 382
dizziness, 143, 208, 231, 271, 273, 334, 339, 340, 343, 350, 398, 421, 423, 428
do no harm, 57, 252, 288
doctors, xiv, 39, 40, 52, 110, 111, 129, 131, 132, 133, 157, 205, 215, 238, 277, 288, 301, 302, 303, 389, 441
Doctors, xiv, 227, 287, 288, 302, 389
Doctors are conflicted, 302
Doctors routinely remove their face masks when talking to a patient, 287
doctors' offices, 227
double mask, 307, 313
drainage of the pericardium, 200
drinking, 150, 244, 253, 407, 409
drop in blood oxygen partial pressure, 273, 337
droplet exhalation, 184
droplets, 185, 191
Drosten, Christian, 44
drowsiness, 143, 148, 205, 208, 240, 272, 334, 350, 383, 421, 423, 428
drowsiness (qualitative neurological deficits), 423
drugs, 155, 247, 257, 304
dry eyes, 389
dry mouth, 371, 373
dryness, 145, 371, 372, 373, 389
dryness in the oral cavity, 373
due to insufficient oxygen intake and excessive carbon dioxide, 304
duration of combined PPE exposure, 238

E

E. coli (Escherichia coli), 191
ear lobe, 379
ears, 21, 49, 98, 145, 379
eating, 109, 150, 198, 253, 409
Ebola, 254, 312, 367
economic collapse, 419
economic lockdowns, 59
EEG (Electroencephalography) changes, 352
elder, high-risk patients with lung disease, 275
elderly, 39, 211, 238, 273, 275, 295, 322, 349, 424
elimination of hazard, 101
elite athletes, 210, 211
elusive authority renders Romans 13 irrelevant, 87
emotional mimicry, 222, 230
emotionality in general is reduced by masking, 230

emphysema, 165
employers, 40, 231, 329
end stage renal disease patients, 271
end-expiratory partial pressure, 211, 235, 272
endocarditis, 142, 198, 200
endocrine, 251
endoscopies, 375
endothelial cells, 104, 175, 199
endothelial dysfunction, 141, 344
end-stage renal disease, 271, 273
ENT (Ear, Nose and Throat), 164, 176
ENT (Ear, Nose and Throat) physicians, 374, 375
Enterobacter, 191
environment hazard, 295
environmental effects, 408
epidemiology, 11, 20, 54, 188, 311
epilepsy, 166, 352, 353
epileptics, 352, 353
epithelia, 175
epithelial damage, 187
epithelial debris, 187
erasing the positive effect of smiles and laughter, 215
ergometer, 269, 323
erythematous, 144, 379
ethanol, 179
ethical guidelines of a physician, 301
ethics, 57, 58, 84, 129, 288, 323
etiquette, 14
ETM (Elevation Training Mask), 210
EUA (Emergency Use Authorization), 22
Europe, 408
evidence-based medicine, 301
Ewing, J.R., 48
exacerbates existing voice disorders, 374
exacerbation of existing cardiopulmonary, metabolic, vascular and neurological conditions, 398
exacerbation of existing conditions, 397
exacerbation of existing conditions and diseases, 399
exacerbation of their pre-existing headache disorders, 238
exaggerating risks, 254
exercise, 97, 103, 106, 114, 139, 140, 148, 149, 158, 165, 210, 211, 261, 263, 264, 265, 266, 267, 268, 269, 270, 278, 279, 281, 332, 333, 349, 350, 351, 393, 403
exercise in face masks, 261
exercise parameters, 332
exercise with face masks is lethal, 281
exercise-induced asthma, 165
exercising with a face mask may increase infection rates, 267
exertion without masks, 268
exhalation resistance, 138, 330
exhaled air, 179, 208, 209, 256, 382, 389
exhaled air blowing upwards, 389
exhaled carbon dioxide equivalents (capnometry), 272
exhaustion, 148, 149, 269, 272, 341, 404, 423, 424, 428
experimentation, xiv, 2, 175, 180
external authority, 62

F

fabric masks, 176, 268, 290
face, xiii, xv, 1, 2, 3, 4, 7, 9, 11, 12, 13, 14, 15, 16, 17, 19, 22, 23, 24, 26, 27, 28, 29, 30, 31, 32, 33, 34, 36, 39, 40, 42, 46, 54, 55, 56, 57, 58, 59, 61, 62, 63, 64, 65, 66, 67, 69, 70, 72, 73, 75, 76, 77, 80, 84, 93, 95, 96, 97, 98, 100, 101, 102, 103, 106, 107, 108, 109, 110, 112, 114, 116, 118, 119, 120, 121, 127, 133, 135, 137, 138, 139, 143, 144, 145, 146, 147, 149, 155, 156, 157, 159, 160, 162, 163, 164, 165, 166, 167, 169, 171, 172, 175, 176, 177, 178, 179, 180, 181, 183, 184, 186, 189, 190, 191, 192, 194, 195, 196, 197, 198, 201, 205, 207, 208, 209, 210, 211, 213, 215, 216, 217, 218, 219, 220, 221, 222, 223, 224, 225, 227, 229, 230, 231, 232, 235, 237, 238, 239,

240, 241, 242, 243, 244, 248, 250, 251, 252, 253, 255, 256, 258, 259, 261, 263, 264, 265, 266, 267, 268, 269, 270, 271, 273, 274, 275, 277, 278, 279, 281, 282, 285, 286, 287, 288, 291, 292, 293, 294, 295, 296, 297, 298, 299, 300, 301, 304, 307, 309, 310, 311, 312, 313, 317, 318, 319, 320, 321, 322, 323, 326, 327, 328, 330, 331, 332, 333, 334, 335, 336, 338, 339, 342, 343, 344, 345, 349, 350, 351, 352, 353, 354, 355, 356, 357, 361, 363, 364, 365, 366, 367, 369, 371, 372, 373, 374, 375, 377, 379, 380, 381, 382, 383, 384, 385, 387, 389, 390, 391, 393, 394, 395, 398, 399, 401, 403, 404, 407, 408, 409, 410, 411, 412, 413, 414, 415, 417, 418, 419, 420, 421, 422, 423, 427, 428, 431, 432, 433, 434, 439, 441, 445, 521
face diapers, 217
face identification, 59
face mask fatalities in kids, 279
face mask reduces social cohesion, 230
face masks, XIII, XV, 1, 9, 11, 12, 13, 14, 15, 16, 17, 19, 22, 23, 26, 27, 28, 29, 31, 32, 33, 34, 39, 40, 42, 54, 55, 57, 58, 59, 61, 62, 64, 65, 72, 96, 102, 103, 107, 108, 112, 118, 119, 120, 127, 133, 135, 137, 138, 139, 143, 144, 155, 157, 159, 160, 162, 163, 164, 165, 166, 167, 169, 171, 172, 175, 176, 177, 178, 180, 181, 184, 186, 189, 191, 194, 195, 205, 207, 208, 210, 211, 213, 215, 216, 219, 220, 221, 222, 223, 225, 227, 229, 230, 231, 232, 235, 237, 238, 239, 241, 242, 243, 244, 248, 250, 252, 256, 258, 259, 263, 265, 266, 267, 270, 273, 274, 275, 277, 281, 282, 285, 286, 287, 288, 291, 292, 293, 294, 295, 296, 297, 298, 299, 304, 309, 310, 311, 312, 313, 317, 318, 319, 321, 322, 326, 327, 330, 331, 332, 334, 335, 336, 338, 342, 343, 344, 345, 352, 353, 357, 361, 362, 363, 364, 367, 371, 375, 379, 381, 385, 389, 393, 394, 403, 404, 407, 409, 410, 411, 412, 413, 420, 421, 423, 427, 428, 433, 434, 439, 441, 521
face masks are harmful for children, 163
face masks cause sore throats, 195
face masks do not work, 9, 11, 13, 15, 17, 19, 22, 23, 27, 29, 31, 40, 189, 313
face masks hurt pregnant women and their babies, 155
face shields, 62, 143, 227, 307
face shields caused fear, 227
face visor, 227
facial hair, 166
facial recognition, 146, 215
facial trauma, 146, 296
failure to recognize hazards, 150, 207
Fairfield University, 105
faith, 2, 4, 89, 96, 110, 367, 438, 439, 440
falsehoods, 6, 64
familial authority, 62
fanaticism of scientism, 92
farmers lung, 170
fasting, 237, 438
fast-twitch fiber size, 148
father, 1, 66, 96, 102, 279, 440, 521
fatigue, 148, 165, 205, 229, 272, 288, 293, 320, 334, 340, 350, 399, 419, 421, 422, 428
fatigue while performing difficult operations, 288, 293
Fauci, Anthony, 33, 42, 43, 44, 51, 177, 309
fear, 4, 20, 42, 50, 56, 96, 100, 102, 150, 223, 227, 251, 254, 287, 290, 299, 367, 399, 411, 440
fear-inducing and often exaggerated media coverage, 254
feeling, 62, 94, 112, 116, 138, 150, 151, 229, 253, 254, 269, 277, 299, 341, 344, 404, 423, 428
    of dampness and heat, 423
    of deprivation of freedom, 150, 253
    of exhaustion, 269, 404, 423
    of heat, 269
fetal–maternal carbon dioxide (CO2) gradient, 158, 160
fetuses, 137, 155, 157, 159, 162
FFP2/N95, 158, 165, 268, 269, 272, 273, 317, 327, 332
FFR, 155
fibroblasts, 172, 175
fibrosis, 140, 142, 172, 174, 175, 176, 198, 375

fibrotic foci, 175
fibrous thickening of peribronchiolar interstitium, 170
find your own voice, 61
Finland, 23, 24, 26, 29
fit protocol, 14
flares of toxins, 142, 198
flesh eating strep, 198
flu, 33, 36, 37, 50, 105, 170, 244, 310, 322, 367, 417, 427
fluid loss through the skin epithelium, 144, 382
fogging-up of glasses, 384
following orders, 66
food chain, 409
force a mask on your child against his will, 74
forced masking of the general population, 259
foreign bodies in the lungs, 139, 171
formaldehyde, 162, 384, 385
Fox News, 12, 15, 304
France, 24, 25, 247, 441
Frank Scale, 339
free will, 64, 65, 90
friable particles, 170, 174
full face mask, 323
fungal balls, 140, 196
fungal fibers, 140, 196
fungal infections of lungs, 196
fungal infestation of the mucous membranes, 146, 373
fungal spores, 196
fungi, 54, 181, 185, 190, 191, 194, 197, 382, 409
fungoid, 183

G

ganglia, 144, 175, 199
gas content for oxygen, 336
gas exchange, 138, 139, 158, 335, 338, 340, 342, 354
gas exchange volume available to the lungs per breath, 340
gateway to neuronal respiratory and circulatory control, 355
gather pollen, 93
Gatto, John Taylor, 68
gene expression, 365
Genentech, 103
general population, xiii, 19, 27, 127, 175, 180, 186, 192, 259, 298, 299, 317, 319, 320, 324, 356, 408
general public, 34, 50, 55, 129, 155, 166, 231, 258, 285, 290, 295, 299, 317, 414, 424
general-population settings, 40
Gerber, Magda, 68
German Industrial Accident Insurance (DGUV), the, 207
German Social Accident Insurance (DGUV), 317
Germany, 24, 25, 247, 317
germ-containing breath, 191
germs (bacteria, fungi and viruses) accumulate on the outside and inside of the masks due to the warm and moist environment, 382
gingivitis, 146, 373
give a good handshake, 222
gliotoxins, 196
global estimates, 419
global suppression of medical information, 209
glomerular filtration rate, 142, 393
gold standard scientists, 15
Gold, Simone, 444
government always seem to be late to the game, 169
gradients, 147, 157, 374
granulomas, 140, 172
graphene in face masks may pose a particular risk, 169
greater vasodilatation, 235
Griesz-Brisson, Margarite, 208, 209
grocery stores, 309
Group A Streptococcus (GAS), 199
group cohesion, 147, 222, 225, 230
gums, 146, 187, 371, 372, 373

Gutentag, Alex, 42, 43, 44, 45, 46, 47, 444
Guy's and St. Thomas' hospitals in London, 104

H

halitosis, 145, 373
Hamburg Environmental Institute, the, 178
hand washing, 13
harmful to eyes, 389
harness a child, 78
headaches, 40, 41, 143, 208, 235, 236, 237, 238, 239, 240,
242, 253, 269, 273, 288, 291, 292, 293, 334, 340, 343,
344, 389, 399, 400, 419, 421
headaches up to four times daily, 235
Health Canada, 169
health care
    community, 40
    facilities, 19
    workers, 19, 20, 27, 220, 235, 291, 309, 311, 363,
    374, 400
health deterioration, 148, 397, 399
health is a state of complete physical, mental and social
well-being and not merely the absence of disease or
infirmity, 294
health-promoting breathing, 282
health-promoting deep breathing, 282
health-related negative feelings, 254
heart
    attacks, 130, 131, 132, 371, 372
    failure, 229, 343
    rate, 141, 165, 270, 272, 273, 281, 332, 337, 338,
    339, 340, 341, 344, 355, 400, 403, 404, 421, 422,
    423, 428
    rate increase, 355, 422
    rate increased by, 400
    rate increased by approximately five
    beats/min, 400
heavy physical exertion, 268
helix, 379
help your child have an allergy to compliance with bad, 67
hemodialysis, 271, 273, 394
herding cats, 78
herding lions, 78
heroes, 1, 320
high bacterial and toxic particle concentration, 399
high blood pressure, 138, 140, 141, 156, 344, 356
high CO2, 398, 399
high fever, 148, 200
high fructose corn syrup, 95
higher overall mortality, 343
hinder babies' acquisition of speech and language,
147, 219
hippocampus, 143, 208
Hippocratic Oath, 288
histiocytes, 172
HIV/AIDS, 248
holistic healing, 282
Holt, John, 68
homeostasis, 139, 148, 251, 364, 399
Hong Kong, 11, 24, 25
hospitalization, 43, 44, 103, 149, 270, 343
how a child's mind develops, 205
human communication, 146, 215, 216, 224, 227
human-to-human connections, 250
humidity, 140, 195, 267, 277, 332, 382, 383, 399, 403
humidity and temperature in the upper airway, 140, 267
Hunt, Beverley, 104
hydrogen sulfide, 179, 343
hygiene, 12, 13, 14, 17, 19, 144, 188, 290, 295, 311
hypercapnia, 34, 141, 160, 236, 240, 256, 263, 275, 334,
335, 338, 349, 356, 365, 394, 397, 398, 399
hypercapnic hypoxemia, 141, 349

hypersensitivities to ingredients of industrially
manufactured masks, 384
hypertension, 140, 141, 165, 198, 344, 355, 356, 398,
399, 420
hypertensive patients, 273
hyperventilation, 139, 321, 352
hypotension, 141, 398
hypoxemia, 34, 271, 273, 393, 397, 398, 399
hypoxemia in nephrons, 393
hypoxia, 141, 164, 236, 240, 263, 266, 338, 356, 357, 361,
364, 365, 393, 394, 399, 419, 428
hypoxia inducible factor-11 (HIF-11), 361

I

iatrogenic harm is believed by some to be the
third leading cause of death in the United
States, 288
Ides of March 2020, 3, 32, 42, 49, 52, 53, 57, 85, 87, 88,
90, 114, 121, 122, 127, 129, 248, 280, 320, 431, 441
idiopathic pulmonary fibrosis, 175
immotile cilia syndrome, 140, 267
immune cells, 105, 361
immune system, 105, 196, 251, 359, 361, 363, 419
immune-mediated inflammatory disorders, 147, 198
immunity, 37, 42, 43, 104, 105, 147, 187, 361, 367
immunity debt, 367
immunosuppression, 147, 196, 252, 397, 399
immunosuppressive toxins, 196
impaired
    cognition, 40, 41, 149, 240, 291, 292, 304
    cognition of healthcare workers, 291
    cognitive performance, 207, 253
    fetal growth, 137, 156
    skin barrier function with acne, itching and skin
    lesions, 424, 428
    thinking, 150, 207, 241, 257, 339, 340
    verbal and non-verbal communication, 59
    vocal cord coordination, 146, 374
impairments and discomfort predominantly affecting the
head and face, 253
importance of the airway resistance, 341
improper mask disposal, 295
improper use of masks, 373
increase acidic environment, 141, 266
increase feelings of insecurity, 221
increase in airway resistance, 341
increase in blood carbon dioxide, 211
increase in brain parenchymal volume measurable under
increased arterial CO2 levels, 242
increased, 17, 26, 46, 51, 56, 104, 137, 138, 139, 140, 141,
142, 143, 144, 145, 146, 147, 148, 149, 150, 151, 156,
158, 160, 164, 166, 179, 190, 198, 210, 211, 220, 230,
235, 239, 242, 248, 250, 256, 257, 265, 268, 270, 271,
272, 273, 275, 278, 290, 293, 295, 310,311, 313, 318, 320,
321, 323, 330, 331, 335, 336, 337, 338, 340, 341, 342,
343, 344, 350, 354, 355, 356, 361, 371, 372, 373, 375,
382, 384, 389, 394, 397, 399, 400, 404, 421
    increased air trapping preventing substantial
    carbon dioxide exchange, 266
    increased airflow causes irritation or
    inflammation, 389
    increased brain volume, 143
    increased breathing
    resistance, 138, 158, 335, 340, 354, 373
    increased breathing frequency, 394
    increased cardiorespiratory stress, 138, 270
    increased cells and blood acidity, 397
    increased cerebral artery flow, 143, 235
    increased dead space is significant, 340
    increased dead space volume, 158, 179, 210, 256,
    335, 340, 342, 354, 423, 428
    increased dry eye symptoms, 145

increased end-expiratory partial pressure of carbon dioxide (PETCO2), 211, 272
increased heart rate, 141, 421
increased heart rates, 268, 344
increased humidity, 382, 383
increased hydration, 382
increased inflammatory substances such as C reactive protein, 148
increased lactate concentration, 141
increased leptin release, 148
increased likelihood of misunderstandings, 146, 215
increased mechanical stress, 383
increased mortality risk, 250, 251
increased muscle tension, 148, 399
increased obesity (BMI), 272
increased oxygen (O2) demand, 156
increased oxygen consumption and demand, 138, 268
increased physiological dead space, 139, 321
increased predisposition for viral and infection illnesses, 399
increased psychosomatic and stress-related illnesses, 150, 254
increased pulse rate, 336
increased resistance of air movement during both inhalation and exhalation process, 398
increased respiratory load, 138, 270
increased respiratory muscle load, 270
increased respiratory rate, 271, 336, 394
increased respiratory work, 268
increased risk for infection, 310
increased risk of disease transmission, 147, 389
increased risk of infection, 190, 311
increased secretion, 375
increased stress hormones level (adrenaline, noradrenaline and cortisol), 399
increased systolic blood pressure, 141, 273
increased tendency to clot, 104
increased the detection of rhinoviruses, 192, 382
increased the number of patients complaining of persistent headaches, 389
increased the risk of infection, 313
increased transcutaneous carbon dioxide, 268
increased use of medication, 149, 270
increased volume of speech, 220
increased work of the respiratory muscles, 341
increased wearing time, 240
index, xiii, 103, 356
India, 23, 25
individual clinicians, 302
Indonesia, 24, 25
induces an artificial version of COPD, 350
industrial workers, 331
infectious, 11, 13, 33, 34, 35, 44, 50, 155, 188, 191, 195, 199, 309, 312
inflammation, 104, 105, 139, 140, 142, 143, 145, 146, 149, 188, 357, 371, 373, 399
inflammation of the gums, 373
inflammation of the lips, 146, 373
inflammatory processes, 365
inflammatory responses, 175
influenza pandemics, 31
influenza viruses, 191, 417
influenza-like illness, 27, 188, 310
influenza-like illness among those who were wearing cloth masks, 310
inhalation of chlorine compounds, 178
inhalation resistance, 138, 330
inhaled carbon dioxide, 298, 320, 321, 322, 325, 330, 336, 338, 344
inhaled CO2 levels, 325, 331
inhaled cotton fibers, 170, 171

inhaled fibers cause pulmonary fibrosis, 174
inhaled mask polypropylene fibers, 139, 375
inhaled synesthetic fibers cause lung disease, 172
innate stress-fear emotion, 251
insomnia, 143, 399, 419
inspiratory and expiratory flow, 350
inspiratory flow, 171, 187, 190, 318
Institute of Health Metrics Evaluation's (IHME), 50
interleukins, 393
internal dryness with external moisture, 373
internal organs, 200
interpret, 118, 120, 222, 230
intracellular level, 365
intracranial pressure, 143, 349
invasive aspergillosis, 196
invasive pathogens, 409
IQ test, 108, 149, 160, 244
irreversible fibrosis in heart tissue, 142, 198
irritation of cervical nerves, 143, 236
irritation of the respiratory tract, 139, 344
ischemic heart disease caused by hypoxic damage to the myocardium, 419
isolation, 106, 147, 221, 238, 250, 251, 419, 423
isolation wards, 238
isoprene, 179
Italy, 24, 25, 29, 59
itch symptoms, 383
itching, 144, 145, 253, 375, 383, 384, 404, 421, 424, 428
itching and swelling of the mucous membranes, 375

J

Japanese, 107, 277

K

Karens, 99
Kennedy, Robert, 49, 444
Kentucky soccer coach, 1
kidneys, 142, 156, 196, 334, 381, 393, 394
Kisielinski, Kai, 32, 164, 165, 166, 176, 179, 180, 191, 192, 211, 215, 216, 235, 253, 254, 256, 257, 268, 272, 273, 336, 338, 339, 340, 344, 354, 355, 356, 365, 374, 382, 383, 384, 385, 409, 421, 423, 424, 427, 445
Kiyosaki, Robert, 68
Klebsiella, 191

L

laboratory confirmed outcomes, 12
laboratory-confirmed influenza, 12, 13, 14
laboratory-confirmed respiratory virus infections, 310
lactobacilli, 187
Lancet, the, 131
large muscle, 104
latent increase in blood gas carbon dioxide levels, 141, 240
legal legitimacy, 302
Legionella pneumonia, 186
Leo, Pam, 68
lesions, 145, 172, 295, 379, 380, 383
liar, xv, 80, 312
life threatening staph infections, 142
lifelong infection, 198
lightheadedness, 143, 271
likelihood for developing a headache during the work shift, 400
Likert scale, 207, 211, 240, 257, 339
limbic part of the brain, 251
limited liability partner, 66
Lincoln Park Police Department, 304
Lincoln Park, New Jersey, 304
linear position transducer, 240

lip-reading, 219
little bees from God, 93
local acne, 144, 253
lockdowns, 1, 16, 39, 43, 45, 46, 56, 103, 106, 244, 248, 419
locus coeruleus, 256, 355
long-term practice of wearing face masks, 419
long-term psychological or developmental negative consequences, 260
look others in the eye, 222
loss mitigation, 101
loss of autonomy, 150, 253
loss of facial expression recognition, 221
loud speech, 147, 220, 374
Louis XIV, 88
low oxygen, 141, 349, 357, 393, 398
lower acceptance of mask-wearing, 257
lower lobes of lungs, 104
lower maximum blood lactate response, 268
lower oxygen availability, 336
lower respiratory reserve, 164
lower respiratory tract infections, 140, 165, 267
lower respiratory tract infections by deep seeding of oropharyngeal flora, 140, 267
lowered health-related self-care, 151, 254
low-grade inflammation, 105
lumen, 164
lung disease, 165, 170, 188, 271, 275
lung function parameters, 138, 268
lung toxicity, 139, 169
lungs, 54, 55, 104, 138, 139, 140, 170, 171, 172, 174, 175, 176, 177, 184, 186, 187, 188, 190, 196, 209, 321, 325, 334, 340, 341, 342, 395
lying sociopaths, 133
lymph, 144, 175, 383, 384

M

MacIntyre, C Raina, 445
Magness, Phil, 51
mainstream, xiv, 56, 125, 327, 442
maintaining own beliefs, 61
Malaysia, 24, 25
mandates of 2020 and beyond, 119
mandating mask wearing is unethical, 301
mandatory masking, 19, 20, 59, 114, 117, 118, 127, 221, 259, 290, 310, 320, 328, 371, 408, 410, 521
manipulated the evidence to score political points, 52
Markham, Laura, 68
Marxist-Leninists, 102
mask, xiii, xiv, xv, 1, 2, 3, 4, 7, 13, 14, 15, 16, 17, 19, 20, 21, 22, 23, 24, 25, 26, 27, 28, 29, 30, 31, 32, 34, 39, 40, 41, 42, 43, 49, 50, 51, 52, 54, 55, 56, 57, 58, 59, 62, 63, 65, 67, 69, 70, 72, 73, 74, 75, 76, 77, 80, 81, 82, 84, 85, 93, 95, 96, 97, 98, 101, 106, 108, 109, 110, 112, 113, 114, 116, 119, 120, 121, 127, 133, 137, 139, 140, 143, 144, 145, 147, 149, 155, 156, 158, 159, 160, 162, 163, 164, 165, 166, 169, 170, 171, 172, 173, 174, 175, 176, 177, 178, 179, 180, 183, 184, 185, 186, 187, 188, 189, 190, 191, 192, 194, 195, 196, 197, 199, 200, 201, 205, 206, 207, 208, 209, 210, 211, 212, 215, 216, 217, 218, 219, 220, 221, 223, 224, 225, 227, 228, 229, 230, 231, 232, 235, 236, 237, 238, 239, 240, 241, 242, 243, 244, 248, 250, 251, 253, 254, 255, 256, 257, 258, 259, 263, 264, 265, 266, 267, 268, 269, 270, 271, 272, 273, 275, 276, 277, 278, 279, 280, 281, 282, 285, 286, 287, 288, 290, 291, 292, 293, 294, 295, 297, 298, 299, 300, 301, 302, 304, 309, 310, 311, 312, 313, 317, 318, 319, 321, 323, 324, 326, 327, 328, 330, 331, 332, 333, 334, 335, 336, 337, 338, 339, 340, 341, 343, 344, 345, 349, 350, 351, 352, 353, 354, 355, 356, 357, 361, 362, 363, 364, 365, 366, 367, 371, 372, 373, 374, 375, 379, 380, 381, 382, 383, 384, 385, 389, 390, 393, 394, 398, 399, 403, 404, 407, 408, 409, 410, 411, 412, 413, 414, 417, 418, 419, 420, 421, 422, 423, 424, 427, 428, 431, 432, 433, 521
and degeneration of brains, 143, 208
as an acoustic filter, 220, 374
as conditioning tool to make your child more compliant, 65
as definitely not suitable for epileptics, 352
as disruptive to basic human communication, 215, 216
as harmful for babies, 163
-associated ocular irritation, 145, 389
-associated skin irritation, 144, 253
does not bring about greater health as defined by the World Health Organization, 294
during exercise, 211
harms teeth and gums, 371
has been visibly misused with largely incorrect popular everyday use, 299
holes, 217
impairs cognition, 291, 305
-induced dental problems, 146, 187
-induced drop in blood oxygen saturation value (SpO2) or the blood oxygen partial pressure (PaO2), 338
-induced exhaustion syndrome (MIES), 415, 423
-induced increased airway resistance, 138, 268
-induced latent drop in blood gas oxygen levels O2, 141, 240
-induced listlessness, 150, 207
-induced restrictions, 268
-induced rhinitis, 140, 375
induces thermal stress, 332
mouth, 145, 371, 373
on pregnant woman should be avoided to protect the unborn child, 160
that is sterile, 298
use impairs vision, 390
-wearers, 56, 177, 187, 188, 210, 211, 235, 254, 255, 268, 273, 290, 299, 300, 318, 336, 338, 340, 344, 365, 375, 383, 389, 422, 423
masking is done in ideal conditions, 298
matrix formation, 174
maximal inspiratory pressure, 139, 318
maximal voluntary ventilation, 139, 318
maximum oxygen uptake, 332
maximum power output, 148, 332
Mayo Clinic, 198, 199
measurable carbon dioxide (CO2) retention (PtcCO2), 269
measurable temperature rise, 382
mechanical skin lesions, 145, 383
mechanistic studies, 12
medical ethics, 57, 58, 288, 323
medical exemptions, 302
medical personnel, 191, 240, 292, 335
Medical Research Council Dyspnea Scale, 272
medically sedated patients, 257
medically trained staff, 298
meditating, 282
meditation, 282
medulla oblongata, 318
men of valor, 81
Mendelsohn, Robert, 68
meningitis, 143, 198
mental health, 46, 252, 253, 349, 419
Merck, 129, 131, 132
mercury, 344
metabolic rate, 148, 323, 324
metabolic syndrome, 344, 355, 356
metabolic system, 155, 158
metabolism, 149, 159, 354, 355, 364, 365, 397
metal fume fever, 170
metastasis, 419
Mexico, 23, 25, 247

Meza, Armando, 195, 445
micro environments, 315
Microbial challenges, 23, 54, 184, 196, 198
Microbial challenges from masks, 23, 54, 184, 196, 198
microbiological, 164, 191
microclimates of the facemasks, 332, 403
Micrococcus, 191
microglia, 199
microplastics, 409
microscopic decay, 409
mild depressive feelings, 150, 254
mild hypoxia, 394
mild pain, 147, 268
mimic the expressions, 222, 230
mimicking negative (frown) emotions, 225
minorities, 45
mistakes and misunderstandings in the operating room, 151, 217
modern life, 63, 116
modernity, 62, 79, 114, 116
moisture retention, 144, 310, 311
mold, 140, 183, 196
Molyneux, Stephan, 68
moment to pause and reflect between input and output, 64
Monroe–Kelly doctrine, 242
Montessori, Maria, 68
mood disturbances, 150, 399, 419
Moore, Alan, 100
morality, 48, 73, 77, 80, 84, 89, 250
morbidity, 35, 156, 356, 397
more than doubled breathing resistance, 354
Morell, Sally Fallon, 68
mortality, 35, 37, 149, 156, 200, 250, 399, 420, 427
mouth, 14, 17, 145, 146, 163, 186, 187, 188, 190, 263, 285, 321, 332, 335, 340, 361, 371, 373, 381, 382, 398, 399, 439
mouth-breathing while wearing a mask, 187, 371, 373
mucosal irritation, 145, 375
mucous membrane, 140, 190
Murray, Christopher, 51
muscle, 138, 142, 148, 200, 210, 268, 270, 276, 350, 354, 398, 399, 419
muscle damage, 148, 350
muscle fiber switch, 350
muscular weakness, 148, 350
myocardial function, 333, 403
myofibroblasts, 175

N

N95 mask, 155, 158, 159, 192, 211, 235, 236, 241, 268, 269, 271, 272, 273, 275, 304, 326, 332, 340, 341, 350, 375, 382, 383, 384, 394, 404
nanomaterial, 155, 169
nanoparticle graphene, 169
naproxen, 130, 131
nasal irrigations, 375
nasal mucosa, 176
nasal obstruction, 166
National Institute of Hygiene and Epidemiology in Vietnam, 311
native English speakers, 217
natural dead space, 335
natural killer cells, 251, 267
nausea, 147, 200, 272, 334
nebulizer, 140, 192, 290
nebulizer effect, 140, 192, 290
negative emotions, 146, 215, 222, 230
negative emotions are amplified, 146, 222, 230
nervous, 143, 175, 242, 251, 325, 354, 355, 364
neuro-adrenalin, 251
neurodegenerative disease, 143, 208

neurological, 143, 151, 164, 166, 199, 205, 209, 240, 242, 257, 326, 339, 343, 344, 398, 423
neurological diseases, 151, 166, 343, 344
neurological disorders, 343
neuromuscular disease, 166
neuropathological, 344
neurophysiologist, 208
neuroprotective, 349
neuro-psychobiological research, 282
New England Journal of Medicine, 19, 20, 129, 132, 228
New Jersey, 304
New Jersey woman, 304
New York, 12, 15, 40, 51, 100, 131, 240, 291, 292, 371, 383, 521
New York Post, 371, 521
New York Times, 12, 15, 51, 100, 131
no one even uses a face mask correctly, 297
non-clinical settings, 227
non-compliance, 41, 83
non-mask wearers, 56, 187
nonsense around masks, 56
nonverbal, 215
noradrenaline, 148, 149, 256
noradrenergic stress response, 149, 355
normal room air, 336
Norway, 24, 25
nose, 11, 17, 48, 140, 145, 163, 164, 166, 190, 199, 285, 297, 321, 332, 335, 340, 361, 371, 375, 382, 383, 398, 414
not only a purely infectiological approach, 299
not science, it is politics, 52
noxious fumes, 164
NPR (National Public Radio), 130, 131
nucleus solitarius, 355
nucleus solitarius in the medulla, 355
numbness, 151, 221
Nuremberg, XIV
Nuremberg Codes, XIV
nurses, 238, 272, 285, 288

O

O2 and CO2 under the masks was determined before and after exercise, 265
obedient to father and mother, 66
obesity, 29, 37, 103, 104, 105, 106, 107, 251, 272, 356
obesity drives Covid, 107
obstructive pulmonary diseases, 333
Occam's Razor, 417
occupational, 164, 207, 311, 312, 317, 318, 326, 327, 331, 394
occupational health regulations, 207
older age, 272
olfactory nerves, 199
one-size-fits-all approach, 56, 57, 110, 311, 324
one-size-fits-all health mandates, 83, 130
operating machinery, 305
operating theater, 28, 151, 240
opioid crisis, 46, 247, 248
opioid epidemic, 247
opioid overdose, 248
opticians, 389
optimal oxygen intake in humans has been calculated in the absence of any obstruction to the airways, 318
oral and nasal environment, 184
oral bacteria, 54, 187, 198, 200, 201
oral diseases, 373
oral dysbiosis, 145, 187, 198
oral flora, 146, 187
oral maxillofacial surgery, 296
oral microbial flora, 55
OSHA considers the micro environment of face masks as, 318
other checks and balances, 86

outside surfaces of surgical masks, 184
outward emotional displays, 146, 225
overall impaired cognitive performance, 207, 253
overlap-COPD sufferers, 275
oxidative stress, 148, 174, 344, 397
oxygen
  availability under the masks, 265
  concentration (% O2), 265
  consumption, 138, 268, 338
  demand, 138, 164, 338
  deprivation, 139, 208, 209
  is essential to life, 318
  saturation dropped by more than 1%, 400
  saturation of the blood (SpO2), 265
  uptake capacity, 158, 210
oxygenation, 104

P

P2, 14
panacea, 19
pandemic, 11, 13, 14, 19, 20, 31, 45, 52, 54, 56, 58, 59,
201, 216, 267, 275, 279, 299, 302, 309, 317, 329, 383,
408, 424
panic attacks, 256, 257
panic disorders, 256, 257
panic reactions and respiratory gases, 256
paramedical staff, 238
parameters, 138, 268, 323, 332, 333, 339
paranoid schizophrenia, 150, 257
parents, xiv, 1, 61, 62, 63, 69, 73, 75, 78, 82, 94, 96, 98,
100, 102, 163, 205, 217, 225, 227, 244, 280, 292, 379, 444
pastors, 40, 75, 87, 88
pathogen reproduction rate, 191
pathogenetic principle, 344
pathogenic bacteria in the mouth, 187
pathogenic synergy, 188
pathological changes, 198, 242, 338, 343
pathological changes inside the skull, 242
pathological consequences, 343, 424
Patient Enablement Instrument (PEI), 215
patient's wound, 285
Pavlov, Ivan, 64
PCR tests, 25, 26, 43, 44, 417
Peale, Norman Vincent, 68
pedagogy, 147, 225
pediatric autoimmune neuropsychiatric disorders
associated with streptococcal infections (PANDAS),
144, 199
peer pressure, 113, 122, 147, 231, 232
peer-reviewed, 11, 15, 44, 103
Penicillium species, 185
perceived interferences of integrity, 253
perception of discomfort, 150, 229, 332, 403
peribronchovascular interstitial thickening, 170
pericarditis, 142, 200
periodontal disease, 146, 187, 371, 372
peripheral blood vessels, 251
permanent disturbance, 253
permanent hyperpigmentation, 145, 385
personal protective equipment (PPE), 55
personality disorders, 257
Pfizer, 95
pharmacies, 309
Philippines, 23, 25
physical activity, 165, 404
physical distancing, 59, 295
physical exertion under an N95 mask, 269
physical inactivity, 251
physical side effects, 59
physical workload, 148, 331
physicians are in a conflict of interest, 302
physiologic dyspnea, 156

physiological feedback mechanisms, 354
Pikler, Emmi, 68
placenta, 157, 158
playground, 100, 101, 102
PMN (polymorphonuclear) neutrophils, 196
pneumoconiosis, 170
pneumonia, 38, 139, 140, 165, 172, 186, 187, 188, 198,
273, 417
poetry, 61
policy makers, 58
political hacks, 15
politicians, 26, 36, 38, 41, 46, 52, 98, 129, 130, 248, 389
polyacrylonitrile, 176, 408
polycarbonate, 176, 408
polyester, 176, 178, 408
polyethylene, 176, 408
polymer fume fever, 170
polymers, 176, 408, 409
polypropylene, 1, 139, 176, 218, 375, 408
polypropylene mask, 1, 218
polystyrene, 176, 408
polyurethane, 176, 408
poor filtration, 190, 310, 311
poor renal artery flow, 393
poor social connections, 250
poor social relationships, 250
poorer clinical outcomes, 147, 419
poorer survival in patients with cancer, 419
positive emotions, 146, 222, 230, 282
positive emotions become less recognizable, 146, 222, 230
postural stability, 151, 349
potentially reduced stigmatization of mask wearers, 254
PPE (Personal Protective Equipment), 55, 143, 147, 238,
239, 288, 293, 312
pragmatism, 84
prayer, 282, 438, 439, 441
precautionary principle, 57, 58
pre-diseased, 211
preeclampsia, 156
pregnant, 137, 138, 155, 156, 158, 159, 160, 162, 275
pregnant healthcare workers, 155
premature mortality, 149, 399
premenstrual dysphoria, 256
pressure, 3, 35, 82, 88, 122, 141, 143, 145, 147, 156, 165,
186, 211, 231, 232, 235, 237, 252, 270, 272, 273, 292,
318, 325, 335, 336, 337, 338, 340, 344, 349, 354, 355,
356, 374, 379, 384, 394, 398, 421, 422, 428
pressure gradients required for undisturbed speech,
147, 374
pressure of carbon dioxide (PETCO2), 211, 272, 273, 336
preterm labor, 137, 156
prevalence of loneliness, 250
preventive measure, 14, 264
Price, Weston, 371, 444
pro-inflammatory state, 252
prolonged hypoxic-hypercapnic state, 419
prolonged mask, 389
prolonged mask use, 40, 159, 242, 256, 291, 292, 355,
385, 389
promote the growth, invasion and spread of cancers, 357
proper use, 17
propionic acid, 179
proprioception, 151, 349
prosthetic devices, 200
protect the surgeon's face from sprays and splashes from
the patient, 285
protecting wounds from surgeons' breath, 299
protozoa, 409
provoke excessively loud speech, 220
Pseudomonads, 191
Pseudomonas species, 185
pseudo-solidarity, 254
psyche, 282
psychiatric, 164, 199, 256, 257

257
evelopmental impact, 259
.irment, 150, 207
port for the general population, 299
>ilities, 339
.gs, 257
., 7, 16, 19, 32, 33, 34, 38, 42, 43, 44, 45,
, 90, 95, 103, 109, 119, 121, 122, 125, 127,
., 164, 178, 192, 193, 201, 218, 254, 280,
.4, 328, 329, 333, 352, 357, 367, 389, 394,

.th organizations, 46
.ds, 413
.ttings, 263, 309
.ary artery pressure, 270
.nary fibrosis, 140, 172, 174, 175, 375
.nary hypertension, 140, 398
.tion of the blood vessels decreases, 242
puric fever, 159
.rsuit of pleasure, 64
.rulent pericarditis, 200

Q

quality of life, 48, 248, 251
quarantine, 102, 419

R

RaeSystems, 336
raised by masked adults, 260
raised by mechanical robots, 260
Rancourt, Denis, 40, 58, 59, 225, 230, 259, 291, 332, 403, 445
randomized controlled trials (RCT), 12, 13, 15, 188, 363
rapid onset of toxic effects, 141, 325
rapport, 222
rashes on the face, 383
rat, 82, 83, 100, 177, 180
    teaching your child to become one, 177
reason and evidence, 98, 418
rebreathing, 138, 179, 208, 242, 256, 320, 335, 338, 350, 354, 399
rebreathing of carbon dioxide, 138, 320, 335, 338, 354
rebreathing our exhaled air, 208
receding gum lines, 146, 187, 372
reduced absorption of oxygen, 343
reduced attention, 150, 211
reduced immune responses, 393
reduced motoric abilities, 150, 240
reduced participation, 149, 254
reduced renal functions, 393
reduced responsiveness, 150, 207, 253
reduces renal blood flow, 393
reduction in O2 intake, 271
release of toxic particles from the mask's materials, 399
release stress hormones, 251
renal metabolic disorders, 344
renal overload, 142, 266
repeated infections in the nasal cavity, 199
reservoirs for respiratory pathogens, 187
resistance during breathing, 210
respiratory burden, 156
respiratory difficulties, 268
respiratory distress, 34, 271, 394
respiratory epithelium, 188
respiratory etiquette and inability to protect against the transmission of respiratory viruses, 14
respiratory frequency and depth, 138
respiratory impairment, 229, 341
respiratory insufficiency, 229
respiratory muscles, 138, 210, 268, 341, 354, 398
respiratory physiology, 138, 158, 165, 211, 275, 340, 354

respiratory protective equipment (RPE), 207, 298, 320, 321, 325, 330
respiratory rate, 159, 271, 272, 273, 277, 336, 337, 338, 340, 344, 352, 355, 394, 423, 428
respiratory rate increase, 355
respiratory syncytial virus, 191
responsible regulation, 101
resulting in generalized nephritis in chronic kidney failure patients, 393
reuse of cloth masks, 311
Review of scientific reports, 40, 58, 59, 219, 222, 259, 291
rheumatoid arthritis, 147, 199
rheumatological, 201
rhinitis, 140, 166, 177, 375
right or left ventricular dysfunction, 142, 398
risk of cancer, 343
risk of suffocation, 138, 163
risk v. reward, 46, 99, 409, 438
Roberge Respirator Comfort Scale, 339
Roberge Subjective Symptoms during-Work Scale, 240
robots, 64, 260
Romans 13, 86, 87, 88, 89
    does not apply to Covid-19, 86
    is a text on moral obligations, not a guide to civic participation, 87
    test was not triggered by Covid response, 89
Rosenberg, Marshall, 68
Ross, Roslyn, 68
RPE (Respiratory Protective Equipment), 320, 321, 325
rubbing their eyes, 389
Rufus, Milan, 93, 445
runny nose, 166

S

saliva, 145, 170, 372, 373
San Francisco, California, 42, 47, 84, 322, 383, 442
sanitizing surfaces, 12
SARS (2004-2005), 27, 31, 33, 271, 313, 363
SARS hype is severely blown out of proportion, 33
Sars-Cov-2, 28, 31, 33, 34, 35, 80, 103, 105, 123, 137, 299, 329, 363, 367, 427
Saudi Arabia, 24, 25
scalp, 237
scar tissue, 174
schizophrenia, 150, 257
school bells, 65
school children, 165, 259
school closures, 45, 59, 248
school-related triggers, 237
science is a process, 92
scientific institutions, 46
scientific method, 7, 15, 46, 64, 92, 120, 127, 286, 309, 329, 418
scientism, 52, 64, 92, 286, 309
scientism as the opposite of science, 52
Score and a Satisfaction Rating Scale, 215
scratching, 150, 253
sebum production, 144, 382
second lockdown, 288
secretion of macrophages, 251
secretory antibodies, 187
seizure, 86, 352, 353
self-contamination, 34, 139, 191, 295, 399
self-identity, 250
self-induced illness, 149, 347
self-induced sleep apnea, 350
self-toxicity, 399
sensations of heat and dampness, 253
sepsis, 142, 198
septic arthritis, 142, 200
seriously sour breath, 145, 187, 372
settled science, 92

shortages of PPE, 312
shortness of breath, 138, 231, 269, 350, 399, 428
sick, v, xiv, 13, 14, 33, 34, 44, 80, 83, 106, 114, 179, 195, 211, 238, 258, 261, 270, 271, 275, 322, 340, 354, 356, 398, 421, 422, 423, 424, 428
Sick Building Syndrome, 421, 422, 423
significant temperature increase, 229
significantly reduced arterial partial oxygen pressure, 394
significantly reduced possible gas exchange volume of the lungs, 342
silicosis, 170
silver bullet, 52
Singapore, 23, 25, 155, 165, 235
single use polymers, 409
single-vehicle crash, 304
Sjogren's syndrome, 199
skin, 29, 40, 41, 56, 141, 144, 145, 146, 162, 178, 184, 253, 291, 295, 339, 344, 373, 379, 381, 382, 383, 384, 385, 424, 428
    as an indicator of the health of the body, 381
    becomes more susceptible to infections and acne, 382
    breakdown, 40, 41, 144, 291
    damage, 383
    irritation, 144, 253, 383, 384
    moisture, 373
Skinner, Burrhus F., 64
Slate, 100
slave, 73
sleep apnea, 149, 156, 186, 275, 349, 355, 356
sleep apnea patients, 275, 356
sleep problems, 237
slowed maximum speed of movement, 148, 211
slowing down of reaction times, 208
slurred speech, 384
smaller airways, 164
smile, 146, 215, 220, 222, 223
smoking, 251
smooth classroom action, 225
sneezing, 11, 166, 194, 375
social bonds, 222
social interaction in schools, 225
social isolation, 250, 419, 420
social medical, 164
social pressure, 231
social withdrawal, 147, 254
socializing of risk, 101
socially isolated, 250
sociological, 164
Solter, Aletha, 68
Sorkin, Aaron, 217
source control, 13, 14, 299
source of plastic and plastic particles for the pollution of all water cycles up to the marine environment, 409
South Koreans, 107
sow seeds of harm in the future, 75
Spain, 23, 25, 29
sphinx, 48
spleen, 105, 175
split plastic tube, 323
spontaneous pneumothorax, 140, 172
spores, 170, 196
sports medicine, 211
standardized hygiene, 290
staph infections, 142, 144, 198, 200, 381
staphylococci, 187
Staphylococcus, 185, 191, 199, 200
Staphylococcus aureus, 191
stem cells, 365
Stepanova, Irena, 217, 444
stigmatization of mask wearers, 254, 299
strap placement, 297
street cleaners, 295
strep pyogenes, 198

Streptococci, 187, 200
Streptococcus, 146, 186, 188, 198, 199, 200
Streptococcus gordonii, 188
stressful for the mentally and hearing-impaired, 221
stressors, 237, 288, 320
stroke patients, 275
strokes, 371, 372, 445
sub pleural ground glass opacities, 139, 170
subacute bacterial endocarditis, 142, 198
subconscious constant distraction, 253
subjective perception of discomfort, 332, 403
subliminal, 158, 344, 354
subthreshold carbon dioxide, 242
subthreshold hypoxia, 356
subthreshold intake of lead is associated with hypertension, 343
subthreshold stimuli, 343
suicide rate, 248
suicides, 419
suit flow rate, 323
Sunnyvale, California, 336
supervisory or caregiving duty, 231
suppress their own needs and concerns, 231
suppressed anger, 150, 253
suppression of emotional signals, 146, 215
suprathreshold stimuli, 343
surface reactivity, 175
surgeons, doctors, and other medical staff in face masks may be more likely to harm patients, 288
surgical face masks were made for surgery and might not even work for that, 285
surgical resection of the pericardium, 200
Sweden, 24, 25
symbol of conformity, 254
sympathetic axis, 355
sympathetic stress response, 151, 355
syncope, 143, 151, 240, 398
    in the operating theater, 240
synesthetic fibers, 172
systemic conditions, VIII, 415
systemic infection, 196
systemic lupus erythematosus, 199
systems of surveillance, 101
Szasz, Thomas, 68

T

T cells, 105
tacit approval, 66, 81
tacit approval of a lie, the, 81
Taiwan, 24, 25
tattle-tale, 82, 83
teach
    a child that reason does not matter, 70
    them to rat out friends, parents, neighbors, strangers, 82
    your child to be a person of preference and not a person of values, 84
    your child to lie, 80
    your child weakness, 78
teachers, 59, 61, 62, 75, 78, 112, 113, 114, 147, 205, 222, 225, 230, 231
teeth, 145, 146, 187, 371, 372
teflon flue, 170
temperature sensation in the face, 229
temperature stress, 315
teratogenic, 162
Thailand, 24, 25
Thalidomide, 157, 159
thermal stress, 148, 332, 403
they will imitate, 93
thiram, 162, 384

Thomas Jefferson's November 13, 1787 letter to William
Stephens Smith, 86
Thoreau, 99
throat, 195, 199, 335, 343
throat irritation, 343
thymus, 105
tighten the nose-clip, 297
tightness of the chest, 138, 334
tissue damage, 105, 198
Tlymphocytes, 361
total volume within the skull always remains
the same, 242
touching, 17, 150, 253, 295, 413
toxic defects of carbon dioxide, 141
toxic shock syndrome, 149, 200
toxicity, 139, 162, 169, 397, 399
trachea, 335
Trader Joe's, 1
tragus, 379
train commuters, 184
trains a dog, 78
transcutaneous, 141, 268, 335, 338
transcutaneous carbon dioxide (PtcCO2) levels, 268
transcytosis, 175, 199
transmission of viral pathogens, 55
trapped air remaining between the mouth, nose and the
facemask is rebreathed, 398
tree of liberty, 49
tremendous psychological impacts, 259
trigger new voice disorders, 374
trigger panic reactions, 256
Trump, Donald, 49
tuberculosis, 45, 367
tumor cell growth, 365
tumor necrosis factors, 267
tumors present some degree of hypoxia, 419
Type 2 alveoli, 175
Type 2 diabetes, 198

U

UAE (United Arab Emirates), 23, 25
ultimately mortality, 397
uncovered part of the face, 253
undermine the sense of trust a child has for you, 75
unemployment, 46, 419
United Kingdom, 24, 25
United States, 24, 25, 34, 43, 47, 53, 86, 87, 88, 107, 109,
121, 129, 137, 201, 220, 277, 280, 317, 326, 336, 417, 521
universal masking, 19, 20, 186, 289
University of New South Wales, 311
University of North Carolina, Chapel Hill, 105
University of Sydney, 311
University of Witten/Herdecke, 205
unqualified for the job, 52
unsolicited electronic recordings, 65
unstudied psychological harm to children, 259
untrained, 211
unwanted individual effects, 301
unwashed mask as breeding ground, 184, 185, 190, 191,
409, 413
upper lobes, 104
urticaria, 144, 384
US Constitution, 86, 87
US Food and Drug Administration, 22
US Occupational Safety and Health Administration
(OSHA), 318
usage time limits, 317
USSR (Union of Soviet Socialist Republics), 102
UV radiation exposure, 344

V

Vainshelboim, Baruch, 33, 34, 250, 251, 252, 310, 394,
397, 398, 399, 400, 419, 445
values, 1, 3, 4, 64, 78, 81, 84, 85, 158, 159, 210, 211, 242,
256, 272, 327, 335
valve breathing, 270
vascular changes, 242
vascular damage, 141, 344
vasoconstriction of visceral blood vessels, 251
vasodilatation, 235, 242
vasodilation, 143, 251
vegetative chronic stress reaction, 365
vegetative noradrenergic neurons, 256
Venker, Suzanne, 68
vertigo, 148, 231
Vietnam, 24, 25, 311
vigorous exercise, 267
violence, 419
Vioxx, 129, 130, 131, 132
viral diseases, 35
viral infections, 139, 197, 361
virtue signally, 292
viruses, 27, 31, 70, 80, 181, 184, 190, 191, 194, 367, 382,
399, 409, 417, 419, 427
virus-infected cells, 105
visceral pleura, 170
visible gap between the mask and skin, 297
visual mask fit test, 297
voice disorder, 147, 220, 374
volatile organic compounds, 179
volume of bacteria shed from the skin, 56
vomiting, 148, 200, 334

W

Walensky, Rochelle, 44
walking while talking, 217
Wall Street Journal, 51
War on Reality, the, 42
warm and humid environment, 190
warm moist environment, 196
waste management issues, 295
we all read lips, 217
We are NOT all in this together, 95
weakened immune systems, 196
wearing of face masks beyond the point of safety, 232
weightlifters, 211
weight-lifting exercises, 211
West Africa, 312
West Coast lockdown, 100, 102
West Wing, the, 217
West, the, 107
Western Europe, 107
white supremacy, 45
WHO (World Health Organization), 17, 33, 264
WHO guidance, 216
widespread medium for microbes, 409
William of Occam, 418
Wired, 100
wisdom, 3, 4, 42, 79, 116, 117, 309, 367, 418
woman of virtue, 81
work endurance time, 330
work rate, 323
working class, 45
workload, 155, 323, 331, 350
World Health Organization, 17, 33, 70, 107, 264, 294, 295

X

Xiao, Jingyi, 11, 12, 13, 14, 15, 16, 17, 20, 21, 188

Y

yeast, 54, 184, 381
yoga, 263, 282
you place your child in the hands of some very twisted
people, 94
you put your child through a class on scientism and not
science, 92
you raise a tyrant, a slave, or both, rather than a healthy
and fully capable adult, 73
you teach a child not to trust you, 72
you teach a child that might makes right, 73
you teach your child tacit approval, 81
you teach your child to misread Romans 13, 86
Younes, Jenin, 50, 51, 52, 53, 444

About The Author

Allan Stevo has been a tireless advocate for more fair treatment of individuals under the law for over two decades. From the disabled to those with severe medical conditions, Stevo has pushed for individualized approaches, rather than the one-size-fits-all treatment our institutions often foist upon those most in need. Stevo's bestselling *Face Masks in One Lesson* demonstrates how and why that individualized, patient-centric approach must be continued for the benefit of those most in need. It provides the ultimate response to mandatory masking, and is an irreplaceable tool for those who will not go masked another day.

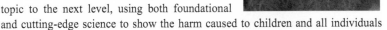

With *Face Masks Hurt Kids*, Stevo takes this topic to the next level, using both foundational and cutting-edge science to show the harm caused to children and all individuals by the one-size-fits-all face mask policies.

Stevo is a nationally syndicated columnist. His work has been widely published by editors at institutions as diverse as *The Daily Caller*, *The Hill*, *The Epoch Times*, The Mises Institute, *Economic Policy Journal*, *The Los Angeles Review of Books*, The Manhattan Institute's *City Journal*, *Emerson Journal*, *The Plain Dealer*, *Lexington Leader,* and *The New York Post.*

He has spoken to audiences at the University of Chicago, MIT, and other top schools in the United States and around the world. In 2012, he became a bestselling author.

Stevo's influential writing has been described as "a precedence of sanity," "the truth in print," and "a beacon of liberty." Stevo has been described as "one of the rare individuals who operate under reason and logic."

"What does Stevo's writing mean to me?" writes Dr. Walter Block "All the world."

He is a graduate of the University of Illinois Urbana-Champaign. He received his Covid-19 contact tracing training from the John Hopkins Bloomberg School of Public Health. A longtime community activist, Stevo's community involvement earned him a "For the Good of Illinois" award. He is the Executive Director of My Body, My Choice, a health freedom organization that has helped thousands fight one-size-fits-all public health mandates in their own lives.

He is foremost a proud father.

After you are done reading *Face Masks Hurt Kids...*

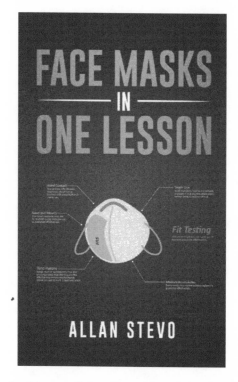

Face mask orders and policies are called mandatory. The truth is millions are exempt from the face mask orders and don't realize it. *Face Masks in One Lesson* provides the ultimate response to mandatory masking, and is an irreplaceable tool for those who will not go masked another day.

Face Masks in One Lesson contains:
- In depth analysis of notable national policies, governmental and non-governmental
- How to never wear a mask again and to do so legitimately
- Points to the most telling studies
- The magic phrases that will get you past virtually any face mask checkpoint
- Fly the friendly sky maskless

Stevo's influential writing has been described as "a precedence of sanity," "the truth in print," and "a beacon of liberty." Stevo's been described as "one of the rare individuals who operate under reason and logic." Reading Face Masks in One Lesson "might be the most important thing you can do for yourself, your family, and your country," writes Professor Robert Wright.

"What does Stevo's writing mean to me?" asks Dr. Walter Block "All the world."

Made in the USA
Las Vegas, NV
09 April 2022

47153187R10307